The Analysis and Valuation of Health Care Enterprises

Readers of this text may be interested in the following related books from the Appraisal Institute: *The Appraisal of Real Estate*, eleventh edition; *Elderly Housing: A Guide to Appraisal, Market Analysis, Development & Financing* by Arthur E. Gimmy, MAI, and Michael G. Boehm; *Hotels & Motels: A Guide to Market Analysis, Investment Analysis & Valuations* by Stephen Rushmore, MAI; and *Market Analysis for Valuation Appraisals* by Stephen F. Fanning, MAI, Terry Grissom, MAI, and Thomas D. Pearson, MAI.

For a catalog of Appraisal Institute publications, contact the PR/Marketing Department of the Appraisal Institute, 875 N. Michigan Avenue, Ste. 2400, Chicago, IL 60611-1980.

THE ANALYSIS AND VALUATION
OF HEALTH CARE ENTERPRISES

by
Arthur E. Gimmy, MAI
with
Charles R. Baumbach

875 North Michigan Avenue
Chicago, Illinois 60611-1980

Reviewers:	James H. Bulthuis, MAI, SRA
	Thomas A. Motta, MAI, SRA
	George F. Silver, MAI, SRA
Senior Vice President, Communications:	Christopher Bettin
Manager, Book Development:	Michael R. Milgrim, PhD
Manager, Design/Production:	Julie B. Beich
Graphic Designer:	Claire Baldwin

For Educational Purposes Only

The material presented in this text has been reviewed by members of the Appraisal Institute, but the opinions and procedures set forth by the author are not necessarily endorsed as the only methodology consistent with proper appraisal practice. While a great deal of care has been taken to provide accurate and current information, neither the Appraisal Institute nor its editors and staff assume responsibility for the accuracy of the data contained herein. Further the general principles and conclusions presented in this text are subject to local, state, and federal laws and regulations, court cases, and any revisions of the same. This publication is sold for educational purposes with the understanding that the publisher is not engaged in rendering legal, accounting, or other professional service.

Nondiscrimination Policy

The Appraisal Institute advocates equal employment and nondiscrimination in the appraisal profession and conducts its activities without regard to race, color, sex, religion, national origin, or handicap status.

Printed in the U.S.A.

99 98 97 96   5 4 3 2 1

Library of Congress Cataloging-in-Publication Data

Gimmy, Arthur E.

The analysis and valuation of health care enterprises / by Arthur E. Gimmy, with Charles R. Baumbach.

p. cm.

Includes bibliographical references.

ISBN 0-922154-32-5

1. Health facilities—Valuation—United States. I. Baumbach, Charles R. II. Title.

RA981.A2G488   1996

362.1'068'1—dc20

96-31795

CIP

TABLE OF CONTENTS

F O R E W O R D

As real estate appraisers seek new avenues of business, the realm of special purpose properties holds a wide range of opportunities for the knowledgeable appraiser. The field of health care in particular comprises numerous types of facilities, each of which has unique markets, property features, and use requirements.

The Appraisal Institute is pleased to publish *The Analysis and Valuation of Health Care Enterprises* because it covers—in one volume—the major types of health care facilities found today. Key chapters discuss traditional general hospitals and nursing homes, but the book also contains chapters on newer health care concepts such as outpatient or ambulatory care centers, assisted living facilities, and psychiatric hospitals. In addition, the book provides discussions on medical office buildings and the adaptive reuse of medical facilities — important in an era when medical technology can make even a recently built facility obsolete for its intended use. The book concludes with chapters on valuing a medical practice, complete with a sample report, or case study, of a business valuation of a family medical practice.

The Analysis and Valuation of Health Care Enterprises joins a long line of publications on special purpose properties published by the Appraisal Institute as a service to the appraisal profession.

Kenneth L. Nicholson, SRA
1997 President
Appraisal Institute

P R E F A C E

Health care reform, costs, and sources of revenues are one of the major issues of the 1990s. With this attention comes the realization that the market or industry is hopelessly complicated and, in many cases, misunderstood. A great variety of property types or classifications serve separate and distinct markets. Political, social, and demographic trends are extremely difficult to identify and quantify, but they have a material effect on markets and the value of facilities.

Specialists are needed to analyze and appraise health care projects for a wide variety of purposes, including purchase and sale, consolidation or merger, financing, tax and estate matters, eminent domain, insurance, disputes, and divorce. The Appraisal Institute has taken the lead in the education process for professionals in this field. This text deals with the most important property types and enterprises in one package.

Readers should reinforce the knowledge gained here with up-to-date information and pertinent data about local and regional trends and markets, specific property type data, transactions, and current statistics. Because health care is currently subject to a variety of wide-reaching influences and factors, medical properties are not likely to stabilize in such a fluid and dynamic environment. Risk factors and other elements are continually changing. A thorough review of current literature is advised. Many excellent texts and treatises are available for those who need or desire in-depth knowledge about specific health care subjects and methodologies. References to some of these are found in Appendix E along with pertinent lists of trade and professional associations, journals, newsletters, and other research publications.

ACKNOWLEDGMENTS

When I first undertook the writing this book, I assumed the task could be accomplished within a one-year time frame. As it turned out, it took over five years. It probably should have been undertaken by an institution rather than a single individual. A lot of data is out there and the trick is finding it (and being able to pay for it). Fortunately, I have been blessed by my daily contacts with a very qualified professional staff that provided me with ideas and data as well as contributed to the content.

Charles R. Baumbach, a fine senior associate and co-manager of our health care appraisal division, wrote the chapter on adaptive reuse of medical facilities (Chapter 9). Wallace W. Reiff, a superb educator, writer, researcher, appraiser, and long-time friend, assisted with the chapters dealing with the valuation of medical practices and related entities (Chapters 10 and 11). I take full responsibility for all of the remaining chapters as well as the Appendix.

I also want to thank Michael L. White for his endless word-processing efforts and Mary G. Gates, J. Gregg Hawthorne, David Betts, and Martin E. Benson, MAI, of the staff of Arthur Gimmy International for their excellent participation in many facets of producing a technical manual that will hopefully assist other analysts and appraisers in the years ahead.

Arthur E. Gimmy, MAI
San Francisco, California
November 1996

ABOUT THE AUTHORS

Arthur E. Gimmy, MAI, is president and owner of Arthur Gimmy International, a real estate appraisal and consulting firm with offices in San Francisco and Newport Beach, California. Mr. Gimmy received the MAI designation in 1965. Mr. Gimmy has been a prolific author, having published nearly 50 articles on a wide variety of appraisal topics and written various books in use by appraisal professionals. Those previously published by the Appraisal Institute include *Elderly Housing; Fitness, Racquet Sports and Spa Projects;* and *Golf Courses and Country Clubs.* He has taught many appraisal courses during his career, including ones at San Jose State, UCLA, SMU, the University of Tampa, and the University of Connecticut. He has also served on numerous local and national committees of the Appraisal Institute, including 10 years as a member of *The Appraisal Journal Board.* A pioneer in the analysis of difficult, unique, or specialized properties, Mr. Gimmy is frequently an expert witness in litigation matters involving complex appraisal issues. He recently received the George L. Schmutz Memorial Award from the Appraisal Institute for his special contribution to the advancement of appraisal knowledge.

Charles R. Baumbach is a senior associate and co-manager of the health care appraisal division of Arthur Gimmy International. He is a graduate of the University of Chicago with bachelor's and master's degrees in accounting and economics as well as a JD degree. He is experienced in right of way appraisal and acquisition and real estate brokerage and development, and has served as a consultant and educator in the fields of legal services, economic development, and education. In addition to hospital and medical building appraisal experience, Mr. Baumbach also has appraised other types of special purpose properties including shopping centers, fitness centers, hotels and motels, and mixed-used properties.

I N T R O D U C T I O N

Health care is an industry in the clutches of change and uncertainty, one characterized by diversity, regulation, competition, and turmoil, all of which factors are likely to continue into the next century. Currently viable facilities will cease to exist or become obsolete, and vast sums of money will be required for new investment. Although financial markets abhor uncertainty, risks will be taken to fund new investment in health care.

The health care market is an enormous one, and the need for qualified appraiser/specialists is expected to grow. At the same time, the valuation problems and types of health care properties to be studied are unique and highly complex. Analysts will have to be trained to deal with the complex factors and programs that affect the marketability and value of these facilities. Appraisers will be expected to perform complicated market analyses and highest and best use studies and convert these data into real estate and going-concern valuations (The latter will be necessary because much of the income and expense data for medically oriented enterprises deals with business operations). Accountants and economists will also be competing for this type of work. To secure a market share, appraisers must be able to provide highly technical analyses that discern the complexities of going concerns, business intangibles, financing arrangements, and detailed contracts as well as to perform conventional, but contemporary valuations.

This book is oriented primarily toward real estate and business appraisers. It aims to provide them with an understanding of, as well as the technical knowledge about, this specialized field. The authors have extensively varied experience in valuing health care facilities ranging from physical asset aspects to business intangibles.

The book will discuss the analysis and valuation of general hospitals, psychiatric hospitals, ambulatory care facilities (primarily surgery centers), convalescent hospitals or nursing homes, assisted living or residential care facilities, subacute care and Alzheimer's units, medical office buildings, abandoned or surplus hospitals, and medical practices. With the possible exception of the last item they all involve real property. Most assignments may require allocations of a variety of assets including personal property and the business component. Even though medical practices have been rarely appraised by appraisers whose experiences are primarily oriented to real property interests, a chapter on medical practices is included because it is important for appraisers to understand the full range of this specialized industry.

Unique Characteristics of Health Care Facilities

A common bond based on similar characteristics or activities extends from one type of health care facility to another. Most are operating businesses; have hospitality, care, social, and recreational elements; are considered to be special purpose in design and function; and appeal to specialized or nontraditional markets. They have overlapping functions relating to various types and degrees of health care as well as common facility characteristics such as administration and property services (e.g., maintenance, facility operations, security). These shared characteristics allow the appraiser/analyst to apply data gathering techniques, analytical processes, and valuation indicators from one property category to another. For example, common threads run through the operating ratios of facilities that provide gerontological services when analyzed on a per bed or per guest/resident basis and adjusted for various levels of care. Another example of this commonality is the value relationship between medical office buildings and related facilities such as surgery, imaging, and urgent care centers, which may involve adjustment or amortization for higher unit construction costs or tenant improvements.

These types of facilities also tend to have limited market data for comparative purposes. Many health care facilities are not commonly traded. The market for facilities may be regional or national in nature, indicating that so-called comparables may need to be obtained from beyond the local jurisdiction. Although this complicates the investigative stage of an appraisal, it allows the appraiser to apply the sales comparison approach in a more thorough manner. A limited number of specialists (corporate executives and investment brokers) may be involved in the application or interpretation of financial data and may communicate their findings in unique formulas or valuation procedures. It is incumbent on the practicing professional appraiser to stay current through published data, seminar presentations, and meetings of industry experts.

This discussion is not meant to provide a definitive list of the unique characteristics of health care facilities. Individual chapters will address specialized aspects of each type of facility. They will also examine existing and emerging factors of obsolescence that can render a property unsuitable for continued occupancy or to be categorized as an uneconomic asset due to continuing and projected future operating losses. A separate chapter dealing with the adaptive reuse of obsolete, abandoned, or surplus facilities will focus on highest and best use considerations and examples of recycled properties where feasible.

Unique Valuation Considerations

The appraiser must recognize that virtually all operating health care facilities represent going concerns whose assets involve land; yard construction; buildings and other structures; furniture, fixtures, and equipment (FF&E); and business or intangible interests. An exception is a medical office building, the analysis of which typically involves a real estate appraisal. However, within the medical office building are tenancies involving medical practices whose value is separate from the real property interests. There are also many examples where medical office buildings are actually clinic or group operations and the property and business are owned as one. In such situations it may be quite complicated to separate the net income attributed to the physical assets from the net income attributed to the medical activities performed by the physicians and support staff.

An appraiser who attempts to perform a real estate valuation of an operating health care enterprise should consult with a business valuation specialist if the appraiser is unqualified to appraise an operating entity or is unable to obtain the necessary experience or advice. In large hospital assignments a team of specialists may be required to appraise the real estate, personal property, and intangibles. Intangibles include patient lists, provider and physician contracts, accounting systems, software, staff in place, and management contracts as well as name, reputation for providing unique and highly successful medical procedures, covenants not to compete, patents, and copyrights. Brief discussions of business valuation techniques that are appropriate to separate categories of health care facilities are included in various chapters.

The appraiser who deals with complex properties that typically include a business or intangible value component faces a formidable research requirement. Specific actions that should be undertaken include interviews with the management of the subject property, competitors (if possible), and experts in the field; investigations of comparable health care property transactions, operating results of competitive properties, and market conditions; and analyses of financial statements, tax returns (if necessary), contracts, leases, and other agreements, including reports by regulatory bodies.

Common Pitfalls

Typically, good comparables will be lacking and competitors will be reluctant to provide insights into the local market. The appraiser may compensate for these factors by extending the geographic area for comparables and obtaining data about the local market from government documents or reports as well as other informed consultants. The appraiser should recognize that examples may have to be drawn from a large geographic area and that considerable research must be accomplished to derive units of comparison and valuation indicators. A typical pitfall is obtaining sale prices for general hospitals on a per bed basis and attempting to use this information without conducting many interviews, developing allocation criteria, or understanding motivation and other considerations.

Appraisers frequently fail to recognize that the concept of market value encompasses a hypothetical sale to an unknown third party, and that the operating history of a current or former operator may not represent the true future financial potential of a facility. Consider, for example, a nursing home with a 91% operating ratio in a competitive market that indicates 82% is typically achievable with good management. An appraisal based on an income approach that does not represent the norm for performance can have a major potential error (e.g., the difference between an 82% and 91% operating ratio can result in a net income available for capitalization that is off by 90%!).

Many appraisers are ill-prepared to compare one medical facility with another. Their analyses tend to be oversimplified and overemphasize the real estate. A relatively new hospital in an overcrowded market can be highly depreciated. Appraisers who specialize in lodging facilities have been able to deal with this problem because of the large number of transactions in recent years at relatively low per-room prices. Where there are no or few transactions (a frequent occurrence in the acute and psychiatric hospital market), the appraiser must do a substantial amount of compensating research to account for this deficiency.

Organization and Methodology of Text

Chapter 1 focuses on the current state of the health care industry and provides an overview of trends in health care, medical costs, and demographic changes. The purpose of this chapter is to provide a general view of the health care market before undertaking more detailed studies of the major health care property types.

Chapters 2 through 8 are devoted to specific health care property types. Chapter 2 deals with medical-surgical (acute) hospitals, Chapter 3 explores the psychiatric hospital situation, Chapter 4 features surgery centers, Chapter 5 is focused entirely on nursing homes, and Chapter 6 deals with the newly evolving assisted living facility. Chapter 7 is concerned with newer types of facilities that can be developed on a stand-alone basis or as part of an integrated health care facility, in particular, subacute facilities. Subacute care is one of the hottest topics in the health care industry. Another specialty program that is drawing attention is the provision of units for those suffering from Alzheimer's disease in a residential care and skilled nursing environment.

A number of other health care property types are not given the status of an entire chapter in this text. Examples include subacute units of a skilled nursing facility, rehabilitation hospitals, and types of freestanding ambulatory care facilities other than surgery centers. However, the methodologies for appraising these types of properties can be derived from a careful reading of the information provided in this text for similar property types and businesses.

Chapter 8 is concerned with medical office buildings and clinics. Chapter 9 deals with the adaptive reuse of medical facilities, primarily hospitals since a large number of them have been closed or abandoned in recent years. The appraisal assignment in an adaptive reuse situation is highly complex and focuses on highest and best use considerations and historical examples of the recycling of hospitals.

Chapter 10 deals with medical practices and related entities and is focused on the non-real estate aspects of appraising these entities. Through proper education and study real estate appraisers can become qualified to appraise various types of intangibles involved in the health care business including medical practices, physical therapy practices, surgery center businesses, etc. To provide the reader with additional assistance in this matter, a complete case study of a business valuation of a family medical practice is provided in Chapter 11.

These chapters comprise the core of this text. A lengthy Appendix provides a glossary of terms, information sources, and other helpful data.

Many potential pitfalls exist in the analysis of health care facilities, especially as the field becomes more complex each year. However, specialization by the appraiser is the means to becoming an expert in a unique technical field.

CHAPTER ONE

Overview and Trends in the Health Care Industry

Despite a sluggish economy the United States spends close to $1 trillion annually on health care at a growth rate of 10% per year. The U.S. health care system has about 7,500 acute hospitals, 750 psychiatric or mental health facilities, 15,900 nursing homes, 10,000 rest homes, and an estimated 300,000 ambulatory care facilities, which include surgery centers, diagnostic facilities, and the whole gamut of medical office buildings and clinics. These figures do not include facilities of nonphysician providers and paramedical personnel such as chiropractors and mental health counselors. These facilities are organized as private for-profit organizations, private not-for-profit organizations, public organizations, and quasi-public organizations. Similarly, they may be operated by individual investors, corporate (closely held and publicly traded) organizations, local government agencies, or a religious denomination, foundation, or some other nonprofit entity.

Growth in the health care field is inevitable even when there is excess capacity. The acute hospital inventory has declined in recent years, and a few new facilities have never opened their doors. Surgery centers have experienced rapid growth in recent years, capturing close to 20% of all inpatient and outpatient cases. Hospitals have countered this threat through acquisitions of these businesses and more efficient use of their own facilities and capabilities. Ambulatory centers, which offer a variety of medical services typically in storefront settings where appointments may not be required, are likely to have tough sledding under health care reform. Their outlook, without some type of affiliation, is unclear at best. Home health care agencies should continue to thrive because their occupancy and staffing requirements are extremely low, but their costs will bear close scrutiny. Diagnostic imaging centers have a clouded outlook due to problems of excess capacity, perceived financial conflicts, and rapidly changing technology. Nursing homes are a good bet for the future due to the well-documented aging of the baby boom generation. Past growth and future outlook in selected health care market segments are summarized in Table 1.1.

Table 1.1	Growth and Outlook in Eight Key Health Care Market Segments				
Provider Type	**1984**	**1987**	**1992**	**1993***	**Sales Outlook****
Hospitals	7,569	7,705	7,441	7,403	++
Surgery centers	330	853	1,690	1,832	++
Ambulatory centers	1,798	3,445	4,285	4,577	+
Home health care agencies	5,337	7,341	9,982	11,507	++
Diagnostic imaging centers	95	489	1,736	1,868	+
HMOs	385	707	562	545	++++
PPOs	115	692	1,036	1,206	++
Nursing homes	13,642	14,285	15,165	15,334	+++

* Estimate
**"Sales Outlook" indicates potential for new or continued growth
Source: SMG Marketing Group, Inc., Chicago, 1994.

Employment Trends

Close to nine million people in the United States work in health services, exclusive of physicians. About five million of them work in hospitals and the balance in medical offices, clinics, and laboratories. Employment has increased 170% since 1980 and 40% since 1985 (see Table 1.2).

The growth rate for physicians, including osteopaths, has been much lower, representing an increase of 41% since 1980 and only 18% since 1985. There were approximately 686,600 physicians in the United States as of 1992. The number of persons employed in health services, however, has been growing at an increasing rate. For every physician there are approximately 13 health care workers as of 1993 compared to 10.85 in 1980.

Facility Problems

The analyst or appraiser must be familiar with macrotrends and microtrends in the health care industry. Macrotrends are defined as those common to all markets while microtrends are generally regional or local in character depending on whether the market is overdeveloped or underdeveloped and on the design sophistication of individual facilities. The matrix in Table 1.3 illustrates some of the key factors that affect the value of health care facilities and that relate to functional and external obsolescence considerations on a major scale.

An interpretation of this matrix would indicate that the general hospitals category represents a substantial number of troubled properties. General hospitals have had enormous financial problems in the last decade or so, most of which have resulted from two factors: the success of American medicine in drastically reducing the length of stay for typical patients and the success of government-based financing programs in developing an excessive number of hospital beds over the past 25 years.[1] As a result, hundreds of hospitals have been closed or abandoned

---

[1] These programs included the Hill-Burton Act, which provided for low-interest rate loans, certain subsidies, and other benefits that allowed existing hospitals to remodel and expand and new hospitals to be created without a proper understanding of market dynamics and future trends in utilization.

Table 1.2	**Employment in the Health Service Industries**				
Industry	**1985**	**1990**	**1994**	**1985-94 % Increase**	
Offices and clinics of MDs	1,028,000	1,338,000	1,562,000	51.9	
Offices and clinics of dentists	439,000	513,000	590,000	34.4	
Offices and clinics of other practitioners	165,000	277,000	389,000	135.8	
Skilled nursing facilities	791,000	989,000	1,170,000	47.9	
Intermediate care facilities	230,000*	200,000	229,000	0	
Other care facilities	190,000*	227,000	233,000	22.6	
General, acute hospitals	2,811,000	3,268,000	3,492,000	24.2	
Psychiatric hospitals	59,000	104,000	94,000	59.3	
Specialty hospitals	126,000	176,000	204,000	61.9	
Medical and dental laboratories	119,000	166,000	202,000	69.8	
Home health care services	152,000	291,000	533,000	250.6	
Other	183,000	265,000	334,000	82.5	
Total	6,293,000	7,814,000	9,032,000	43.5	

* Estimated by author.

Source: U.S. Bureau of Labor Statistics, Bulletin 2445, and *Employment and Earnings* (monthly, March and June issues).

Table 1.3	**Obsolescence Characteristics of Health Care Facilities**					
	Property Type and Rating					
Major Obsolescence Factors	**General Hospitals**	**Psychiatric Hospitals**	**Nursing Homes**	**Assisted Living Facilities**	**Surgery Centers**	**Medical Office Buildings**
Excess beds	1	1	3	3	3	4
Overly competitive market	1	1	2	3	2	2
Outmoded design	2	2	1	3	3	2
Inadequate demographics	2	1	2	2	2	2
Marginal or no profit	2	2	3	3	3	3
Neighborhood deterioration	2	3	2	3	3	2

Legend: 1 = Likely; 2 = Possible; 3 = Unlikely; 4 = Not Applicable
Source: Arthur Gimmy International

in recent years to the extent that a separate specialization or discipline has arisen to deal with the valuation problems of surplus facilities (see Chapter 9).

Other health care property types are newer in nature and less likely to be subject to the destructive forces of overbuilding and excess competition. Newer concepts such as assisted living facilities and surgery centers are difficult to organize and develop and involve complicated financial structures and management organizations. They are much less likely to suffer from depreciation attributed to obsolescence than older properties that have not kept up with state-of-the-art technology and have become duplicative in function within defined markets.

Major Influences

Health care properties are unique among commercial property types because their utility and therefore their value are subject to technological changes and evolving services, to the integration of delivery systems, and to the influence of government.

Technological Change and Evolving Services

Health care activities, by definition, involve rapidly changing technology which requires new construction, reconfiguration of existing buildings, and installation of very costly fixed and movable equipment installations. An example is the rapid development of magnetic resonance imaging (MRI) facilities in the past decade. MRI equipment requires a special enclosure for the powerful electrical and magnetic fields created by the diagnostic process. Hospitals added MRI nodules or remodeled sections of radiological departments at great expense. Hundreds of millions of dollars were invested in MRI installations. Then freestanding MRI plants and portable, trailer-type MRI units were developed that could be moved from one hospital to another or permanently stationed in a hospital parking lot. Now even newer and superior forms of imaging are available that may be less costly, are more technically proficient, and reduce patient exposure to huge electrical and magnetic forces. The appraiser must consider the declining contribution of existing MRI facilities as well as the degree of obsolescence of the support facilities.

The appraiser/analyst must be aware of new technological developments and services provided to patients, residents, guests, or tenants that affect the income-producing potential of subject properties as well as competitors. In comparing the capabilities of a subject hospital with competing facilities, for example, a checklist might be used to indicate the medical specialties that are provided. The prestige or status of a hospital within a local community is partially based on its provision of popularly recognized and publicized medical procedures, e.g., open heart surgery or the treatment of exotic cancers. Facilities that lack certain capabilities may acquire the services of well-known medical specialists to improve their competitive position, or hospital management can decide to add additional facilities or engage in contractual relationships with outside medical groups or practices that accomplish the same result.

In analyzing the future income-producing potential of a certain property the appraiser must consider whether the subject has the capability to expand its bundle of services or engage in facility alterations that can correct functional deficiencies. Obviously, a consultant must have the specialized experience and knowledge of current and future medical services and technology to analyze such issues.

The rapid decline in the unit prices paid for general hospitals in the past decade is illustrative of the principle of volatility. Appraisers should be constantly aware that health care properties, especially hospitals, are "moving targets" and the element of risk must be accorded appropriate weight in the process of yield capitalization and estimates of external depreciation.

Integrated Delivery Systems

Health care can be described as a realm of continuous specialized services that can operate independently or on an interdependent basis depending on the circumstances of the services required (see Figure 1.1). This continuum of care can involve all of the types of facilities included in this textbook, which begin and end at the home or in a long-term care environment. The care elements are all integrated, beginning with the individual physician and ending with a well person or one who is confined to a nursing home. More and more emphasis is being placed on efficiencies and practicalities.

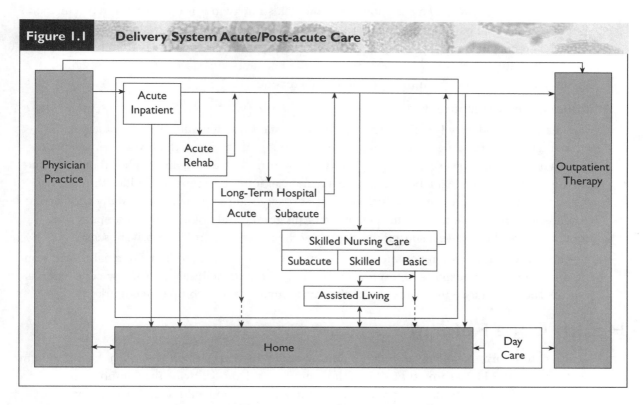

Figure 1.1   Delivery System Acute/Post-acute Care

One way to develop an integrated delivery system is through the provision of joint ventures. Arrangements typically involve acute care hospitals, subacute providers, nursing homes, rehabilitation facilities, and assisted living projects. The following five models are the most common joint venture strategies.[2]

Joint Ownership. Under this arrangement, a hospital and skilled nursing facility develop and jointly own a subacute facility in the form of a long-term care hospital, freestanding skilled nursing facility, rehab hospital, or rehab unit. The hospital and nursing facility both put in capital and share governance.

Leasing Model. Under this model, the hospital or nursing facility will lease a floor or unit to a subacute provider, whose program will function separately and have its own license and provider number although housed within the hospital. This model must be closely examined because of the hospital-within-a-hospital issue.

Management Model. The most common joint venture model involves a hospital that sets up a skilled nursing facility as part of its system and contracts with a subacute provider to oversee administration, program development, billing and collection, staffing, and operations. In

---

[2] Tim McDowell and Harvey Brown, "Integrated Delivery Systems," *Transitions*, vol. 1, no. 1 (July/August 1994), 10-11.

exchange the hospital receives a management fee that may range from 7% to 20% of revenues. The hospital is able to retain hospital-based status for the skilled nursing facility, which is able to provide subacute services without the capital costs of setting up a freestanding facility. The nursing facility is also not competing directly with the hospital.

Shared Services Arrangement. Under this strategy, a hospital and skilled nursing facility each agree to provide certain designated services, resources, and personnel. Typically, these services are offered within one of the two facilities. This is a low-cost option, but it also presents control issues.

Bed Reserve Agreement. This is a low-cost, low-risk strategy, but it is limited. It has real use in situations where a hospital experiences difficulty placing some patients in a long-term care setting. The hospital can contract with a skilled nursing facility to reserve certain beds for such patients. In return for paying a reservation fee, the hospital gains access to units providing higher skilled care, and the nursing facility gains revenue.

Influence of Government

The health care industry is highly regulated by local, state, and federal government agencies. These regulations have significant impacts on revenues and expenses and involve virtually all aspects of operations by establishing standards and controls. Medicare and Medicaid programs are the most well known. Regulations can have a beneficial impact on property values through the enhancement of revenues, especially in the case of Medicaid reimbursements. Many convalescent hospitals that benefit from this public sector program could not otherwise compete with nursing homes that derive a substantial portion of their revenues from the private sector.

The analyst/appraiser must know about applicable programs and their financial impacts on the operation of the business enterprise and management of facilities. This knowledge extends to proposed health care programs and their future impact on the competitive market.

Health Care Reform

Health care reform has received much publicity in recent years. When 15% of the population in the United States lacks some type of health insurance and almost twice that number are underinsured, reform initiatives are likely to be instituted. The health care crisis and various reform initiatives at the federal and state levels have been described in literally thousands of publications in the past few years. It is not the purpose of this book to review and digest the various plans and proposals. Rather, an attempt will be made to discuss trends and factors in the U.S. health care system that will significantly impact valuation assignments. These considerations include demographic factors, health care financing, newly developing services and facilities, utilization performance trends, and other factors.

The private sector has struggled to deal with future unknowns that will result from national health reform. Evolving entities such as health maintenance organizations (HMOs) and preferred provider organizations (PPOs) are extending their regional market penetration to even national geographic coverage. On the local and regional level, a process of consolidation, affiliation, and vertical integration is occurring, primarily among primary hospitals, in an attempt to solidify market share and improve bargaining positions.

Reform will have a great impact not only on those who pay the bill but also on most categories of providers. Even efficient operators are not likely to thrive but at least they will survive; smaller and older entities will need a heroic management effort to avoid falling by the wayside, and many obsolete facilities will close for good. The costs to achieve competitive efficiencies are excessive in the health care industry because of government mandated design and construction requirements and other unique factors.

Both business and government mostly agree:

that reform of the U.S. health care system should seek to accomplish the following objectives: 1) provide cost-effective health care services that will reduce overall spending levels; 2) design a comprehensive health care system that will include the 37 million Americans who are currently uninsured; 3) assess the effects of an ever-greater reliance on modern medical technology; 4) review the impact of managed care on health care expenditures; 5) examine the accessibility of various socio-economic groups to health care services; 6) improve levels of health care in rural America; 7) reduce cost of malpractice liability; 8) determine what characteristics best assess quality of service; 9) restructure the Medicare program and fold Medicaid into the reform process; 10) improve medical education; 10) assess health care planning; and 11) enhance the use of preventive, primary and patient-centered care. [3]

Accomplishing several or all of these goals will affect the valuation of health care facilities. Most of these goals are assumed to be beneficial; however, actual impacts will not be known for many years. The appraiser/analyst must be aware of these and other considerations to properly assess the impacts on future revenue streams and the risk related to the possible achievement of financial objectives.

Efforts to Control Medical Costs

If there has been one significant trend during the past decade affecting the operation of hospitals, it has been the effort by the government and HMOs to control medical costs which historically have been virtually uncontrolled. Real or inflation-adjusted per capita health spending in the U.S. increased by 86% from 1980 ($1,926) to 1995 ($3,579). This resulted in health care spending growing 3.3 percentage points faster than the nation's total economic output to the degree that it now consumes 12.6% of the gross domestic product.

Prospective Payment System (PPS)

Due to rapidly growing Medicare spending for inpatient hospital care and forecasts that the hospital insurance component of the Medicare program would be bankrupt by the mid-1990s, Congress enacted Title VI of the Social Security Amendments of 1983. This legislation, which took effect on October 1, 1983, replaced Medicare's hospital cost reimbursement system with a Prospective Payment System (PPS). Formerly, Medicare essentially reimbursed hospitals for any money spent in treating Medicare beneficiaries. Under PPS, hospitals are paid a prospective rate for a Medicare patient, depending on the Diagnosis-Related Group (DRG) to which a patient is assigned. A hospital receives a fixed DRG rate for each hospital patient or the number of ancillary services furnished. Hospital insurance plans, including Blue Cross, also implemented DRG plans to stem escalating health insurance premiums.

PPS has slowed the rate of Medicare spending, resulting in a decline in Medicare profits and increased competition among hospitals. DRG payments began well below the cost of services and have not kept up with the rising cost of providing care. Side effects from PPS have included the choking off of patient and financial information among hospitals, encouragement of patient dumping, expansion of hospital-related services on a vertically integrated basis, development of new, lucrative Medicare services, and establishment of cooperation among hospitals shortchanged by Medicare. In essence, DRGs were an effective tool in controlling Medicare spending

---

[3] *The Comparative Performance of U.S. Hospitals: The Sourcebook* (Baltimore, MD: Health Care Investment Analysts, Inc., and Deloitte & Touche, 1993).

on inpatient care. After Medicare gave hospitals big pay increases in fiscal 1984 and 1985, the annual increase in PPS operating payments per discharge averaged a little more than 5% over the next six years. As shown in Table 1.4, losses to general, acute care hospitals from treating Medicare patients became a significant factor in the late 1980s and reached a high point in 1990. Since that time they have remained relatively constant.

Table 1.4	Hospital Payment to Cost Ratios for Medicare, Medicaid, and Private Payers, 1980-1993						
Payment to Cost Ratio				Payment to Cost Ratio			
Year	Medicare	Medicaid	Private	Year	Medicare	Medicaid	Private
1980	0.96	0.91	1.12	1987	0.98	0.83	1.20
1981	0.97	0.93	1.12	1988	0.94	0.80	1.22
1982	0.96	0.91	1.14	1989	0.91	0.76	1.22
1983	0.97	0.92	1.16	1990	0.89	0.80	1.27
1984	0.98	0.88	1.16	1991	0.88	0.82	1.30
1985	1.01	0.90	1.16	1992	0.89	0.91	1.31
1986	1.01	0.88	1.16	1993	0.89	0.93	1.29
				1994	0.97	0.94	1.24

Note: Payments and costs include both inpatient and outpatient services. These ratios cannot be used to compare payment levels because both the mix of services and the cost per unit of service vary across payers. They do, however, indicate the relative degree to which payments from each payer cover the costs of treating its patients. Due to reporting inconsistencies related to Medicaid disproportionate share payments and provider-specific taxes, there are significant margins of error for the numbers related to all payers in 1992 and 1993.
Source: ProPAC analysis of data from the American Hospital Association Annual Survey of Hospitals.

Hospital losses from the Medicaid program also accelerated in the late 1980s, reaching a high point in 1989. This was partially due to expanding enrollment and payment limitations in some states. In the early 1990s, however, many state Medicaid programs began to use taxes and donations to attract more and larger federal payments to hospitals serving a disproportionate share of low-income patients. Thus, the losses decreased.

Hospitals have historically survived through a concept known as "cost shifting," wherein losses from federal programs are compensated by generating additional revenue through raising charges to the private sector, particularly insurance companies. Before PPS, hospital payments to cost ratios were between 112% and 116%. By 1993, however, when Medicare and Medicaid reimbursed only 89% and 93% of hospital costs, respectively, the private payer's percentage of costs had increased to 129%.

Because of their payer mix, not all hospitals have been able to generate additional revenue to cover losses from uncompensated care and below-cost payments from Medicaid and Medicare. Hospitals situated in low-income areas or those with limited capability to attract privately insured patients have had little opportunity to cost shift. However, hospitals serving affluent populations where the service area is not overbedded have been successful in this process.

There is a limitation to cost shifting because businesses, which pay most of the premiums, are also in a highly competitive environment. In response to pressure from insureds, insurance companies have adopted aggressive utilization review programs and stricter payment constraints to transfer more of the financial risk to hospitals. Insurance companies have also turned to management organizations to implement comprehensive approaches to control costs.

Hospitals have responded to the profit margin squeeze by instituting drastic cost-cutting programs and searching for revenues in other settings, for example, post acute and ambulatory care facilities as well as outpatient care.

Health Care Provider Trends

Managed care plans or health maintenance organizations (HMOs) and preferred provider organizations (PPOs) or managed fee for service plans are replacing all other forms of health insurance and currently serve more than 60% of Americans. This dominance is expected to reach over 80% by 1997. The magnitude of hospital revenues from HMOs and PPOs by category in 1993 is shown in Table 1.5.

Table 1.5	Hospital Net Patient Care Revenues from HMOs and PPOs, 1993					
		Percentage of Net Patient Care Revenues				
Hospital Category	Number of Hospitals	0-10%	11-25%	25-50%	Over 50%	
Total	1,495	64.1%	24.5%	7.8%	0.9%	
Atlantic	400	65.5%	25.5%	6.0%	2.0%	
East Central	391	60.6%	30.2%	7.2%	—	
West Central	404	75.4%	14.9%	5.9%	1.0%	
Far West	300	51.7%	29.0%	13.3%	2.3%	
Urban	736	43.6%	37.8%	14.1%	1.5%	
Rural	759	84.1%	11.7%	1.6%	0.3%	
Teaching	233	59.7%	33.0%	3.9%	0.9%	
Non-teaching	1,262	65.0%	22.7%	8.5%	0.9%	

Note: Rows may not add to 100% due to survey item nonresponse.
Atlantic includes the New England, Middle Atlantic, and South Atlantic Census divisions. East Central includes the East North Central and East South Central Census divisions. West Central includes the West North Central and West South Central Census divisions. Far West includes the Mountain and Pacific Census divisions. Teaching hospitals are those with more than 5% professional time spent teaching.
Source: Health Care Financing Administration, U. S. Department of Health & Human Services.

The growth in managed care systems is attributed to soaring health care expenditures, which are motivating more and more firms to drop traditional health hospitalization insurance plans in favor of less costly plans. Currently, the average HMO's hospital reimbursement rate is about 40% less than that of a typical indemnity plan.

Managed competition is a market-driven, multifaceted approach to health care reform that creates incentives for insurers and providers to deliver the most effective care in terms of price, quality, and benefits. Managed competition includes a series of elements: group purchasing, a standard benefits package, open enrollment, community rating, a national health board, uniform data reporting, and competing provider/insurer entities. Managed care derives its revenue from prepaid patients, which is known as a capitated system. Capitation is a payment mechanism that seeks to reduce the financial incentive to increase services. Few providers have been able to prove they can control health care costs without having strict rules about delivery imposed by an outside insurer or payer.

Physician groups will be profitable if they do not unduly strain the applicable delivery systems, particularly costly elements such as emergency services and highly specialized treatment programs. Emphasis will tend to be on the prevention of disease and disability. Healthier insureds, especially when they are clustered into capitated groups, invariably generate more profit.

As managed care steadily attracts more enrollees and expands its share of the U.S. health care market, individual primary care physicians will draw patients from a decreasing pool of fee-for-service covered persons. Few doctors will be able to generate enough business by themselves to achieve economies of scale and competitive performance ratios. Since quality and quantity are intertwined, it will be mandatory for primary care physicians to join some kind of group. Those groups that deliver quality patient care within the capitated cost reimbursement limitations will likely be the survivors in the managed care health environment of the late 1990s.

The consequences of this trend, as far as the appraiser is concerned, include lower future rates of hospital revenue and inflation, implementation of cost-cutting programs, continued consolidation of facilities, termination and failure of weak entities, greater uncertainty regarding market share for marginal hospitals, and steady downward pressure on certain hospital values.

Vertical Relationships in the Health Care System

A valuable framework for understanding the health care system is the organizational structure of patient care in terms of levels of complexity. This framework is illustrated in Figure 1.2. These levels are generally referred to as primary care, secondary care, tertiary care, and quaternary care.

1. *Primary care* is the base that supports the more complex levels of care. It typically is provided in physicians' offices, clinics, and home settings and involves the provision of basic services such as general examinations, treatment of minor or routine illnesses, and preventive services. Primary care services performed in a general hospital are typically routine medical and surgical procedures, diagnostic tests, and obstetrical services.

2. *Secondary care* involves a higher degree of specialization and technological sophistication. Physician care is provided by specialists such as specialized surgeons (e.g:, urologists and ophthalmologists) or specialized internists (e.g:, cardiologists and oncologists). Secondary care is provided in hospitals with more complex technological backup, physician specialist support, and ancillary services.

3. *Tertiary care* deals with the most complex surgical and medical conditions. Frequently, a single hospital may not be sufficient to provide tertiary care; a "medical center" may be required. However, secondary facilities are increasingly performing what were previously considered tertiary procedures. The "routinization" of previously uncommon procedures reflects to a great extent improvements in technology and in the increased number of specialists with advanced surgical training.

4. *Quaternary care* involves highly complex procedures such as organ transplants and complicated trauma cases. Some of these procedures, however, are now being performed at tertiary facilities.

	Figure 1.2	Levels of Patient Care

	Procedure	Site	Physician
		Quarternary Care	
	Organ transplant	Multi-institution medical centers	Teams of super-specialist physicians
	Complex trauma		
		Tertiary Care	
	Specialized surgery	Large-scale comprehensive	Physician sub-specialists
	Complex medical cases	hospitals with extensive	
		technological support	
		Secondary Care	
	Moderately complex	Moderate-scale hospitals	Physician specialists
	surgical and medical	Some freestanding surgery	
	cases	and diagnostic centers	
		Primary Care	
	Routine care	General hospitals	Primary care physicians
	Standard tests	Clinics	Physician "extenders" (e.g., nurse
	Simple surgery	Physician offices "urgicenters"	practitioners, physician assistants,
	Prevention		nurses)

Complexity
Severity
Specialization

Source: Demography of Health and Health Care, Plenum Press (1992), p. 39

The vertical integration of the health care system (where provider entities are increasing their market share through the development and acquisition of related, specialized facilities) can offer appraisers opportunities to provide market studies, financial feasibility reports, and valuations.

Subacute care is a current example of the above concept. Subacute care facilities (see Chapter 7) have grown rapidly in recent years in response to changes in health care coverage and reimbursement. They offer care to patients who no longer need acute care services but still require highly skilled nursing care and access to technologically advanced therapies. An off-site subacute care facility enables a primary care hospital to discharge a patient into a facility that is licensed as a nursing home. Subacute care facilities can be developed and operated at a much lower cost than is required for a primary care medical surgical hospital. Moreover, subacute reimbursement rates are substantially higher than those attributed to typical skilled nursing care.

Hospitals have also expanded their capacity to furnish ambulatory surgery (see Chapter 4) and other outpatient services and have developed specialized units to provide inpatient psychiatric care and rehabilitation. Some hospitals also offer subacute nursing care as well as home health care and other community-based services.

Demographic Changes and Impacts

The nation's health care system has been shaped by demographic processes related to the nation's living standards, its educational level, and its lifestyles. Demographic factors include fertility, mortality, population growth, migration, age distribution, sex distribution, racial and ethnic diversity, marital status, family and household structure, educational level, occupational/industrial distribution, and income distribution. A discussion of all of these factors is beyond the scope of this text. Readers are referred to recent books entirely devoted to the relationship between demography and health care (see bibliography).

The most publicized demographic trend involves the change in the U.S. age pyramid (see Figure 1.3). During the 1990s the median age will increase from 33 to 36 years. The bulk of the population is now concentrated in the 30-plus age cohorts, with no net growth expected for the under 45 population during the 1990s. Population increases will be recorded among the 45-plus population. This trend is not expected to diminish until well into the 21st century. Increases in the elderly population have resulted in the increased use of hospitals by those over 65 and a drop in usage among the younger age groups. This tends to mean a "sicker" patient load, which can have a negative effect on the financial results for a hospital as well as increased work for hospital staff. The elderly not only need more care but they need different care. Examples of such care include the development of assisted living facilities (see Chapter 6), those dealing with mental decline such as specialized Alzheimer's facilities (see Chapter 7), and gero-psychiatric facilities. These projects all require market analyses, financial feasibility studies, and appraisals for investment and financing purposes.

In conclusion, demographic trends point to increases in the demand for pediatric services, "maintenance" services, geriatric services, and rehabilitation services as well as preventive care, fitness, and wellness programs. By the year 2000 there will be fewer demands for obstetrical services, acute care relative to chronic care, invasive surgical procedures or diagnostic tests, inpatient psychiatric (including substance abuse) services, and trauma services related to violence and accidents. New outpatient construction and expansion/renovations (see Table 1.6) are a response to some of these trends.

Allocation of Medical Resources

The allocation of medical resources in terms of the geographic location of physicians, dentists, and nurses is quite uneven in the United States (see Table 1.7). In 1992 there were 224 physicians and 731 nurses for every 100,000 people nationwide. However, by individual state, the ratio ranges from a low of 129 physicians in Idaho to a high of 353 physicians in Massachusetts per 100,000 civilian population.

This type of information is valuable in studying the demand for services and space. It illustrates the problem of providing a fair share of medical care to states that are less developed. Suppose, for example, that it is determined that a particular hospital or medical market area should have a ratio of 250 physicians per 100,000 civilian population. By comparison with the actual inventory of physicians within a particular trade or a service area, the differential rate can be used to estimate the necessary amount of medical office space (based on a known factor of so many square feet per physician) the market can support. This measure of demand can then be compared to the supply to indicate the likely marketability of a proposed project. Chapter 8, which deals with medical office buildings and clinics, will show how the desired number of physicians per capita can be used to estimate the amount of building space for a particular service area. These data will also assist in estimating the feasibility of developing new hospitals and related care facilities in underserved markets.

In addition to its geographic unevenness, the amount of medical care being dispensed to the population is also unequally distributed by age group, race, and sex (see Table 1.8). These data also can be used in feasibility studies to measure demand for services and space through an analysis of the demographic composition of a service area. The estimated number of potential

Figure 1.3   U.S. Age Pyramid

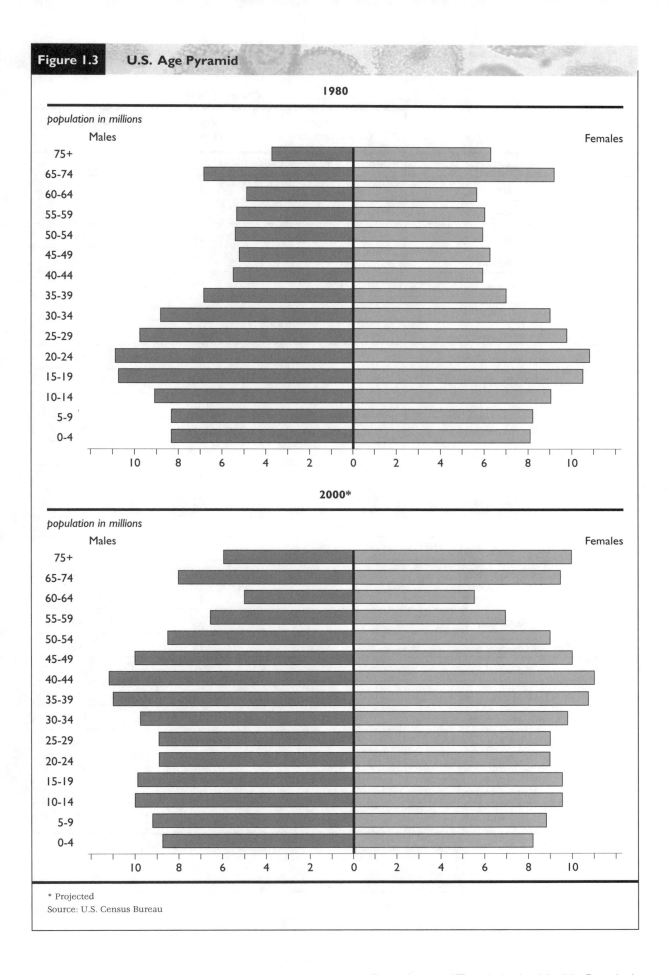

1980

population in millions

Males   Females

* Projected
Source: U.S. Census Bureau

Table 1.6

New Outpatient Construction and Hospital Expansions/Renovations by Type of Service

Service	Project Phase in 1994		
	Completed Construction	Broke Ground	Completed Design
Adult day care	19	12	39
Adult independent living	17	12	51
Ambulatory care	286	222	382
Assisted living	36	27	102
Birthing center	116	77	128
Cancer center	106	79	111
Cardiology services	162	112	136
Diagnostic imaging center	318	189	269
Emergency medicine	101	143	255
Home health/mobile outreach	17	14	55
Intensive-care unit	160	104	166
Medical laboratory	200	121	204
Medical office building	255	166	296
Parking garage	69	34	69
Pediatrics unit	95	63	114
Pharmacy	122	99	149
Physical therapy/sports	113	89	127
Psychiatric wing/unit	74	41	107
Rehabilitation wing/unit	98	53	107
Renal dialysis	67	45	67
Research building/unit	43	37	68
Subacute care	69	36	118
Substance abuse	25	15	32
Surgery center/suite	279	176	302
Utility building/unit	74	50	90
Waiting/lobby/entrance	326	249	421
Wellness center	40	29	63
Women's health center	113	54	126

Figures are derived from the number of projects reported by architecture and design/building firms. Projects reported by construction management firms and general contractors have been excluded to avoid duplication.

Source: *Modern Healthcare,* March 27, 1995.

Table 1.7 — Active Non-Federal Physicians and Nurses, by State: 1992

(Nurses as of March; Physicians as of Jan. 1. Excludes doctors of osteopathy. Federally employed persons and physicians with addresses unknown. Includes all physicians not classified according to activity status)

State	Physicians Total	Physicians Rate*	Nurses Total	Nurses Rate*
United States	568,132	224	1,853,024	731
Alabama	6,913	168	27,717	673
Alaska	748	133	3,583	637
Arizona	7,461	196	27,093	711
Arkansas	3,855	161	14,001	587
California	73,713	241	173,973	568
Colorado	7,431	217	26,697	780
Connecticut	10,383	318	30,918	946
Delaware	1,420	207	6,137	894
District of Columbia	3,908	677	11,352	1,968
Florida	28,379	212	94,591	707
Georgia	12,000	179	43,386	647
Hawaii	2,740	249	7,674	697
Idaho	1,366	129	5,702	537
Illinois	26,395	228	93,069	804
Indiana	9,318	165	39,602	700
Iowa	4,393	157	25,838	922
Kansas	4,549	183	19,773	794
Kentucky	6,644	178	24,552	659
Louisiana	8,526	201	24,233	570
Maine	2,325	189	10,584	861
Maryland	16,695	342	38,170	783
Massachusetts	21,129	353	63,751	1,066
Michigan	18,265	194	65,441	694
Minnesota	10,379	232	39,876	893
Mississippi	3,539	136	13,415	516
Missouri	10,722	207	42,035	812
Montana	1,359	166	5,848	715
Nebraska	2,964	187	13,257	834
Nevada	1,928	145	7,135	538
New Hampshire	2,324	209	10,743	964
New Jersey	20,277	260	64,519	827
New Mexico	2,987	191	9,393	600
New York	60,171	333	159,297	881
North Carolina	13,332	198	47,602	708
North Dakota	1,157	185	6,300	1,007
Ohio	22,709	206	89,799	816
Oklahoma	4,865	153	16,972	534
Oregon	6,246	210	23,992	808
Pennsylvania	30,090	251	108,663	907
Rhode Island	2,680	269	9,665	971
South Carolina	6,091	172	20,684	584
South Dakota	1,062	151	6,828	973
Tennessee	10,396	208	35,318	706
Texas	31,374	179	92,810	528
Utah	3,384	187	9,831	545
Vermont	1,503	263	5,199	910
Virginia	13,366	215	42,519	684
Washington	11,054	217	38,698	761
West Virginia	3,240	179	11,875	657
Wisconsin	9,733	195	39,883	799
Wyoming	644	140	3,032	658

* Per 100,000 civilian population. Based on U.S. Bureau of the Census estimates as of July 1, 1992.

Source: Physicians: *Socioeconomic Characteristics of Medical Practice* and *Physician Characteristics and Distribution in the U.S.*, American Medical Association, copyright 1994. Nurses: U.S. Dept. of Health and Human Services, Health Resources and Services Administration, unpublished data.

Table 1.8 Physician Contacts, by Place of Contact and Selected Patient Characteristics, 1992

Characteristic	Number (1,000)					Visits per Person				
	All Places[a]	Telephone	Office	Hospital[b]	Other	All Places[a]	Telephone	Office	Hospital[b]	Other
All Persons[c]	1,513	181	834	222	266	6.0	0.7	3.3	0.9	1.1
Age										
Under 5 years	136	20	80	19	16	6.9	1.0	4.1	1.0	0.8
5-17 years	164	23	94	25	20	3.5	0.5	2.0	0.5	0.4
18-24 years	101	11	48	19	22	4.1	0.4	2.0	0.8	0.9
25-44 years	436	57	248	61	67	5.4	0.7	3.1	0.7	0.8
45-64 years	349	42	191	55	59	7.2	0.9	3.9	1.1	1.2
65-74 years	179	17	98	26	36	9.7	0.9	5.3	1.4	2.0
75 years and over	149	12	74	16	46	12.1	1.0	6.0	1.3	3.7
Sex										
Male	624	66	338	106	110	5.1	0.5	2.8	0.9	0.9
Female	889	115	496	115	156	6.9	0.9	3.8	0.9	1.2
Race										
White	1,286	161	728	174	216	6.1	0.8	3.5	0.8	1.0
Black	181	15	83	38	42	5.8	0.5	2.6	1.2	1.3
Income										
Under $10,000	192	20	83	42	46	7.8	0.8	3.4	1.7	1.9
$10,000-$19,999	255	30	128	42	53	6.6	0.8	3.3	1.1	1.4
$20,000-$34,999	299	38	162	45	53	5.8	0.7	3.2	0.9	1.0
$35,000 or more	515	74	318	60	59	5.7	0.8	3.5	0.7	0.6

Notes: a = Includes unknown place of contact; b = Excludes contacts while an overnight patient in a hospital; c = Includes other races.
Source: U.S. National Center for Health Statistics, *Vital and Health Statistics*, series 10, No. 189.

Table 1.9

Table 1.9 Physician and Dental Contacts, by Patient Characteristics, 1970 to 1992

| Type of visit and year | Total Visits (mil) | | | | Visits per Person per Year | | | | | | | | | |
| | Sex | | Race | | Sex | | Race | | Age (years) | | | | | |
	Male	Female	White	Black	Male	Female	White	Black	Under 5	5 to 17	18 to 24	25 to 44	45 to 64	65 and over
Physicians:														
1970	396	531	832	87	4.1	5.1	4.8	3.9	5.9[a]	2.9[b]	4.6[c]	4.6	5.2	6.3
1980	426	610	903	115	4.0	5.4	4.8	4.5	6.7[a]	3.2[b]	4.0[c]	4.6	5.1	6.4
1983	470	694	1,018	126	4.3	5.8	5.2	4.6	6.5[a]	3.2[b]	4.0[c]	4.7	5.8	7.6
1985	498	733	1,074	132	4.4	6.1	5.4	4.7	6.3[a]	3.1[b]	4.2[c]	4.9	6.1	8.3
1986	515	756	1,110	131	4.5	6.2	5.5	4.6	6.3	3.3	4.2	4.7	6.6	9.1
1987	523	765	1,118	140	4.5	6.2	5.5	4.9	6.7	3.3	4.4	4.8	6.4	8.9
1988	530	774	1,139	136	4.5	6.2	5.6	4.6	7.0	3.4	3.8	5.1	6.1	8.7
1989	552	771	1,148	140	4.7	6.1	5.6	4.7	6.7	3.5	3.9	5.1	6.1	8.9
1990	558	806	1,178	148	4.7	6.4	5.7	4.9	6.9	3.2	4.3	5.1	6.4	9.2
1991	589	842	1,243	152	4.9	6.6	6.0	4.9	7.1	3.4	3.9	5.1	6.6	10.4
1992	624	889	1,286	181	5.1	6.9	6.1	5.8	6.9	3.5	4.1	5.4	7.2	10.6
Dentists:														
1970	133	171	283	17	1.4	1.7	1.6	0.8	0.5[a]	1.9[b]	1.8[c]	1.7	1.5	1.1
1980	158	207	333	26	1.5	1.8	1.8	1.0	0.5[a]	2.3[b]	1.6[c]	1.7	1.8	1.4
1983	183	239	382	31	1.6	2.0	1.9	1.1	0.5[a]	2.6[b]	1.6[c]	1.9	2.0	1.5
1986	210	256	416	37	1.9	2.2	2.1	1.4	0.7	2.4	1.7	2.0	2.2	2.1
1989	221	271	441	34	1.9	2.2	2.2	1.2	0.5	2.4	1.6	2.0	2.4	2.0

Notes: a = Under 6 years; b = 6 to 17 years; c = 17 to 24 years
Source: U.S. National Center for Health Statistics, *Vital and Health Statistics*, series 10, No. 189, and earlier reports; and unpublished data

physician or dental visits per person can be combined with an average charge per person and the number of physicians or dentists to project potential revenues for a particular medical activity or group practice, for example, to provide an indication of economic or financial potential.

Most medical business (55%) is conducted in physicians' offices, but a significant amount is also done by telephone (12%), at hospitals (15%), and the balance of 18% in other locations (e.g., at home, business, or accident site). The ratios of visits per person by place of contact (see Table 1.9) vary significantly by age, sex, race, and incomes groups. These statistics are also helpful in macroestimates of future space needs.

C H A P T E R
T W O

Medical and Surgical (Acute) Hospitals

From the viewpoint of an appraiser a hospital is an extremely complex, highly regulated, special purpose property that lacks the normal requisites for marketability and complicates the application of traditional appraisal techniques. Hospitals have been described as the equivalent of small cities wherein functions such as residential (permanent housing as well as transient housing for patients), commercial (retail, restaurant, offices), industrial (scientific laboratories, research, processing, repairs), and institutional (educational, medical, clinical) activities take place.

This chapter will deal with the analysis and valuation of acute care general hospitals, which differ from psychiatric, rehabilitation, and other specialized hospitals. Such hospitals have entirely separate and unique considerations, which will be covered in later chapters. This chapter focuses on specific trends in medical and surgical hospitals and the application of appropriate analytical and valuation procedures and techniques.

Appraisers may typically provide valuations of physical assets including real estate and personal property, going-concern values wherein intangibles may be considered, and estimates of fair market rental value. Possible assignments might also involve market studies and appraisals of components of a medical center such as a surgery center, outpatient clinic, ambulatory care center, convalescent facility, or medical office building. Vertical integration by primary hospitals is spurring this type of assignment. The need for expert real estate services is considerable because of the large number of these facilities in the United States, the relatively small number of available experts, and the monumental changes taking place in health care that are affecting property values.

Current Trends

The American hospital industry is suffering from financial instability, overcapacity, a declining rate of inpatient utilization, a nursing shortage, the AIDS crisis, and shrinking Medicare profit margins. These vital factors affect hospital property values. Although the industry has been swept by dozens of mergers and shows slight signs of improvement in profitability, serious questions remain about its aggregate productivity.

Hospitals are business enterprises whether they are investor owned or operated on a not-for-profit basis. Currently there are roughly four nonprofit, nongovernment hospitals for every profit-motivated operation in the United States. This factor has been relatively stable even though not-for-profit hospitals are becoming more important in the hospital takeover game. Investor-owned hospitals appear to control a slightly increasing number of beds and ratio of beds (currently almost 1:6). Consolidation in the industry is led by Columbia/HCA. At the end of 1995 it controlled a reported 337 hospitals and received about $17 billion in revenue that year. It has managed to dominate the business by delivering profits (up 41% to $267 million in the first nine months of 1995 compared with the same period in 1994) through tight quality and cost controls.

Supply Considerations

At the end of 1993 the total number of hospitals of all types registered by the American Hospital Association was 6,467, down from a 1980 total of 6,965. An inventory of U.S. hospitals covering the period 1980-1993 appears in Table 2.1. The typical hospital either was constructed during the past 20 years or has been extensively remodeled on several occasions. In some recent years, hospital closures have exceeded the rate of new construction. About 250 acute care hospitals have closed in the past five years.

According to the American Hospital Association, in 1993 hospital ownership was divided as follows: 3,338 hospitals (52%) were owned by religious orders or other nongovernment, non-profit entities; 1,708 (26%) were owned by local agencies and operated on a not-for-profit basis; and 1,105 (17%) were owned by corporations, real estate investment groups, or individuals. These latter are proprietary operations that were developed initially to provide not only health care but a return on invested capital and resources. A balance of 316 facilities was owned by the federal government.

Approximately half of all hospitals now belong to or are operated by a larger organization or system. Larger, older, and well-established hospitals tend to dominate a market although some of them are in a delicate economic position due to their higher costs of operation and lack of profitability. Stand-alone operations are the least profitable. It is believed that virtually all hospitals will be involved in a merger, acquisition, or consolidation in the near future.

Some hospitals are assuming nonprofit status now because they are losing money. For the industry as a whole, however, all measures of hospital profitability showed slight signs of improvement in recent years. The median total profit margin for all U.S. hospitals was 4.23% in 1993, up from 4.22% in 1992. Overall improvements in profitability were primarily the result of hospitals holding down expenses. For example, a major 500-bed medical center in one of the nation's largest MSAs has discontinued high-tech surgical specialties such as organ transplants, deeply cut its educational and training programs, and eliminated its university-style research efforts. The goal is to reformulate the region's largest private hospital into a "first class" community hospital. (For additional specific information on current trends affecting the financial and operating performance of hospitals, see Appendix A.)

Bed Trends

There are about 920,000 medical and surgical hospital beds in the United States situated within 5,261 "community"[1] hospitals. While only 6% have more than 500 beds and 70% have less than 200 beds, the larger hospitals (over 500 beds) account for about 24% of admissions and 28% of gross revenues. The average hospital has about 115 beds in service, and the average investment (book value) is $90,000 per bed.

Hospitals are using fewer beds every year. Occupancy rates nationally declined to an average of 47% in 1994. Typical is a hospital with 200 licensed beds, of which 116 are set up for use (58%) and 54.5 (or 47% of the 116) are normally occupied. Many former patient wings have been converted to outpatient or other services and some have just been shut down.

---

[1] Community hospitals exclude medical and surgical units of institutions but include nonfederal, short-term general, and some specialty hospitals.

Hospital Category	1980	1985	1990	1993	Percent Change 1980-1993
All hospitals	6,965	6,872	6,649	6,467	-7.2%
Short-term	6,407	6,339	6,141	6,040	-5.7
Long-term	558	533	508	427	-23.5
General medical and surgical	6,105	5,961	5,566	5,369	-12.1
Psychiatric	558	629	774	760	36.2
Tuberculosis and other specialty	302	282	309	338	11.9
Community*	5,830	5,732	5,384	5,261	-9.8
Noncommunity	1,135	1,140	1,265	1,206	6.3
Number of beds:					
6-24	327	267	301	290	-11.3
25-49	1,209	1,134	1,095	1,065	-11.9
50-99	1,674	1,666	1,633	1,554	-7.2
100-199	1,567	1,618	1,562	1,582	1.0
200-299	802	848	830	834	4.0
399-399	484	507	503	471	-2.7
400-499	334	301	276	253	-24.3
500+	568	531	449	418	-26.4
Voluntary	3,505	3,544	3,388	3,338	-4.8
Proprietary	891	1,052	1,139	1,105	24.0
Federal government	359	343	337	316	-12.0
Nonfederal government	2,210	1,933	1,785	1,708	-22.7
Residency training	1,257	1,232	1,249	1,197	-4.8
Medical school affiliation	997	1,120	1,238	1,177	18.1
Council of Teaching Hospitals member	406	454	387	394	-3.0

* Community hospitals include nonfederal short-term general and some specialty hospitals.

Source: American Hospital Association, *Hospital Statistics,* 1994 edition. Copyright by the American Hospital Association. Reprinted with permission.

Average Length of Stay (ALOS)

One measure of the success or efficiency of health care is the trend in average length of stay. The average stay for all patients dropped from 8.0 to 7.3 days between 1970 and 1980. A more dramatic change occurred between 1980 and 1986 when the ALOS reached 6.4 days. After that the average stayed virtually unchanged through 1991, ranging between 6.4 and 6.5 days. By 1993 it had reached 6.0 days. When pediatric discharges are included, the ALOS was 4.79 days in 1993. ALOS is an important statistic for comparing hospitals since it is a key indicator of utilization and clinical management.

Continued reductions in ALOS are consistent with incentives provided under Medicare and private insurance payment policies. Advances in modern technology have also facilitated this trend. In general, rural hospitals have shorter ALOS than urban hospitals; teaching hospitals have the longest ALOS.

Utilization rates of inpatients discharged from noninstitutional, short-stay hospitals, exclusive of federal hospitals, are shown in Table 2.2.

New Projects

Hospital construction has shown a stable and optimistic market despite a general surplus of beds in the industry, the uncertainty over health care reform, and financing difficulties. Table 2.3 summarizes projects by construction phase in 1994. A total of 34,652 acute, rehabilitation, or specialty beds were in the pipeline or completed in 1994, while another 46,642 beds were involved in hospital expansions or renovations. For new or replacement acute hospitals the average construction cost was $304,000 per bed. Much of the expansion was driven by technological change and a shift to more outpatient care.

Characteristics of Medical-Surgical Hospitals

An acute care general hospital is an extremely complex institution. There are few typical hospitals anymore. They differ in size, services and specialties, ownership, age, location, market conditions, competition, reputation, professional staff, and degree of obsolescence. Facilities and services provided by community hospitals are set forth in Table 2.4. Physical assets typically involve land, yard improvements, buildings, fixed equipment, movable equipment, minor equipment, and rolling stock.

Hospitals are frequently bought, sold, and leased by private sector hospital management and investment firms and less frequently by nonprivate entities. Prices paid for hospitals are extremely volatile. Within a short period of years price conditions may range from one of rapid escalation to one of stagnation in revenues and extreme drops in prices. In the latter context the appraiser must be able to understand the degrees to which management can deal with hospital operating inefficiencies and provide for a continuing evolution in services to derive new revenue sources and maximize market penetration.

Frequently, hospitals will add high-technology services even when clinical indications for their appropriate use are largely unstudied or when they are duplicating costly facilities available at a nearby hospital. Computerized tomography (CT) scanners are an example of excessive equipment acquisitions. CT scanners first appeared about 1973; by 1985 almost all community hospitals with more than 300 beds had a CT unit, even though the typical cost was about $500,000. See Table 2.5 for other examples of the growth in high-tech (and extremely costly) services and equipment.

Table 2.2 Hospital Utilization Rates: 1970 to 1993

Selected Characteristic	Patients Discharged (1,000)	Patients Discharged per 1,000 Persons*			Days of Care per 1,000 Persons*			Average Stay (Days)		
		Total	Male	Female	Total	Male	Female	Total	Male	Female
1970	29,127	144	118	169	1,122	982	1,251	8.0	8.7	7.6
1980	37,832	168	139	194	1,217	1,068	1,356	7.3	7.7	7.0
1985	35,056	148	124	171	954	849	1,053	6.5	6.9	6.2
1986	34,256	143	121	164	913	817	1,003	6.4	6.8	6.1
1987	33,387	138	116	159	889	806	968	6.4	6.9	6.1
1988**	31,146	128	107	147	834	757	907	6.5	7.1	6.2
1989**	30,947	126	105	145	815	741	884	6.5	7.0	6.1
1990**	30,788	124	102	144	792	704	875	6.4	6.9	6.1
1991**	31,098	124	103	144	795	715	869	6.4	7.0	6.0
1992**	30,951	122	101	142	751	680	818	6.2	6.7	5.8
1993 Total*	30,825	120	98	141	720	644	792	6.0	6.5	5.6
Age:										
Under 1 year old	710	181	206	156	1,155	1,265	1,041	6.4	6.1	6.7
1 to 4 years old	654	41	46	37	163	169	157	3.9	3.7	4.3
5 to 14 years old	777	21	22	20	108	110	105	5.1	5.1	5.2
15 to 24 years old	3,088	87	37	138	309	204	416	3.5	5.5	3.0
25 to 34 years	4,655	113	53	171	446	313	575	4.0	5.9	3.4
35 to 44 years old	3,457	85	72	99	431	424	438	5.1	5.9	4.4
45 to 64 years old	6,283	127	132	123	785	831	742	6.2	6.3	6.1
65 to 74 years old	4,890	262	284	245	1,927	2,033	1,844	7.4	7.2	7.5
75 years old and over	6,130	446	476	430	3,665	3,746	3,609	8.2	7.9	8.4
Region:										
Northeast	6,965	136	119	152	952	876	1,023	7.0	7.4	6.7
Midwest	7,097	116	98	134	706	638	771	6.1	6.5	5.8
South	11,580	131	104	156	749	658	771	6.1	6.5	5.8
West	5,138	93	72	114	473	419	527	5.1	5.8	4.6

* Based on Bureau of the Census estimated civilian population as of July 1. Estimates for 1980-90 do not reflect revisions based on the 1990 Census of Population.
** Comparison beginning 1988 with data for earlier years should be made with caution as estimates of change may reflect improvements in the design rather than true changes in hospital use.

Source: U.S. National Center for Health Statistics, *Vital Health Statistics*, series 13; and unpublished data (pediatrics are excluded).

Table 2.3 — Projects by Construction Phase in 1994

	Completed			Broke Ground			Designed		
	No. of Projects	Completed No. of Beds	Construction Cost**	No. of Projects	No. of Beds	Construction Cost**	No. of Projects	No. of Beds	Construction Cost**
New or replacement acute care hospitals	29	4,391	$1,136.1	35	7,809	$4,008.0	60	11,685	$6,370.1
New or replacement rehabilitation hospitals	26	1,140	$125.7	6	286	$34.5	19	997	$143.2
Other new or replacement specialty hospitals	25	1,833	$554.0	27	3,322	$1,329.2	30	3,189	$1,185.5
Hospital expansions or renovations	2,149	18,472	$6,068.8	992	9,676	$4,222.3	2,023	18,494	$8,392.8
Parking garages (multilevel)	62	—	$326.2	26	—	$138.3	59	—	$281.7
Total	2,291	25,836	$8,210.8	1,086	21,093	$9,732.3	2,191	34,365	$16,373.3

* Beds are new or replacement.
** All dollar figures are reported in millions.
Note: Freestanding outpatient facilities may be on or off campus. If on campus, such facilities may be independent or connected to the main hospital through a skyway or tunnel, for example, but not physically part of it. Figures are derived from the number of projects reported by architecture and design/build firms. Projects reported by construction management firms and general contractors have been excluded to avoid duplication. Figures include projects completed in the United States.
Source: *Modern Healthcare*, March 27, 1995.

Service		Hospitals with Service	Percent of Total
Adult day care program		362	7.5%
Alzheimer's diagnostic/assessment		475	9.8
Angioplasty		1,055	21.8
Alcoholism/chemical dependency outpatient services		1.025	21.2
Birthing rooms		3,228	66.6
Blood bank		3,382	69.8
Cardiac rehabilitation		2,374	49.0
Computerized tomographic (CT) scanner		3,750	77.4
Emergency department		4,460	92.1
Extracorporeal shock wave lithotripter		516	10.7
Genetic counseling services		501	10.3
Geriatric services		3,147	65.0
Hemodialysis		1,358	28.0
Histopathology laboratory		3,105	64.1
Home health services		2,047	42.2
Hospice		964	19.9
Hospital auxiliary		3,861	79.7
AIDS inpatient care		3,564	73.6
AIDS outpatient care		326	6.7
Magnetic resonance imaging (MRI)		1,507	31.1
Open-heart surgery facilities		908	18.7
Outpatient surgery services		4,541	93.7
Patient representative services		2,739	56.5
Trauma center		810	16.7
Ultrasound		4,115	84.9
Volunteer services department		3,356	69.3
Women's center		1,364	28.2
Rehabilitation outpatient department		2,802	57.4
Reproductive health services		2,130	44.0
Psychiatric services:	Emergency	1,694	35.0
	Outpatient	1,130	23.3
Radiation therapy:	X-ray	967	20.0
	Radio-active implants	1,231	25.4
Radio isotope facilities:	Diagnostic	2,988	61.7
	Therapeutic	1,288	26.6
Therapy services:	Occupational therapy services	2,688	55.5
	Physical therapy services	4,143	85.5
	Recreational therapy services	1,751	36.1
	Respiratory therapy services	4,420	91.2

Source: American Hospital Association, Chicago, IL, *Hospital Statistics, 1994-95* and *1993 Annual Survey of Hospitals* (copyright).

Table 2.5	High-Technology Services Provided by Hospitals, Selected Years						
Year	Cardiac Catheterization	CT Scan	Lithotripsy (ESWL)	Magnetic Resonance Imaging	Megavolt Radiation Therapy	Open-Heart Surgery	SPECT
1981	14.8%	21.4%	—	—	14.5%	9.6%	—
1985	16.8%	48.5%	0.8%	—	15.2%	11.1%	—
1990	24.1%	61.1%	5.4%	15.6%	17.0%	14.7%	16.2%
1992	27.6%	65.9%	7.2%	21.3%	17.5%	16.0%	24.0%

Note: CT = computerized tomography. ESWL = extracorporeal shock wave lithotripsy. SPECT = single photon emission computerized tomography. Includes all Federal, nonfederal, general acute care, long-term care, and psychiatric hospitals as well as hospital units of institutions.

Source: American Hospital Association, *Hospital Statistics, 1981,* and *Annual Survey of Hospitals,* 1985, 1990, and 1992.

Describing the Hospital

Normal property descriptions as detailed in *The Appraisal of Real Estate* must be combined with descriptions and explanations of unique design considerations, special purpose facilities, and special health and safety requirements. This information can be obtained from building plans as well as from the hospital's architect, engineer, or building maintenance personnel. Regulatory agencies may also be of assistance regarding health and safety requirements. Factors unique to hospitals can increase costs up to 75% of normal construction for a comparable class and quality of building. Specialized requirements can include:

- gas/liquid lines
- toxic/other waste handling facilities
- emergency controls
- electronic monitoring and sensing systems
- internal conveying systems
- internal communication and recording systems
- specialized storage capabilities
- specialized insulation requirements
- seismic stressing
- specialized wall, floor, and other coverings

Hospital buildings have construction criteria that are generally superior to all other types of buildings. For example, in seismically active zones, requirements for bracing and sizing of columns and beams as well as oversized foundations can easily add 20% to the basic construction cost. Additional seismic requirements pertain to flexible linkages and other expensive fittings in all of the systems mentioned above. An example of a component description of a hospital is shown in Table 2.6.

Design Considerations

Hospital design is controlled by overall financial feasibility, which may require stringent budgeting of space for cost control purposes. At the same time the design must allow for flexibility to enable a facility to adjust to future changes in technology, health care procedures, and hospital codes. Flexibility also relates to building systems, levels of care, and staffing ratios.

System/Component	Specifications	Unit
Foundations		
Footings & foundations	Poured concrete; strip and spread footings and 4' foundation wall	S.F. Ground
Excavation & backfill	Site preparation for slab and trench for foundation wall and footing	S.F. Ground
Substructure		
Slab on grade	4" reinforced concrete with vapor barrier and granular base	S.F. Slab
Superstructure		
Columns & beams	Fireproofed steel columns	L.F. Column
Elevated floors	Concrete slab with metal deck and beams	S.F. Floor
Roof	Metal deck, open web steel joists, beams, interior columns	S.F. Floor
Stairs	Concrete filled metal pan	Flight
Exterior Closure		
Walls	Face brick and structural facing tile (70% of wall)	S.F. Wall
Doors	Double aluminum and glass and sliding doors	Each
Windows & glazed walls	Aluminum sliding (30% of wall)	Each
Roofing		
Roof coverings	Built-up tar and gravel with flashing	S.F. Roof
Insulation	Perlite/urethane composite	S.F. Roof
Openings & specialties	Gravel stop and hatches	S.F. Roof
Interior Construction		
Partitions	Gypsum board on metal studs with sound deadening board	S.F. Partition
Interior doors	Single leaf hollow metal (90 SF Floor/Door)	Each
Wall finishes	40% vinyl wall covering, 35% ceramic tile, 25% epoxy coating	S.F. Surface
Floor finishes	60% vinyl tile, 20% ceramic, 20% terrazzo	S.F. Floor
Ceiling finishes	Plaster on suspended metal lath	S.F. Ceiling
Interior surface/exterior wall	Glazed coating (70% of wall)	S.F. Wall
Conveying		
Elevators	Six passenger elevators	Each
Mechanical		
Plumbing	Kitchen, toilet and service fixtures, supply and drainage (1 fixture/275 SF Fl.)	Each
Fire protection	Sprinklers	S.F. Floor
Heating	Oil fired hot water, wall fin radiation	S.F. Floor
Cooling	Chilled water, fan coil units	S.F. Floor
Electrical		
Service & distribution	3600-ampere service, panel board and feeders	S.F. Floor
Lighting & power	Fluorescent fixtures, receptacles, switches and misc. power	S.F. Floor
Special electrical	Alarm systems, communications systems and emergency lighting	S.F. Floor
Special Construction		
Specialties	Conductive flooring, oxygen piping, curtain partitions	S.F. Floor
Sitework		

Source: R.S. Means

When a facility is planned, it is sometimes difficult to foresee the ultimate future use of a room because its function may change dramatically in less than a decade. One approach is to design rooms slightly larger than normal to allow for additional equipment, storage, furnishings, or people. For example, a standard 100-square-foot examination room may be designed to contain 140 square feet so that it can eventually be used as a procedure room. Building systems must also respond to changing activities within the building. Large interstitial spaces, vertical structural expansion, and extra conduit for future telecommunications can greatly aid the future flexibility of a building.

Staffing ratios and level of care must also be considered in the design. Staffing ratios are one of the most challenging variables in the design process. Nursing models frequently change and nursing shortages are not uncommon. Acuity of care also rises and falls during an average patient's stay. Therefore, nursing units should be designed to take advantage of varying nurse-to-patient ratios. Features that add flexibility include single patient rooms, sub-chart areas, glass windows that allow viewing into rooms, and beds placed in small, even-numbered clusters. Such elements, however, can add as much as 20% to the square footage of a nursing unit. A typical medical-surgical space may contain 550 square feet per bed, while a design that has all single patient rooms and features to optimize staff flexibility may require 650 square feet per bed.

Determining future levels of care is difficult because reimbursement levels are changing, competition is increasing, and the acuity of patients' illnesses is growing. Planning for the future can often involve the provision for unfinished space. It is much cheaper to finish shell space when additional space is indicated than to add to a structure or move a new department into an obsolete space configuration.

The following example illustrates the economic feasibility of providing flexibility for future space utilization. A typical hospital addition of 50,000 square feet at $175 per square foot may cost $8,750,000 in today's dollars. An equipment budget is set at 25% of the building cost, or $2,200,000, bringing the total budget to $11,000,000. During the design process the hospital sets aside additional shell space at a cost of $100 per square foot and a larger than currently necessary nursing area of 4,000 square feet at $175 per square foot, or $700,000. With other incidentals such as extra conduit, HVAC, and transport space, the total additional cost comes to $1,800,000, or 16% of the current building and equipment budget. However, to retrofit or expand at a later date is likely to cost as much as three times that amount when expense is considered in terms of inflated dollars, loss in revenue, disruption to operations, and delays in schedule.

Market Analysis

Market studies should be performed in all instances, whether the appraiser is involved in a proposed facility or an existing hospital. Typical commercial market analysis techniques that deal with demographics, characteristics of competitive and proposed facilities, degree of bed utilization, and future trends can be applied.

Bed requirements are somewhat crudely measured on a per capita basis. Years ago a rule of thumb was five beds per 1,000 persons. Today there are about 3.5 beds per 1,000 persons in community hospitals, but the actual level of need is as low as two and may decrease even more in the future. There is no exact, applicable ratio of beds per capita for any one location.

Demographic factors relative to the population's age, income, general health rating, and proximity to major medical centers have a tremendous influence on bed needs and hospital utilization in a primary market area. Another factor to consider is the ability of health maintenance organizations (HMOs) to control where members can seek hospital services. This may range from referrals to selected hospitals in a region to the use of only an HMO-controlled hospital.

A preferred technique for measuring market acceptance of hospital beds is known as "penetration analysis." This type of study considers differences in hospitalization requirements by categories of age, income, and even occupation. An example of a market penetration analysis for a proposed 130-bed hospital is shown in Table 2.7.

Table 2.7	Market Penetration and Demand Analysis of a Hypothetical 130-Bed Medical-Surgical Hospital

1. Estimate of Bed Demand (by Age and Sex)

Sex	Age Group in Years	Number	Likely to Be Hospitalized	Total Est. Bed Days*
M	under 15	27,400	1,264	7,584
M	15-44	58,500	6,110	9,165
M	45-64	30,200	2,999	10,497
M	65 & over	14,000	2,119	14,833
F	under 15	26,400	903	5,418
F	15-44	58,900	15,857	31,714
F	45-64	31,000	3,075	13,838
F	65 & over	20,700	4,059	32,472
Total		267,100	36,386	181,930

2. Bed Needs Satisfied by Competitive Hospitals

Hospital	No. of Beds	Occupancy Rate	Total Bed Days
A	118	48%	20,674
B	240	61%	53,436
C	82	38%	11,373
D	198	56%	40,471
Total	638	54%	125,954

3.	Bed needs satisfied by regional medical centers — Estimate 15%	27,290
4.	Unsatisfied bed need (No. 1 – No. 2 – No. 3)	28,686
5.	Average estimated occupancy of subject	60%
6.	Total additional beds needed (28,686 ÷ 365) = 78.59 ÷ 0.6 =	130

* Calculated by multiplying the ALOS of each category times the number of persons likely to be hospitalized.
Caveat - This is a hypothetical example drawn from national statistics that are believed to be reliable. Each market is unique unto itself. The analyst should derive actual local experience from discharge data and other sources to accurately measure the unsatisfied demand, if any, in the market to be studied.

Sources of Data

A great deal of statistical information is available to the appraiser from a wide variety of sources. Health Care Investment Analysts, Inc. (HCIA), of Baltimore, Maryland, maintains a national database for hospitals throughout the United States and publishes a wide variety of operating statistics and financial data on an individual hospital and group (local, regional and national) basis. Among its annual publications is *The Comparative Performance of U.S. Hospitals: The Sourcebook,* which relies on Medicare cost reports filed by general, acute care hospitals as its primary data source. For a single hospital the firm can provide information on over 500 data elements using a standard profile or a user-defined custom profile. The information is available on-line or by facsimile. HCIA also provides hospital performance overviews, patient origin and destination reports, admission studies, and provider analyses. Patient origin and destination reports include data on strategic planning, marketing, physician relations, finance, program and facilities planning. Examples of other HCIA services are included in the Appendix. Other data are available from a variety of governmental sources as well as industry publications, especially those of the American Hospital Association.

In an individual assignment the analyst or appraiser may be overwhelmed by the amount of statistical information available for analysis. It may not be necessary to purchase a standard profile or user-defined customer profile since key data may also be available on a statewide basis through the applicable regulatory agency.

Financial Feasibility

Analyzing financial feasibility basically involves comparing the present value of projected net revenues with an estimate of the development cost per project. Typically the analyst will project revenues and expenses by operating departments and functional categories for a sufficient period into the future to allow the project to reach a stabilized level of operation, if this is possible. The net income stream is then discounted to the date of commencement of the hospital and is combined with the present value of the reversion (otherwise known as the residual value or terminal value) to indicate the total value of the future benefits. A three- to five-year period is a minimum amount of time for the projection, while a maximum time will likely be 11 years because many discounted cash flow programs are established on this basis and investors are familiar with this length of time. Also, it is reasonable to consider a holding period of seven to ten years, a yardstick commonly used in the past.

An example of a simplified projection of market penetration and financial performance for a projected 130-bed hospital is shown in Table 2.8. All of the unit factors used to estimate number of bed days, number of discharges, operating revenue and expenses per discharge, and cash flow per discharge are derived from published data in *The Sourcebook* and the U.S. National Center for Health Statistics. In this example, assuming a 15% capitalization rate is appropriate, the budget limitation for the proposed project would amount to $200,000 per bed for all facilities.

Relative to cost indicators, the median total building area per bed in general hospitals is 1,035 square feet with a typical range of 630 to 1,600 square feet. Community hospitals, particularly teaching and newer hospitals with a high percentage of private rooms, tend toward the high end, while investor-owned hospitals and older, public hospitals with more ward areas tend toward the lower end of the range. The costs per bed of completely equipped general hospitals,

Table 2.8	Estimated Market Penetration and Financial Performance for a Projected 130-Bed Hospital in an Underserved Market		
		Male	**Female**
1.	**Estimate of total potential discharges**		
	a) Service area population	118,853	123,607
	b) Days of care per 1,000 persons	680	818
	c) Annual bed days (a ÷ 1,000 x b)	80,820	101,110
	d) Average stay in days	6.7	5.8
	e) Number of discharges (c ÷ d)	12,063	17,433
	f) Percentage captured by proposed 130-bed acute hospital (based on services to be provided)	29.0%	25.0%
	g) Annual discharges for subject (e x f)	3,498	4,358
2.	**Estimates of hospital financial performance**		
	h) Gross patient revenue per discharge		$11,180
	i) Deductions from gross patient revenue		47.2%
	j) Operating revenue per discharge		$5,902
	k) Operating expenses per discharge (net of depreciation and interest charges)		91.7%
	l) Cash flow per discharge		$490
	m) Total cash flow (g x $490)		$3,849,440
3.	**Capitalized value of hospital**		
	n) Total value: $3,849,440 ÷ 15%		$25,662,933
	Rounded		$26,000,000
	o) Value per bed		$200,000

including Group I and II equipment[2] but excluding extremes, at designed capacity appear in Table 2.9. Figures are not adjusted for time or location.

In summary, a state-of-the-art hospital in a typical location can range in total cost (excluding land and Group III equipment) from approximately $120,000 to nearly $240,000 per bed,

---

[2] Group I equipment is permanent equipment installed in or attached to the building, part of the general contract, and included in typical quoted unit cost figures.

Group II equipment is equipment often installed and becoming part of the real property, but typically not part of the general contract, such as autoclaves, permanent surgical lights, and other equipment.

Group III equipment is movable personal property such as furniture and instruments.

Table 2.9	Total Costs of Acute Hospitals, Including Group I and II Equipment	
Class	Average Cost per Bed	Typical Upper Cost Range
A & B	$152,000	$240,000
C & D	$120,000	$195,000

Source: *Marshall Valuation Service*, Marshall & Swift, 1995.

depending on a variety of factors including type of construction, site conditions, inspection fees, and governmental approval.

The financial feasibility analysis may represent the entire report provided by the appraiser. Combined with a market study and estimated development costs, conclusions can be reached as to overall project feasibility, size modification, specialized services that should be offered, and timing of construction phases. If a full appraisal of the hospital is being made, the income and expense projections become an integral part of the income approach.

In addition to detailed information on hospital revenues and operating expenses by departmental and functional category, the appraiser must obtain information relative to market trends and the performance of competitive facilities. Market trends include future bed requirements, future additions to or deletions from supply, and unique factors affecting revenue production such as development of freestanding surgery centers or other ambulatory care facilities, for example. Recent data measuring hospital performance appears in Table 2.10.

Financial Rating of Hospitals

Financial investment rating firms such as Standard & Poor's and Moody's Investors Service grade hospital debt based on the likelihood of repayment of principal and debt to bondholders. The AA rating usually is the highest ranking a freestanding hospital, hospital system, or group practice can achieve. Only insured bonds and refunding issues secured by U.S. Treasury securities in escrow carry S&P's AAA or Moody's Aaa ratings.

In recent years some hospitals have watched their credit ratings slip as net revenues dropped or losses were incurred. Those hospitals that have retained their ratings generally dominate or command a strong share of their local or regional markets and are well-known tertiary-care teaching facilities. A recent study pointed out the following characteristics of ratings.

Standard & Poor's estimates that of 590 hospitals it has recently rated, about 8% are in the AA category (AA+, AA, AA-) and about 13% are in the A+ (see Table 2.11 for S&P rating data). When S&P assigns an AA rating, the firm believes the organization will maintain that distinction over a 30-year life of a bond. AA-rated providers are characterized by

- a large number of beds
- consistently high occupancy rates with a wide patient draw
- dominance in local or regional market
- research facilities with strong medical school affiliations
- high quality medical staffs
- strong managers/management systems
- minimal debt

Table 2.10

Table 2.10   Measuring Hospital Performance, 1990-1994

Performance Measures	Median Standards				
	1990	1991	1992	1993	1994
Occupancy rate (for beds in service)	51.4	50.3	49.1	47.3	46.6
Average length of stay, case-mix adjusted	5.13	5.08	4.95	4.81	4.57
% Medicare inpatient days	5.26	53.7	55.3	56.2	57.5
% Medicaid inpatient days	8.3	9.3	10.1	10.1	10.2
% Outpatient revenue	26.6	29.0	31.1	33.0	35.0
Average age of plant (years)	8.07	8.21	8.36	8.52	8.80
Long-term debt to capitalization	0.41	0.40	0.40	0.39	0.38
Debt service coverage ratio	2.63	2.90	3.40	3.47	3.67
Days in accounts receivable	77.4	75.6	71.6	68.8	69.0
Days cash on hand	38.4	39.3	42.7	44.7	49.4
Operating profit margin	2.17	2.42	2.88	3.06	3.45
Total profit margin	3.77	4.00	4.20	4.25	4.52
Cash flow per bed	$17,841	$20,558	$23,021	$24,013	$26,307
Discharges per bed, acute care	33.58	34.57	34.81	34.95	35.96
FTE personnel per 100 adjusted discharges, case-mix adjusted	5.30	5.26	5.22	5.17	5.03

Sources: *The Comparative Performance of U.S. Hospitals: The Sourcebook,* Health Care Investment Analysts, Inc., 1995; and American Hospital Association National Hospital Panel Survey.

- high reserves
- profitability

Multihospital systems exhibit benefits from central management, beneficial distribution of facilities, and economies of scale.

Long-term debt as a percentage of total assets for the median AA-rated hospital has been stable in recent years (about 29% in 1994). Those facilities whose ratings were BB+ or lower had a median debt ratio of 49% in 1994. AA-rated hospitals generally had a median operating profit margin of 5.94% of total revenues while BB+ and lower hospitals had a median of only 1.30%. Size is also a factor in financial success: the median AA-rated hospital had 540 beds while the median BB+ and lower rated hospital had 155 beds in service.

Table 2.12 provides selected statistics for S&P bond-rated hospitals by percentile for 1994. The statistics show certain financial characteristics that distinguish successful hospitals from those that are less fortunate. Overall, the financial and operating health of the industry shows improvement (i.e., the operating revenue per discharge increased more than the operating expense per discharge).

Table 2.11	Standard & Poor's Rating Categories		
Rating	**Description**	**%**	**Number of Hospitals**
AA(+/-)	Debt rated "AA" indicates a hospital has a very strong capacity to pay interest and repay principal, and differs from the highest rating issues only in a small degree.	7.8%	46
A (+/-)	Debt rated "A" indicates a hospital has a strong capacity to pay interest and repay principal, although it is somewhat more susceptible to the adverse effects of changes in circumstances and economic conditions than debt in higher rated categories.	46.3%	273
BBB (+/-)	Debt rated "BBB" indicates a hospital is regarded as having an adequate capacity to pay interest and repay principal while it normally exhibits adequate protection parameters; adverse economic conditions and circumstances are more likely to lead to a weakened capacity to pay interest and repay principal in this category than in higher rated categories.	37.6%	222
BB, B, CCC, or CC	Debt rated "BB," "CCC," or "CC" indicates a hospital is regarded as predominantly speculative in its capacity to pay interest and repay principal in accordance with the terms of the obligation. "BB" indicates the lowest degree of speculation and "CC" the highest. While such debt is likely to have some quality and protective characteristics, these are outweighed by large uncertainties or major risk exposures to adverse conditions.	8.3%	49

Note: The ratings from "AA" to "CCC" are typically modified by the addition of a plus or minus sign to show relative standing within the major rating categories.

Source: *The Comparative Performance of U.S. Hospitals: The Sourcebook,* Health Care Investment Analysts, Inc., 1996.

Standard & Poor's is one of three independent organizations that evaluate and rate the creditworthiness of debt issues. Most hospitals that raise capital through the use of tax-exempt revenue bonds rely on one or more of the rating agencies to assign a rating to the bonds. Bond ratings enhance the marketability of the issue by summarizing credit quality for purposes of investment decisions; these credit ratings have achieved acceptance among investors.

The S&P bond ratings can be a guide for appraisers in terms of analyzing the risk element of an overall capitalization rate as well as the future cost of capital and the quality rating for comparative sale price or competitive market position analyses.

Valuation Methodology

In many sales or leases of hospitals professional valuation assistance is often obtained from a small group of practitioners who specialize in these projects and tend to monopolize the market. Systematic procedures for conducting analysis are virtually nonexistent and the quality of work is highly variable. For example, some analysts believe that the only applicable approach is a cost approach; this work is typically deficient because of weak treatment of all the potential aspects of obsolescence, especially external obsolescence.

	Table 2.12 Selected Statistics for Standard & Poor's Bond-Rated Hospitals, 1994								
	Percentile	AA	A+	A	A-	BBB+	BBB	BBB-+	BB+ (and lower)
No. of Beds in Service per Hospital	75	670	529	290	300	243	258	211	208
	50	511	365	238	195	181	158	140	135
	25	387	238	167	150	118	101	97	78
Long-Term Debt to Total Assets	75	.35	.42	.42	.47	.48	.50	.51	.59
	50	.29	.32	.35	.38	.40	.41	.41	.49
	25	.22	.25	.28	.30	.30	.31	.32	.37
Debt Service Coverage Ratio	75	11.12	8.17	6.92	5.30	5.12	4.19	3.27	3.00
	50	5.74	4.19	4.88	3.96	2.89	2.65	2.25	1.98
	25	4.24	2.80	3.30	2.83	2.24	1.95	1.71	1.43
Operating Revenue per Adjusted Discharge ($000)	75	10.8	8.5	6.4	6.6	6.6	6.8	6.1	6.1
	50	8.2	7.0	5.4	5.5	5.2	5.2	5.1	4.7
	25	6.6	5.5	4.6	4.4	4.4	4.0	3.9	3.8
Operating Expenses per Adjusted Discharge ($000)	75	10.9	7.9	6.2	6.3	6.2	6.7	6.1	6.3
	50	8.0	6.6	5.2	5.0	4.9	4.9	5.1	4.6
	25	6.1	5.3	4.3	4.1	4.3	3.9	3.7	3.8
Operating Profit Margin (%)	75	8.36	8.36	7.15	7.02	5.81	5.07	4.77	2.57
	50	5.94	4.45	4.28	3.79	2.79	2.00	2.47	1.30
	25	2.33	2.78	2.25	1.55	1.10	(0.12)	0.56	(1.82)

Note: Favorable values are below the median for the long-term debt to total assets and operating expense per adjusted discharge categories. Favorable values for all other financial categories are above the median. Operating profit margins include depreciation charges and interest payments as expenses.

Source: *The Sourcebook*, Health Care Investment Analysts, Inc., 1996.

Primary emphasis is generally given to the cost and income approaches in valuing hospitals. The income approach should be given the most emphasis to reflect market factors. The cost approach is useful where specialized value assumptions such as value-in-use are considered or in situations where an allocation of value components is needed or the cost of replacement is of major consideration because of a lack of alternative facilities. Except under extraordinary circumstances, the sales comparison approach is only suitable for indicating a range in value or showing trends. The variables between hospitals are so great that they tend to defy reasonable quantification. Nevertheless, a sales comparison technique is commonly referred to by buyers and sellers, especially if a significant number of transactions are available for analysis.

Cost Approach

In the past, primary emphasis was given to depreciated replacement cost because of the special purpose nature of hospitals and because many were developed for noneconomic reasons. Traditional cost approach procedures are applicable; however, the appraiser should be aware of the necessity to consider all forms of physical assets, especially furniture, fixtures, and equipment. There are three classes of hospital equipment:

- Group I: fixed to the building

- Group II: major movable items

- Group III: minor equipment items that in many cases are considered on a group basis

It is important to consider the distinction between minor equipment items and inventory/supply. The latter is part of operating capital when appraising a hospital as a going concern.

Special factors that may affect the value of the land site usually relate to the developed density of the hospital rather than to specific zoning designations. Many hospitals are situated in zoning districts with a unique designation such as government or public that are established on a spot basis for a particular project. Since in these cases no similar vacant land designations exist, it is necessary to identify land comparables with a type of zoning that otherwise would be applicable to hospital activities. Typically, this is multiple residential but sometimes it is low-density residential or commercial. Sound judgment has to be applied to recognize these considerations and to estimate the appropriate level of adjustments for size differences and factors such as location, density, and use limitations.

Hospital construction costs have traditionally been among the highest for all types of structures. Primary sources of information include, in order of preference,

- actual bids

- contractor's detailed estimate

- detailed component estimate by the appraiser or cost estimator

- adjusted historical cost

- unit cost on a per-square-foot or per-bed basis.

Table 2.13 summarizes the March 1995 figures for general hospitals for various construction categories. The cost estimates in Table 2.13 do not include Group II and III equipment categories. These typically range from $12.50 to $33.25 per square foot or $12,938 to $34,414 per bed (utilizing 1,035 square feet per bed as typical).

In summary, a state-of-the-art hospital in a typical location can range in total development cost from approximately $150 to nearly $300 per square foot. Factors affecting this range include type of construction, site conditions, inspection fees, governmental approval costs, length of approval process, specialty departments and equipment, and architectural embellishments. Generally, lower costs are found in investor-owned projects located in a suburban environment, while the most costly structures are those involving teaching and research institutions in an urban context.

Within the cost approach, the real challenge to the appraiser is estimating depreciation. Our discussion will concentrate on functional and economic factors. Some obsolescence factors were identified in Table 1.3 in Chapter 1.

Functional depreciation exists in virtually every hospital due to technological change. The majority of hospitals have grown like an old French farmhouse, a wing at a time, over the past 10 to 40 years. The portions of a hospital that are more than 20 years old are generally obsolete by today's standards. This is reflected in changing requirements for built-in systems and the

Table 2.13	Cost Estimate for Typical Midwest City Hospital**
Class/Quality*	**Typical Unit Cost**
Class A excellent	$196
Class A good	$157
Class A average	$126
Class B excellent	$189
Class B good	$151
Class B average	$122
Class C excellent	$162
Class C good	$127
Class D good	$117

* Class A = steel frame; Class B = reinforced concrete; Class C = masonry and wood; Class D = wood framed. Cost estimates exclude Group II and III movable equipment.
** Time adjustment of 1.00, location adjustments of 1.02 and 1.03 (Kansas City).
Source: *Marshall Valuation Service,* Marshall & Swift, 1995.

housing of equipment, regulations stemming from the Americans with Disabilities Act, floor-to-floor heights, and sizing of patient rooms as well as in changing functions for whole floors of facilities and individual departments. For example, changes in surgical suite design have occurred because of specialty procedures and the proliferation of freestanding surgery centers.

Aging environmental systems such as heating and lighting may have substantial deficiencies. Some may violate current fire safety and health care codes but are allowed to operate due to grandfather clauses. Hospitals are a popular focus of government involvement, and building and related standards are constantly changing so that a "new" (two- to three-year old) structure may be out of compliance with current codes in some ways. Many obsolescence factors are readily apparent in the high rate of remodeling that has taken place in recent years. Departments within hospitals always seem to be on the move and construction activities never end. Much of this work is done by the maintenance or building department staff and may not be fully reflected in the balance sheet or property accounts.

An additional difficulty may be encountered regarding the book value of equipment. Accounting predictions of equipment life when new are often upset by the introduction of better technology before the full write-off.

Economic depreciation is seriously evident in many hospitals in the United States because of the dramatic decline in average occupancy rates and profitability. It is also evidenced by numerous closings and well-publicized bankruptcies that have occurred in recent years. Counties have gone out of the hospital business and major hospital chains have disposed of facilities on a mass basis. However, it seems that buyers are always available for nearly all of these properties. These buyers may be acting from civic and charitable motivations as well as the pursuit of economic gain, sometimes in an alternative use scenario. Some buyers may be pursuing a different set of medical services and proposing a cost containment program based on newly established medical service contracts. Motivation to preserve a medical center may transcend economic considerations, resulting in a greater challenge to the appraiser. External obsolescence is also due to the emergence of competing independent surgery centers and other ambulatory and urgent care facilities that drain off outpatient revenue from hospitals.

As a starting point in estimating external obsolescence it may be considered that most hospitals were designed and costed on the basis of achieving an average occupancy of 70% or higher. The difference between projected and actual bed days, quantified and capitalized on a net basis, is a crude technique for estimating one aspect of external obsolescence. A simplified example of the application of the depreciated replacement cost estimate for a relatively new facility is shown in Figure 2.1.

Income Approach

Theoretically the physical assets of a hospital can be appraised on a capitalized lease basis where there is an existing lease or sufficient evidence is available to estimate the rental value of the facility. Hospitals, however, are rarely leased on an open-market basis. Where they are leased, many complications relative to third-party relationships can materially affect income-producing capabilities over a projected time interval.

The income approach traditionally deals with net business income, and either a discounted cash flow (DCF) procedure or direct capitalization process is applied. A DCF procedure is recommended because of short-term variances in operations and the need to allow for the effect of future capital improvement programs; this is particularly true for older facilities. For a new hospital a DCF is necessary to allow time to reach stabilized occupancy and varying levels of revenue, expenses, and net income or losses.

Hospital revenues must be estimated on a department or functional category basis. Generally, the major item listed is "inpatient revenue." Within that category may be numerous sources of revenue from various departments that may need analysis.

Typically, hospital revenues are reported and analyzed on a gross or operating revenue per adjusted discharge basis. They can also be analyzed on a per inpatient day basis by dividing the operating revenue per adjusted discharge by the average length of stay (ALOS). For example, in 1994 the median urban hospital of 400 beds or more had gross patient revenue per adjusted discharge of $11,599 and an ALOS of 5.73 days. This means that the gross patient revenue per inpatient day was $2,024. Median gross patient revenue per adjusted discharge for the same category of hospitals in 1990 was $8,045, or $1,236 per inpatient day. Many hospitals produce $2,000 or more of operating revenue per inpatient day. Under such circumstances the facility is normally specializing in high-cost procedures (e.g., open heart operations, transplants) wherein a single operation can involve a fee in excess of $250,000. In any event, reference to the appropriate statistical source will provide a ready range of unit revenues on a categorical basis. Published information is available for individual hospitals from licensing and other regulatory agencies and from private data sources.

Once the gross patient revenue has been estimated and projected, it is necessary to make deductions for contractual allowances and discounts, bad debts, and charity care. Total deductions from gross patient revenue are divided by gross patient revenue and expressed as a percentage. The median value for deductions for gross patient revenue as a percentage of gross revenue for all U.S. hospitals continued to increase from 30.32% in 1990 to 35.72% in 1994.[3] Steady increases in deductions result from increasing payer differentials and the greater prevalence of managed care organizations, which negotiate discounts from charges. In general, larger

---

[3] The *Comparative Performance of U.S. Hospitals: The Sourcebook* (Baltimore, MD: Health Care Investment Analysts, Inc., 1996), 134.

Figure 2.1   Cost Approach Example

Hospital

Region:	Western
Climate:	Mild
Age:	1972
Class:	D
Quality:	Good - Good stucco with good entrance and ornamentation. Plaster or drywall interior walls with vinyl, ceramic tile and carpet floors. Includes signal system, oxygen piping, good lighting and plumbing, and complete HVAC.
Condition:	Excellent
No. of Stories:	One — 12-foot height
Area:	77,926 sq. ft. (gross)

Cost Estimate

Base Cost:	$115.13 (3/95)
Sprinklers:	$1.80/sq. ft.
Adjusted base cost:	$116.93/sq. ft.
Story multiplier:	1.0
Floor area	
Perimeter multiplier:	.915
Combined height and size multiplier:	.915
Refined cost:	$106.99/sq. ft.
Current cost multiplier:	1.01
Local multiplier:	1.11
Final cost factor:	$119.95/sq. ft.
Area:	77,926 sq. ft.
Replacement cost new:	$9,347,224
Depreciation:	Effective Age - 15 years
	Economic Life - 40 years
	Indicated Depreciation - 20%

Replacement cost new less depreciation:		$7,477,779

Canopy Entrance/Portico:

Cost: 5,147 sq. ft. x $42.50/sq. ft.	$218,748	
Current cost and local multiplier:	1.2768	
Replacement cost new:	$279,297	
Less depreciation @ 20%	(55,859)	
Indicated replacement cost new less depreciation		$223,438

Parking Lot

Cost: 330 parking spaces @ $950 each, including paving, striping, lighting, landscaping, etc.	$313,500	
Current cost and local multiplier:	1.2768	
Replacement cost new:	$399,963	
Less depreciation on 25 year life @ 48%	(191,982)	
Indicated replacement cost new less depreciation		$207,981

Landscaping (estimated as is):

		$120,000
Summary of replacement cost new less depreciation:		$8,029,197
Rounded		$8,050,000

---

* All references to costs and depreciation are from *Marshall Valuation Service,* Marshall and Swift, Section 15, pp. 22-23 for costs and Section 97, p. 16, for depreciation.

hospitals and those in urban settings experience significantly higher ratios of deductions from gross patient revenue (up to 47.72% for all urban hospitals at the 75th percentile).

While revenues on a unit basis may be extremely high relative to what is commonly encountered in real estate appraisals, operating expenses are similarly high, sometimes exceeding 90% of revenues. Obviously, a very accurate estimate of expenses is necessary because a 1% difference (say, 85% compared to 86%) can amount to a difference in value of as much as $21,900 per bed when revenues are $1,500 per patient day ($1,500 per patient day x 1% = $15 x 365 days x 60% occupancy factor = $3,285 capitalized at, say, 15% = $21,900 per bed). For a hospital typically valued at $180,000 per bed, this 1% difference in expenses could amount to a valuation error of slightly more than 12%.

Investment revenue in some instances can be an important source of net income for a hospital (e.g., not-for-profit hospitals generated $2.8 billion in investment income in 1994). However, it may not be part of a hospital's assets to be appraised. The appraiser should investigate this aspect of a balance sheet and handle the contribution of investment revenue in an appropriate manner.

Some examples of cash flow margins are set forth in Table 2.15. In addition to investment income, profit margins may include philanthropic contributions, endowment revenue, government grants, and other revenue and expense not related to patient care operations. Consultation with hospital officials should enable the appraiser to consider these special factors properly in the projection of the net operating income (*NOI*) to be utilized for valuation purposes.

A discounted cash flow valuation example is shown in Table 2.16. The annual net incomes are discounted and capitalized to indicate a total property value which takes into account all elements of the business. These include the value of the staff in place, covenants not to compete, medical records, contracts, and licenses, etc., if appropriate.

Supporting data for estimates of discount and capitalization rates are derived from nontraditional sources since detailed financial information (i.e., capitalization rate, discount rate, target IRR, etc.) for hospital transactions is extremely difficult to obtain and not uniform in presentation. Thus, a capitalization rate may be impossible to derive from the hospital market itself.

It is absolutely essential to support the selection of a discount and capitalization rate through interviews with industry representatives. The appraiser should also investigate such financial indicators as price/earnings ratios and returns on invested capital of publicly traded health service and management organizations. With such data, supplemented by information from lenders, the appraiser can construct a capitalization rate by the band-of-investment technique. *OAR*s and discount rates for successful entities are typically 300 to 700 basis points higher than similar rates for typical commercial investments. Examples of equity valuation factors for publicly traded hospital management companies are shown in Table 2.17. Individual properties will have much higher yield requirements.

In place of a capitalization rate the most common standard in today's market is a multiple times *EBITDA* (earnings before interest, taxes, depreciation, and amortization). Most investor-owned chains consider a range of three to six times *EBITDA* as desirable, but most acquisitions of profitable hospitals will be at multiples between four and seven. In cases where hospitals are marginally successful and the buyer expects it could operate the facility more profitably, the appropriate multiple could be as much as 20 times trailing *EBITDA*.

The income approach, as applied to the hospital's *NOI* or cash flow (net income plus depreciation, amortization, and debt service), results in a valuation of the hospital as a going concern. The business value may be separately estimated on a total basis or by components, or it can be allocated or isolated by reference to the cost approach estimate.

Table 2.15	Cash Flow Margins, 1994 (cash flow as a % of operating revenue)		
	Percentiles		
Investor-Owned Hospitals	**75th**	**50th**	**25th**
All	21.5%	16.6%	11.1%
25-99 Beds	20.2%	14.2%	10.4%
100-249 Beds	22.6%	17.7%	10.0%
250-399 Beds	23.1%	17.0%	17.3%
400 and over	22.2%	19.0%	16.2%
Urban	20.8%	16.7%	9.8%
25-99 Beds	17.1%	11.1%	4.9%
100-249 Beds	22.2%	15.5%	11.1%
250-399 Beds	23.1%	17.3%	17.0%
400 and over	22.2%	19.0%	16.2%
Rural	26.3%	20.2%	13.7%
25-99 Beds	23.7%	16.2%	11.6%
100-249 Beds	29.7%	26.7%	19.8%

Note: The publication does not set forth the above ratios. Total cash flow is derived by multiplying cash flow per bed times the number of beds in service for each category. Total operating revenue is derived by dividing operating revenue per discharge by the average length of stay to get operating revenue per inpatient day, which figure is then multiplied by 365 days, the number of beds, and the percentage of occupancy.

Source: *The Comparative Performance of U.S. Hospitals: The Sourcebook,* Health Care Investment Analysts, Inc., 1996.

Separate techniques for estimating the business value of a hospital are set forth in a later section of this chapter.

Sales Comparison Approach

As typically applied, the "market" approach is analyzed on the basis of price per bed. Admittedly a crude technique for reasons already expressed, it has been used by buyers and sellers as an authentic indicator and is seriously considered as an appropriate measure by many industry analysts.

For a historical perspective the reader should know that when hospital prices peaked in the mid 1980s, they reached heights of $300,000+ per bed for relatively new properties possessing excellent future outlooks, albeit on a short-term basis. In some cases, actual current profits supported the investment. Most properties that were sold at that time were at prices that reflected the current cost of replacement plus a large dose of intangible value and an optimistic outlook for future property value inflation. Capitalization rates were on the low side.

In the market of the mid 1990s, many transactions are in process, mostly by wealthy, not-for-profit institutions. They are typically 1) large, freestanding, not-for-profit hospitals that have amassed a large amount of capital from profits during past years or 2) not-for-profit, often religious, hospital systems that want to expand and have the financial resources to do so.

Table 2.16   Example of Income Approach Using Discounted Cash Flow

Description	Year 1	Year 2	Year 3	Year 4
Gross revenues	$24,521,498	$24,726,433	$26,380,907	$31,465,529
Estimated % growth in gross revenue	13%	0.80%	7.00%	19.00%
Estimated patient days - adult	15,859	16,161	15,268	16,736
Estimated patient days - pediatric	1,750	1,697	1,826	1,327
Total patient days	17,609	17,858	17,094	18,063
Estimated gross revenue per patient day (GRPPD)*	$1,393	$1,385	$1,543	$1,742
% Increase (decrease) in GRPPD		-1%	11%	13%
% Occupancy (patient days/138 ÷ 365)	35%	35%	34%	36%
Estimated deductions:				
Bad debt	$191,648	$281,776	$369,581	$574,573
Contractual:				
Medicare	$5,875,610	$4,737,596	$6,014,464	$8,471,019
Medicaid	$837,554	$617,626	$1,007,133	$991,802
Other	$332,674	$318,313	$646,361	0
Total	$7,237,486	$5,955,311	$8,037,539	$10,037,394
Other allowances	$182,410	$300,716	$353,573	$1,470,179
Estimated net patient operating revenue	$17,101,602	$18,470,406	$17,989,795	$19,957,956
% of bad debt & contractual to net revenue	43.4%	33.9%	46.6%	57.7%
Total other revenue	$122,437	$78,381	$77,000	$175,089
Estimated total operating revenue	$17,224,039	$18,548,787	$18,066,795	$20,133,045
Estimated operating expenses	$13,737,413	$12,613,520	$13,966,912	$16,919,084
% Change	6.7%	-8.2%	10.7%	21.1%
Expense ratio	80%	68%	77%	84%
Estimated net operating income:				
(Revenue-expense)	$3,486,626	$5,935,267	$4,099,883	$3,213,961
% Change in NOI	-11%	70%	-31%	-22%
Discount rate/capitalization rate:	18%/15%			
Appraised value				
1. Present value of income stream	$9,712,700			
2. Present value of reversion**	$13,040,773			
3. Total	$22,753,473			Called: $22,750,000

*   This is a blended rate reflecting separate rates for adult care and pediatric care.
** No allowance is made for selling costs because hospital sales are usually between two corporate entities.

Table 2.17	Yield Rates for Publicly Traded Companies	
Company	**After Tax P/E Ratios (1994)**	**Estimated Before Tax Cap Rate***
A. Acute Care		
American Medical Holdings	16.4	9.38%
Columbia/HCA Healthcare Corporation	17.3	8.89%
Community Psychiatric Centers	32.0	4.81%
Universal Health Services	12.6	12.21%
B. Health Care REITS		
American Health Properties	—	9.9%
Healthcare Realty Trust	—	10.0%
Meditrust	—	11.6%
National Health Investors	—	10.6%
Nationwide Health Properties	—	13.2%
C. Long-Term Care/Nursing Homes		
Beverly Enterprises	16.6	9.27%
Genesis Health Ventures	21.4	7.19%
Health Care and Retirement	21.1	7.29%
Hillhaven	20.9	7.36%
Living Centers of America	15.2	10.12%
Manor Care	21.4	7.19%
Multicare Companies	17.1	9.00%
D. Niches/Emerging Growth		
Continental Medical Systems	17.8	8.64%
Lincare Holdings, Inc.	17.4	8.84%
Medical Care America	12.6	12.21%
Pyxis Corporation	25.3	6.08%
Surgical Care Affiliates	15.3	10.05%

* Conversion based on average corporate income tax rate of 35%.
Source: Investext, April 1, 1994.

For example, in the third quarter of 1995 the number of hospital mergers and acquisitions rose 39% to 43%, compared with 31 closures in the previous quarter.[4] According to a recent report,[5] of 43 hospital deals, 25 involved mergers between not-for-profit hospital systems. Of the 18 deals that involved for-profit chains, nine included Columbia/HCA Healthcare Corp. Columbia's largest deal announced in the quarter was its $250 million offer to the Medical University of South Carolina, Charleston. Columbia offered $90 million for the hospital's assets and $8 million in annual lease payments, which amounts to $160 million over a 20-year lease. In other deals in which prices were disclosed, according to the same report:

- Columbia agreed to buy Good Samaritan Health System, San Jose, California, for $165 million. The deal involves four tax-exempt hospitals and a medical foundation that is affiliated with 400 physicians.

- OrNda HealthCorp, based in Nashville, Tennessee, agreed to buy Houston Northwest Medical Center for $153 million. OrNda already owns a $74 million stake in the hospital and is buying the remaining interest.

- Sierra Health Services, Las Vegas, agreed to buy Mohave Valley Medical Center, Bullhead City, Arizona, for $11 million.

- Vencor, Louisville, Kentucky, agreed to buy shuttered Physicians' Community Hospital, St. Petersburg, Florida, for $5.5 million.

- The largest chain deal announced in the quarter was the acquisition of Brim, a Portland, Oregon, based chain of rural hospitals, by Paracelsus, based in Pasadena, California. Paracelsus will emerge with 90 facilities in 27 states and annual revenues of about $700 million.

Many analysts have commented on the irony of not-for-profits capitalizing on the financial desperation of investor-owned hospitals that formerly tried to build an empire on the problem-plagued not-for-profit organizations.

Prices quoted in 1988 by a representative of a Chicago-based investment banking firm indicate that hospitals with a daily census of 20 to 40 patients (a remarkably small number and therefore not general hospital size) "are selling for at least $60,000 to $90,000 per bed, and hospitals with a daily census of 100 patients are selling for at least $125,000 per bed...."[6] More hospitals will be sold because investor-owned systems are revising their strategic plans, restructuring their operations, and focusing on more profitable service areas.

An example of a sales comparison approach grid is shown in Table 2.18.

Business Valuation

As an operating enterprise, a general hospital has the capability of supporting a separate value for the intangibles over and above the valuation of the physical assets. Business value in this instance is defined as the ability to produce excess profits. It should also represent the extra value afforded by the assemblage of all of the components of production in one location where, even if the profit producing potential is minimal, a valuable and virtually irreplaceable service is being performed. On the whole, however, it should be considered that a business value exists except where a hospital is losing money and is likely to continue doing so in the future.

---

[4] *Healthcare Merger and Acquisition Report* (New Canaan, CT.: Irving Levin Associates).

[5] *Modern Healthcare*, December 4, 1995, 8-12.

[6] David Burda, "Changing Ownership," *Modern Healthcare*, May 7, 1988.

| Table 2.18 | Summary and Analysis of Hospital Sales |

Item	Sale No. 1	Sale No. 2	Sale No. 3	Sale No. 4	Subject
Name	A	B	C	D	Presbyterian
Location	CBD	Suburb	Suburb	Edge City	Edge City
Type	Acute	Acute	Acute	Acute	Acute
Age	28 yrs.	17 yrs.	12 yrs.	15 yrs.	20 yrs.
Licensed beds	350	180	100	88	220
Operating beds	110	140	78	60	88
Square feet	245,000	118,800	82,000	46,200	158,400
Land (acres)	3.2	10.6	6.1	2.1	8.7
Parking spaces	1,080	890	425	310	1,221
Code status*	3	1	1	2	1
FF&E	Included	Included	Included	Excluded	Included
Date of sale/value	2/92	3/94	10/89	4/95	7/95
Price ($000)	$23,800	$25,200	$14,100	$3,960	
Terms	Cash	Cash	Seller Carry	Cash	
Price/licenced bed	$68,000	$140,000	$141,000	$45,000	
Price/operating bed	$216,363	$180,000	$180,769	$66,000	
Price/sq. ft.	$97.14	$212.12	$171.95	$85.71	
Oper. rev. mult.	0.65	0.53	0.47	0.40	
Cap. rate	12.6%	22.6%	9.6%	(3.4%)	

* Code Status: (1) = conforming   (2) = needs minor work   (3) = needs structural work

A hospital's success is not only derived from the services performed and the assembled workforce plus other intangible factors, it is also a function of site or location. Location, however, is not a guarantee of success because other factors have to be considered such as competition and management. Accordingly, when valuing the business component of a hospital, separate and unique procedures must be followed and analytical techniques applied that are somewhat unique to this particular property type.

Intangibles may be appraised by separate techniques, among which are the following:

1. Excess profits.

2. Individual categories of intangible value.

3. Comparison of the results of the income approach with the results of the cost approach.

4. Other techniques such as a) a percentage deduction from net income to allow for entrepreneurial return and b) analysis and sales of hospital business opportunities and leaseholds.

The individual methodologies are briefly discussed below.

Excess Profits

Comparison of the operating performance of the subject in terms of key financial factors with industry standards can indicate the relative percentile rating of an individual hospital and its productive differential as compared to the median or any other percentile selection (if appropriate). These financial factors include

- gross patient revenue per adjusted discharge
- operating revenue per adjusted discharge
- operating expense per adjusted discharge
- deductions from gross patient revenue as a percentage of gross patient revenue
- operating profit margin
- cash flow per bed

Through such comparisons the excess profit can be indicated as a percentage and in terms of total aggregate dollars. The last step is to capitalize that excess profit figure into a total value for the business component of the property.

Selection of the capitalization rate requires considerable skill and research since no published data are available for its derivation. It is generally considered to be a function of the number of years in the future for which these excess profits can reasonably be expected to be received, but this time period should not be excessive due to the volatility of this business and uncertainty about the future. For example, if the excess profits can reasonably be expected to be received for three years in the future, the capitalization rate would be 33%.

Valuation of Excess Profits

Operating profit margin for all hospitals (same state, size bracket, and ownership type)	17.7%
Subject operating profit margin	20.2%
Subject operating revenue	$17,700,000
Subject excess profits (2.5% x $17,700,000)	$442,500
Net profit multiplier for excess profits	2.5
Valuation of excess profits	$1,106,250

By Individual Category

This is the most difficult methodology to employ because it requires multiple, individual valuations of factors such as assembled workforce, medical records, name, and contracts as well as extraordinary factors such as covenants not to compete with other hospitals in the service or trade area for control over groups of physicians. After all of the individual categories of intangible value are identified, they can be separately appraised through careful analysis. The value of an assembled workforce can be determined by calculating the cost and time of finding, employing, and training new personnel to the degree that they can perform the functions of the existing staff. The value of medical records can be determined by estimating the hospital's ability to retain a certain percentage of patronage that might normally be lost due to competition and conditions such as distance from the hospital, preferred provider list, etc. This type of calculation must reflect the fact that medical records become obsolete for a period of time; the cost to assemble them may be the easiest technique for estimating their productive value.

Comparison of Approaches

A simple technique for identifying a broad range of business value is to deduct the valuation estimate by the cost approach (assuming it reflects all of the physical and other assets of the business) from the value indicated by the income approach. The differential figure derived can logically be deemed to represent the financial advantage attributable to the hospital due to its ability to produce a yield on investment in excess of depreciated replacement cost for all other tangible components of the property. This is a commonly used technique and, if properly employed, deserves recognition as a logical application of appraisal techniques. The disadvantage is that it does not explain the sources of intangible value.

Other Methodologies

Based on input from financial executives in the hospital industry, it may be possible to derive a percentage reduction from net income (prior to its capitalization into a value of the physical assets) that represents a fair allowance for the entrepreneurial component of the property. In the application of the income approach, this technique results in an appraisal of physical assets. The valuation of intangibles can be then determined by applying a separate capitalization rate to the portion of the net income allocated to the business. In many ways this technique resembles an excess profit methodology except that a determination of the percentage allotted to the business enterprise is from industry sources rather than published operating results for a wide array of similar hospitals. This technique should be viewed with skepticism unless it is supported by strong indications from the market such as the opinions of financial executives and unbiased experts.

It is also possible to analyze sales of hospital business opportunities combined with leaseholds since hospital companies may acquire entities where the leasing of physical facilities is separate from the operating entity. These leaseholds may be transferred or assigned under circumstances that represent reasonable arm's-length transactions. If such price data are available, it is necessary to analyze the financial and other capabilities of the entire hospital entity to derive appropriate adjustments and therefore units of comparison that can be applied to a subject property. Such units of comparison may be a multiplier, price per bed, percentage of total value, or percentage of total potential net revenue.

There is no dispute about the potential for a medical surgical hospital to produce a substantial business or intangible value. In periods of economic uncertainty, however, the projection of such a business value into the future must be carefully considered. Because of the volatility of the business, hospital financial results can vary drastically from year to year. Actual sale prices are the best indicator but they are few and far between and extremely difficult to disassemble. For future taxation purposes the argument of the separate salability of intangibles might have to be considered. Appraisal of intangibles by separate components along with an estimate of their remaining or productive life can be quite beneficial for depreciation and therefore taxation purposes. Experts must be aware of all of these circumstances.

C H A P T E R
T H R E E

Psychiatric Hospitals

Psychiatric hospitals are limited purpose but moderately complicated medical treatment facilities that flourished in the 1970s and 1980s but during the 1990s have been experiencing tough financial times. Recently facilities have been plagued by insurer and patient lawsuits, declining occupancies and average lengths of stay, reduced treatment programs, oversupply, and capitation of fees. That the industry is undergoing a competitive shakeout is evidenced by declining values, minimal new construction, and implementation of managed care programs controlled by third-party networks of mental health professionals and insurance companies. Of all the health care enterprises discussed in this text, psychiatric hospitals have the poorest future outlook and the highest degree of risk.

Psychiatric Hospital Services

Acute inpatient psychiatric services are provided to individuals who require the specialized resources of a hospital for the diagnosis and/or treatment of an acute mental disorder. This includes chronically ill patients who may have acute episodes and need intensive patient care. A wide variety of conditions may indicate the need for acute psychiatric hospitalization, including (in the order of principal diagnosis)

1. effective disorders

2. schizophrenia

3. substance related

4. alcohol related

5. anxiety/somatoform/dissociative

6. preadult disorders

7. organic disorders

8. personality disorders

9. other nonpsychotic

10. other psychotic

Acute inpatient psychiatric care is appropriate for patients who are severely and acutely mentally disordered and who may also have medical problems. Patient admissions may be voluntary or involuntary. Patients are characterized by marked impairments, e.g., violent or suicidal, requiring restraints, medication, or intensive treatment. The need for acute care is determined by physician specialists according to the severity of the dysfunction.

There are two basic types of facilities in which inpatient acute psychiatric services may be offered. One is a psychiatric unit or wing of a general acute care hospital. The other is a free-standing, acute psychiatric hospital. Each has its own license category. The major difference between the two categories is that a general acute hospital is required to provide more compre-hensive ancillary and supporting services than a freestanding facility. A freestanding facility is restricted by federal law from receiving Medicaid reimbursement for patients between the ages of 21 and 65.

Among the required services are immediate, 24-hour, intensive crisis care and treatment with clear medical direction and orientation, including comprehensive medical examination at the time of admission. Psychiatric hospitalization offers a combined medical and psychiatric approach to the treatment of psychiatric conditions where a clear organic condition underlies the psychiatric disorder.

An acute psychiatric hospital has a duly constituted governing body which has overall administrative and professional responsibility and an organized medical staff which provides 24-hour inpatient care for mentally disordered, incompetent, or other patients. Staffing require-ments are typically outlined in government statutes or codes. In practice, however, the organi-zation and staffing of inpatient psychiatric services vary widely.

Inventory and Categories

A multitude of institutions and organizations provide inpatient or 24-hour care in a hospital setting. According to the U.S. Substance Abuse and Mental Health Services Administration, Center for Mental Health Services, in 1990 there were 5,284 facilities that provided inpatient and outpatient mental health care (see Table 3.1). Of these 270 were freestanding state and county mental hospitals, 967 were private mental health hospitals, 1,674 were general hospitals with separate psychiatric services, and 141 were Veterans Administration hospitals. The 5,284 facilities had 272,200 inpatient beds (a rate of 111.5 beds per 100,000 population), 229,700 inpatients (at a rate of 93 per 100,000 population), and a total patient care staff of 471,800. These facilities accounted for a total of $28.4 billion in expenditures ($116.30 per capita).

This chapter is concerned with the freestanding, privately owned and operated psychiatric hospitals. There are about 550 in the nation, accounting for about 45,000 beds and with annual expenditures of inpatient care of about $5.5 billion. About 350 of these freestanding facitilies are operated by health care systems such as Magellan Health Services (formerly known as Charter Medical), CPC, Columbia/HCA Healthcare Corp., Ramsay Health Care, Healthcare America, and Universal Health Systems. Most are owned or leased facilities (97%); the remaining 3% are operated under management agreements. An inventory of the facilities controlled by the major systems, excluding substance abuse facilities, appears in Table 3.2.

Table 3.1

Table 3.1   Mental Health Facilities—Summary, by Type of Facility: 1990

[Revised 1990 data. Facilities, beds, and inpatients as of year-end 1990; other data are for calendar year or fiscal year ending in a month other than December since facilities are permitted to report on either a calendar or fiscal year basis. Excludes private psychiatric office practice and psychiatric service modes of all types in hospitals or outpatient clinics of Federal agencies other than U.S. Dept. of Veterans Affairs. Excludes data from Puerto Rico, Virgin Islands, Guam, and other territories]

Type of Facility	Number of Facilities	Inpatient Beds		Inpatients		Average daily inpatients (1,000)	Inpatient care episodes[2] (1,000)	Expenditures		Patient care staff[4] (1,000)
		Total (1,000)	Rate[1]	Total (1,000)	Rate[1]			Total (mil. dol.)	Per capita[3] (dol.)	
Total	5,284	272.2	111.5	229.7	93.0	224.4	2,260.9	$28,357	$116.3	471.8
Mental hospitals:										
State and county	270	98.4	40.3	90.3	37.0	89.7	365.7	7,705	31.6	112.8
Private[5]	967	75.0	30.7	60.3	24.7	58.4	509.0	8,093	33.2	99.6
General hospitals[6]	1,674	53.5	21.9	38.3	15.7	38.6	997.6	4,662	19.1	80.7
Veterans Administration[7]	141	21.7	8.9	17.2	7.1	17.3	215.6	1,480	6.1	29.7
Freestanding psychiatric outpatient clinics[8]	743	(X)	(X)	(X)	(X)	(X)	(X)	671	2.8	14.3
Other[9]	1,489	23.6	9.7	23.6	8.5	20.4	173.0	5,746	23.5	134.7

X Not applicable [1] Rate per 100,000 population. Based on Bureau of the Census estimated civilian population as of July 1. [2] "Inpatient care episodes" is defined as the number of residents in inpatient facilities at the beginning of the year plus the total additions to inpatient facilities during the year. [3] Based on Bureau of the Census estimated civilian population as of July 1. [4] Full-time equivalent. [5] Includes residential treatment centers for emotionally disturbed children. [6] Nonfederal hospitals with separate psychiatric services. [7] Includes U.S. Department of Veterans Affairs (VA) neuropsychiatric hospitals, VA general hospitals with separate psychiatric settings and VA freestanding psychiatric outpatient clinics. [8] Includes mental health facilities which provide only psychiatric outpatient services. [9] Includes other multiservice mental health facilities with two or more settings, which are not elsewhere classified, as well as freestanding partial care facilities which only provide psychiatric partial care services. Number of facilities, expenditures, and staff data also include freestanding psychiatric partial care facilities.

Source: U.S. Substance Abuse and Mental Health Services Administration, Center for Mental Health Services, unpublished data.

Table 3.2	Psychiatric Facilities in the U.S. Operated by Systems, 1995			
Type	**Number of Systems**	**Number of Hospitals**	**Beds**	**%**
Investor-owned	25	301	26,030	88.9
Secular nonprofit	16	19	1,865	6.4
Catholic	11	14	1,119	3.8
Other religious	2	3	205	0.7
Public	1	1	70	0.2
Total	55	338	29,289	100.0

Source: *Modern Healthcare,* May 20, 1996.

Background

Private, freestanding psychiatric hospitals are a recent phenomenon. Historically, most psychiatric care has been provided in government-controlled facilities, and as of 1990, there were 270 state and county operated facilities attending to over 90,000 residents. In the past three decades, however, with the proliferation of employer-paid health insurance programs and the increasing incidence of mental disorders, the private sector moved rapidly into this market. Illustrative of this growth is industry leader Community Psychiatric Centers, which grew from a small number of beds in 1970 to 8,285 beds in 1990. In that year the publicly traded firm achieved revenues of $382,000,000.

In the late 19th and early 20th centuries a movement developed in the United States to provide more humane treatment and care for mentally disordered individuals. A principal outcome of this movement was the development of a system of state supported hospitals or asylums, which provided varying degrees of treatment and custodial care for individuals deemed mentally disordered. The development of this system established the pattern of institutionalization and hospital-based care as the principal modality of treatment.

The introduction of tranquilizers in the early 1950s opened up the possibility of community-based programs as an alternative to hospitalization. The fact that these drugs controlled agitated and excited behavior made it possible to treat and maintain the mentally ill in the community rather than in a hospital. The trend in mental health services since the mid-1950s has been toward the noninstitutional treatment of the mentally ill.

The most dramatic evidence of the shift toward nonhospital-based treatment of the mentally ill is the decrease over a 20-year period in the percentage of patients treated in inpatient settings. In 1955, 77% of the 1.7 million patient care episodes in the United States were treated on an inpatient basis and 23% as outpatient. By 1975, the situation had completely reversed, with 24% of the 6.9 million episodes in inpatient care and 76% in outpatient settings.

The shift from state hospital care to community-based care has resulted in part from the steady decline in funds allocated to state hospitals for mental health care—from 98.9% in 1957-58 to 30.1% in 1977-78. Such shifts represent a deliberate attempt to decrease the resident populations of state and county mental hospitals and return those residents to their own communities.

Impact of Health Care Industry Changes

Occupancy rates are a good barometer of the status of the industry. In 1988, the median occupancy rate for psychiatric hospitals was 70.1%; in 1994 it was 55.97%, a decline of 20.2%.[1] Overcapacity has affected the psychiatric hospital industry just as it has affected acute care or medical surgical hospitals.

Until the mid 1980s the growth and development of private psychiatric hospital facilities was largely attributed to liberal employee benefit programs that encouraged workers to obtain psychiatric care on an inpatient basis. The stigma attached to such hospitalization was mostly a thing of the past. Mental health awareness and burgeoning substance abuse programs fueled a growing need for specialized facilities and treatment. Under most insurance plans, hospitals had no incentive to release patients before their policy benefits expired, which enabled psychiatric hospital chains and programs to overmaximize their profits. In addition to the anticipation of high profit margins, a construction frenzy in urban markets was also driven by the fact that state governments dropped the requirement that hospital owners prove a definite need for facilities to obtain a license.

The cost of mental health program benefits was growing at annual rates of 30% or more, or at least twice the rate of overall health care costs. As a result businesses and government began to tighten their insurance policies and cut health care costs. By 1990, the boom was over and the market was saturated with private hospitals as well as mental health and chemical dependency treatment centers.

Negative publicity, accusations of fraud, and shrinking profits are also reshaping the psychiatric care field. Patient abuse stories have stretched the credibility of those who work in the psychiatric hospital industry to the extent that the informed public has responded with a major vote of no confidence.

One approach to cut the cost of health care is that of "managed care." Major corporations have contracted with insurers or third-party intermediaries to consolidate all the elements of mental health and substance abuse services, from referral and treatment to case management and claims management. Prudential's Total Psychiatric Management (TPM) program is an example of this new format. The implementation of managed care plans has reduced the number and type of inpatient treatments, because they mandate outpatient care: In metropolitan areas where TPM or similar programs are in force, there has been a one-third reduction in required beds. The managers of these programs claim that they have reduced treatment costs by 6% to 8% of total plan costs.[2]

Another approach to cost containment is a government-sponsored concept known as a "gatekeeper," in which a patient's private health plan contracts directly with a psychiatrist, who directs all aspects of outpatient care. A gatekeeper program revises the traditional, hospital-managed mental health care program, whereby patients were diagnosed by a nurse or other professional and directed to a psychologist for both inpatient and outpatient care. The alleged advantage of this concept is that a psychiatrist diagnoses and directs care, thus reducing potential malpractice liability. Recent reductions in both private and Medicaid reimbursements to psychiatrists have prompted them to promote the "gatekeeper" program to protect their market share.

Another government "cost-saving" promotion involves a Medicaid waiver that allows states to extend health coverage (including psychiatric care) on a more limited scale to more people,

---

[1] "Psych Chains Had Another Tough Year," *Modern Healthcare*, May 22, 1995, 64, and *The Comparative Performance of U.S. Hospitals: The Sourcebook* (Baltimore, MD: Health Care Investment Analysts, Inc., 1996), 71.

[2] Howard Larkin, "Managed Mental Health Moves Patients Out," *Hospitals*, April 20, 1989, 64.

while containing costs through mandated managed care arrangements. States that have adopted this approach include Arizona, Hawaii, Kentucky, Ohio, Oregon, Rhode Island, South Carolina, and Tennessee.

For psychiatric hospitals all of these factors have led to fewer patients and a decline in the average length of stay. Nationwide, the median length of stay decreased about 38%, from 23.79 days in 1988 to 12.35 days in 1994[3]. The downward trend in number of patients and average length of stay is expected to continue for the foreseeable future. One industry expert states that "between 40% and 70% of the people now in psychiatric hospitals don't need to be there."[4]

Current industry strategies involve the closing or selling of freestanding substance-abuse treatment centers, suspension of psychiatric and substance-abuse treatment and acute general hospital-based units, and consolidation of services at certain principal hospitals. These strategies are aimed at positioning the psychiatric care industry to succeed in a managed-care environment. For some hospitals, the effect of managed care plans has been positive because revenues from new outpatient programs have helped offset declines in inpatient utilization.

Texas illustrates the difficulties the psychiatric hospital industry has faced. The 1980s was a boom time for the construction of psychiatric hospitals. The number of hospitals in the state dropped from a peak of 75 in 1990 to 49 as of this writing. Throughout the country the number of facilities that dropped out of the business in just one year (1994) was estimated to be in the 5% to 10% range.

In retrospect, 1993 was the year psychiatric providers had hoped would bring relief after two years of falling profits and bad press. Unfortunately, little relief came, and future prospects are clouded by the uncertainties of health care reform. Some business groups wanted to see mental health deleted from a basic benefits package, charging that the benefit would lead to uncontrollable costs. By 1994, inpatient business continued to erode; and industry losses were reported at $209.1 million, more than double losses of $102.5 million in 1993.[5]

While in 1994 patient revenues for the 324 freestanding psychiatric hospitals reported an increase in patient revenues of 8.8% to $1.8 billion,[6] increased revenues don't necessarily mean increased or any profits, because the average revenue per patient is declining. This increase came on top of a 6.9% decrease in the number of system-operated, freestanding psychiatric hospitals.[7] Industry leader Charter Medical Corp. reported a loss of $59.6 million for its fiscal year ended September 30, 1994.[8]

Little construction is taking place at this time. In 1994 construction or renovation was completed on 74 psychiatric wings within acute care hospitals; 41 projects broke ground; and 107 were in the design phase. During the same period 25 substance abuse projects were completed, 15 broke ground, and 32 had completed designs.

Emerging Trends

After several years of falling profits and bad press, psychiatric providers had been looking forward to relief. Unfortunately, this has not happened and future prospects are clouded by the uncertainties of health care reform. A worst-case scenario would delete mental health from a

---

[3] Op. cit., *The Comparative Performance of U.S. Hospitals: The Sourcebook*, 73.

[4] John H. Taylor, "Tranquilizers, Anyone?," *Forbes*, December 10, 1990, 214.

[5] Op. cit., Larkin, 64.

[6] Ibid.

[7] Ibid.

[8] Ibid.

basic benefits package. At the writing of this text it is too early to know what the outcome will be. Many other shifts in the business have taken place in recent years that are likely to continue. Some psychiatric hospitals are moving into long-term care where the average length of stay is much more than 25 days and patients typically have brain injuries or neurological disorders. Long-term care is more profitable to the hospitals because when the PPS system was conceived, psychiatric, rehabilitation, cancer, children's and long-term hospitals were exempted, leaving them to be reimbursed on the generally more lucrative cost-based system. One subsidiary set up to provide long-term intensive care estimated an ALOS of 70.5 days (as compared to 14.7 days for psychiatric services) and a net revenue per patient day of $787.49 (compared to $450.90 for a psychiatric service).

The Health Care Financing Administration is recommending a moratorium on the new long-term hospitals. The government is concerned that primary hospitals will open long-term facilities within their walls simply to get higher reimbursement for certain patients. Operators of these facilities, which are also known as "Vencor-type" hospitals, argue that payers are saving money since the rates are 40% to 50% below the cost of similar treatment in intensive care units of acute care hospitals. Following are some other emerging trends.

1. Some psychiatric hospitals wil0l close and few new ones will be built, based on a diminishing growth in demand and resistance from payers.

2. Utilization review and managed care will be increased. Payers and providers alike are talking about "continuum of care" as the new paradigm. This includes outpatient, partial hospitalization, and residential treatment programs. In 1990, 26% of psychiatric patients received treatment through inpatient facilities, 5% through partial hospitalization, and 69% through outpatient care, according to federal government figures. Psychiatric providers must create alternatives so that treatment operations are under a single management structure.

3. Current high management turnover will stabilize. Hospital administrator turnover has been as high as 31% annually in recent years. This is due to the financial crises that have affected the industry, the inability of administrators to reach target budgets, and the inability of individuals to adapt to the new market-driven managed care business. A corporate objective should be to design a compensation system that rewards initiative without encouraging over-zealous pursuits.

4. Outcomes research will allow hospitals to provide data to third-party payers, enabling them to analyze their effectiveness. One technique is for patients to be graded at admission, at discharge, and in three-, six-, and 12-month intervals after discharge to determine the outcome. Use of services will be closely scrutinized and controlled and inpatient programs will likely be adjusted.

5. Declining lengths of stay and fewer admissions will reduce demands for inpatient accommodations and many inpatients will be hospitalized briefly for little more than diagnosis and stabilization. Activity therapies are likely to be limited during these short stays.

6. Technological advances will result in greater emphasis on sophisticated imaging and laboratory testing. This trend, added to the growth of med-psych, neuro-psych, and gero-psych programs, may require more sophisticated building systems that are not now commonly found in private psychiatric facilities.

7. Patients requiring long-term, overnight care will be treated in subacute residential-type facilities with fewer staff than traditional inpatient units. Other patients not requiring 24-

hour staff supervision will be placed in intensive outpatient or partial-hospitalization settings. The facility master-planning implications of these trends are significant.

8. The focus of care may shift from the nursing unit as a traditional hub of care to multiple treatment program components with an "activities core" of group, occupational, recreational, and other related therapies. This activities core may require a range of accommodations for outpatient, partial hospitalization, acute inpatient, subacute, and residential patients.

Operational Statistics

The following data on psychiatric hospitals are from *The Comparative Performance of U.S. Hospitals: The Sourcebook.*[9] Another data source is the National Association of Private Psychiatric Hospitals (NAPPH), which compiles an annual survey on the nation's nongovernmental, freestanding specialty hospitals. The survey can be of valuable assistance to appraisers and analysts in this field.

1. *Beds in service.* The typical hospital has 80 beds in service, down from 87 in 1991 and 86 in 1990. It is likely that the trend to smaller units has stabilized.

2. *Total discharges.* The total number of patients discharged in one year is one measure of the utilization of acute care inpatient services at a psychiatric hospital. Total discharges have been increasing since 1988. The typical hospital had 849 in 1989, 908 in 1990, 899 in 1991, 977 in 1992, 1,027 in 1993 and 1,127 in 1994. This recent growth has not been significant enough to reverse the trend toward an overall decline in inpatient utilization.

3. *Occupancy rate.* Occupancy rate is another measure of utilization. As mentioned earlier, occupancy rates have been steadily declining. For the median hospital they were 70.0% in 1989, 65.0% in 1990, 60.3% in 1991, 55.9% in 1992, and 52.5% in 1993.

4. *Average length of stay.* ALOS is predictive of the average resources used by the hospital per patient discharge. As mentioned previously, ALOS has been steadily declining. For the typical hospital it was 23.79 days in 1988, 23.07 in 1989, 20.69 in 1990, 18.85 in 1991, 16.63 in 1992, 14.60 in 1993, and 12.35 in 1994. This is a decline of 48.1% in six years.

5. *Medicare and Medicaid days as a percentage of total acute care days.* As a measure of payer mix, these elements are representative of the psychiatric hospital industry's increased reliance on government funding. It has increased for the typical hospital as follows: 12.36% in 1989, 14.33% in 1990, 15.09% in 1991, 20.97% in 1992, 26.35% in 1993, and 31.51% in 1994. "Continued growth in the proportion of Medicare and Medicaid patients at the typical hospital, who are reimbursed under less generous payment methods, is an unfavorable trend for the U.S. hospital industry, especially in light of the fact that future reform will likely bring further cuts in Medicare and Medicaid spending for hospital services."

6. *Average age of plant.* Calculated as total accumulated depreciation on all plant, property, and equipment, divided by total current depreciation, this ratio measures the average accounting age of a hospital's capital assets such as buildings, fixtures, and major movable equipment. The typical hospital is slowly getting older because little construction has taken place in this field. The median age of the typical hospital went from 3.99 years in 1988 to 6.86 years in 1994. The entire business is characterized by relatively new facilities.

---

[9] Op. cit., *The Comparative Performance of U.S. Hospitals: The Sourcebook,* 1995.

7. *Full-time equivalent personnel per adjusted average daily census.* The total number of full-time equivalent (FTE) personnel at the hospital divided by the hospital's adjusted average daily census is a measure of the staffing level of a hospital and its efficiency. This factor has been relatively stable for the typical psychiatric hospital in recent years. It was 2.29 in 1988 and 2.62 in 1994. Due to mandated FTEs by regulatory agencies, there is slight variance within the entire industry. It should be noted that a higher FTE level may indicate the facility is providing a higher quality of service, which differentiates it from its competitors. Thus the higher FTE may not represent a negative financial factor.

Market Analysis

Based on current trends, estimating the future market for inpatient psychiatric beds should not be undertaken by someone without specialized training or an understanding of the industry. Determining the level of need with any degree of precision is difficult. In most cases, actual data will not be available on a local basis, and broader estimates of need will have to be made. A number of models have been developed to estimate and project the demand for a particular service, and model data must be used in projecting future levels of need. Typically the level of need is expressed as a rate or percentage of the population or a segment of the population. The most common measures of need are prevalence and incidence rates used by epidemiologists and public health officials.

After the general level of need has been identified for the estimated trade or service area, one may estimate the number of potential cases. A high prevalence rate by itself does not ensure a meaningful market. Health care requires a large number of bodies to support any service.

Statistics regarding mental illness indicate that about 15% of Americans over the age of 18 meet the diagnostic criteria for at least one alcohol, drug abuse, or mental disorder. Two out of five adults may expect to have a diagnosable mental illness (22.5%) or a serious drug (6.1%) or alcohol abuse (13.5%) problem at some point in their life. It is reported that more than 2,000,000 Americans over the course of their lifetimes will be stricken with schizophrenia. As many as 14,000,000 children and adolescents experience mental disorders, many of which persist into adulthood. Some 200,000 to 300,000 suffer from autism; childhood depression ranges from 1.7% in prepuberty to 4.7% in adolescence; attention deficit hyperactivity disorder affects 3% to 5% of the pediatric population; and fetal alcohol syndrome occurs in 10 to 30 cases per 10,000 live births. It has been shown that 3,000,000 children in this country are seriously mentally ill, defined as having a duration of more than one year and as being known to more than two social service agencies serving children. Other estimates of mental illness for those under 18 range from 12% to 22%.

In the health care market, however, having a potential number of cases does not mean that services will actually be desired or acquired. According to Thomas[10], the market is "composed of those who need services and want them, those who need services and do not want them (or cannot or do not obtain them for some reason), those who do not truly need the services but want them, and those who neither need nor want the services." Possible combinations of needs, wants, and consumption are illustrated in Figure 3.1.

Other steps involved in the market analysis include the determination of such factors as the distribution of cases, level of interest, ability to pay, and adjustments for competition. All of these steps are extremely difficult to undertake for psychiatric services. Obviously, it is important to conduct an in-depth analysis of location relative to population and competition. Considerations of patient affluence will also influence the outcome of the analysis.

---

[10] Richard K. Thomas, *Health Care Consumers in the 1990s* (Ithaca, NY: American Demographic Books, 1993), 91.

| Figure 3.1 | The Interface of Need and Want for Health Care Consumers |

Possible Consumer Segments

1. Need services, but do not want or consume them
2. Need and want services, but do not consume them
3. Want services, but do not need or consume them
4. Want, need, and consume services
5. Need and consume services, but do not want them
6. Want and consume services, but do not need them
7. Consume services, but do not need or want them

Orientation to Health Care Services

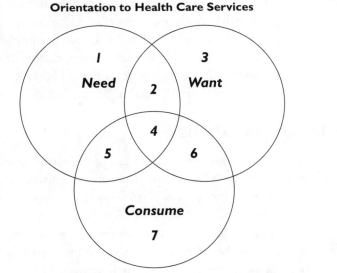

Source: Richard K. Thomas, *Health Care Consumers in the 1990s,* American Demographic Books (1993).

Since the level of need within the target population may not correspond with the level of interest, it is important to determine the extent to which the population really wants the service. This information can only be obtained by practical research, such as a consumer focus survey. Many programs have been unsuccessful because the actual level of interest in the target population was much lower in reality than it was on paper. An increasingly important factor in health care marketing is a consumer's ability to pay. It is necessary to determine the potential payer mix of the target population to estimate the level of reimbursement expected for a particular service. Historically, psychiatric costs were provided for the most part by commercial insurers, followed by Medicare, Medicaid, self-pay, and other. Given the fact that different payers offer different levels of reimbursement, the payer mix determines the actual level of payment.

Lastly, analysis of competition is extremely important, especially in light of current low occupancy trends and the extensive marketing efforts of similar facilities. The quality of the competition, its proposed facilities and services, and its strengths and weaknesses compared to the subject property must be assessed. A example of a market survey of competitive facilities is illustrated in Table 3.3.

Design and Development Considerations

Psychiatric hospital designs are unique because of the special needs of mental patients. In the past patient rooms and other spaces were predominantly characterless in nature, providing few clues to patients for appropriate behavior. This pattern existed throughout the facility from individual rooms to the building and its overall surroundings. Design specialists now recognize the importance of varying the physical elements such construction materials, paint colors, textures of surface finishes, and the size and shape of spaces. Sensitive design can help patients in their recovery process. Behavioral goals and patient needs, however, are still not being adequately translated into architectural guidelines.

Table 3.3   Sample Market Survey Of Competitive Psychiatric Hospitals

Name	City	Type Of Control	Peer Group Assignment Type	Type of Care	1989-90		1990-91		1991-92		1992-93		Remarks
					Avg. # of Beds	Avg. % OCC	Avg. # of Beds	Avg. % OCC	Avg. # of Beds	Avg. % OCC	Avg. # of Beds	Avg. % OCC	
Hospital A	Brea	Investor	Acute Psych	S T Psych	142	31.70%	151	19.80%	151	21.80%	161	19.20%	Closed 11-93
Hospital B	La Habra	Investor	Mod Psych	S T General	299	18.30%	274	32.70%	274	28.80%	274	30.60%	# Psych Beds?
Hospital C	Yorba Linda	Non-Profit	Acute Psych	S T Psych	106	27.40%	80	49.80%	80	40.90%	80	33.70%	# Psych Beds?
Hospital D	Stanton	Investor	Mod Psych	S T General	110	37.90%	122	21.00%	110	17.50%	Closed		Closed 7-92
Hospital E	Fountain Vly	Investor	Acute Psych	S T Psych	287	67.40%	120	18.70%	120	13.50%	Closed		Closed 5-92
Hospital F	Santa Ana	Investor	Acute Psych	S T Psych	100	45.00%	100	33.50%	100	38.40%	100	34.50%	
Hospital G	Orange	Investor	Acute Psych	S T Psych	103	49.90%	103	17.50%	Closed		Closed		Closed 3-91
Hospital H	Newport Beach	Investor	A & D Rehab	S T Psych	68	74.90%	68	65.10%	68	68.20%	Closed		Closed 2-93
Hospital I	Costa Mesa	Investor	A & D Rehab	S T Special	59	60.90%	70	40.50%	70	27.50%	70	20.90%	Costa Mesa
Hospital J	Laguna Hills	Investor	Psych H.F.	S T Psych	DNE		DNE		DNE		5	48.70%	
Hospital K	Laguna Hills	Investor	Acute Psych	S T Psych	78	27.50%	78	40.50%	78	29.20%	78	21.50%	
Hospital L	Dana Point	Investor	Acute Psych	S T Psych	98	49.20%	82	45.60%	98	49.70%	98	42.90%	Subject
Hospital M	Mission Viejo	Investor	Acute Psych	S T Psych	DNE		80	17.30%	80	18.40%	80	36.00%	
				Total	**1,450**		**1,328**		**1,229**		**947**		
				Average	132	44.55%	111	33.50%	112	32.17%	105	32.00%	
				High	299	74.90%	274	65.10%	274	68.20%	274	48.70%	
				Low	59	18.30%	68	17.30%	68	13.50%	6	19.20%	
				Demand (OCC Patient Days)	225,143		151,242		135,133		102,704		
				% Of Demand Change	N/A		-32.82%		-10.65%		-24.00%		
				Subject Demand (OCC Patients Days)	17,599		13,648		17,778		15,345		
				Subject % Demand Change	N/A		-22.45%		30.26%		-13.68%		

General guidelines addressing the needs of mental patients specify that patients must not be overcrowded or overconcentrated, which forces them to interact with too many people. Patients must have a private place of their own and be given the opportunity to retreat physically when they feel threatened. They also must have the opportunity to form beneficial relationships. These concepts have has been defined as the "four dimensions of environmental differentiation": 1) differentiation of patients' territorial constraints and freedom, based on their level of functioning; 2) differentiation of space for a variety of behaviors; 3) differentiation of personal and group territory; and 4) differentiation in the degree of responsibility patients are expected to take for their environment.[11]

The following specific design guidelines have been developed from the literature[12] and from experience in designing environments for psychiatric hospitals:

- *Provide a clear indication of a room's intended use.* Rooms should present a clear visual message about their function. For example, a design scheme for patients with schizophrenia may not be optimal for patients with depressive disorders. A hospital should also include rooms such as living rooms, kitchens and dens that provide environments that relate to activities in the home.

- *Provide distinct visual differentiation between building parts.* Walls, floors, and ceilings should be differentiated by the use of different colors, dark baseboards, or changing textures to eliminate ambiguity and confusion. Doors, windows, and architectural details should also be clearly identifiable so their relationship to the entire room is evident.

- *Provide a variety of spaces to support social interaction.* Because the desire to congregate with others varies from patient to patient and over time, settings of appropriate size should be available to meet their changing psychosocial needs.

- *Use distinctive colors to enhance activities and space.* Colors have several functions in hospital design; they can be used to cue behavior, to improve the quality of the environmental setting, and to differentiate various architectural elements of a room. For example, warm colors can be used to identify spaces for active social programs, while cool colors could be used for counseling or sleeping areas.

- *Use a variety of materials to provide different tactile and visual experiences.* Materials can be used to suggest the behavior expected in a setting as well as to enhance the space. Carpeting, for example, can be used to indicate a quiet atmosphere or a nonsmoking area in addition to providing a soft walking surface.

- *Use lighting to help define space.* All spaces should be lighted in ways that enhance their intended use.

- *Enhance spaces that have special meanings to patients.* Lobbies can be designed as living rooms and furnished with residential furniture rather than with common institutional pieces. Patients can relate to the space as an important place for meeting family and friends.

The trend in building layouts has been toward modular or village type of designs. A central service area provides public access, support services, and connections to living quarters that are clustered into a neighborhood with an educational center at the hub. Functional zones such as adult, child and adolescent, recreation, visitor, outpatient and service areas must be identified to create appropriate separations that can be integrated in the building and site design. Separate

---

[11] Morton B. Gulak, "Architectural Guidelines for State Psychiatric Hospitals," *Hospital and Community Psychiatry,* July 1991, 706.

[12] Ibid.

zones provide privacy and remove nonpatient facilities (such as service buildings) from inpatient or outpatient areas. Separating visitor areas from patient outdoor recreation areas also contributes to patient privacy.

Because buildings are naturally inflexible and require renovation for a change in function, constructing flexible buildings is difficult. Nevertheless, construction features such as nonload-bearing walls, adequate floor-to-floor heights, and flexible engineering systems allow easier and less costly renovation. A key feature is a centralized activity core, which should be designed with space for occupational therapy, daily living activities, exercise, group therapy, education, consultation, and testing. It should be convenient to all patients (inpatient, residential, partial-hospitalization, and outpatient) to encourage extensive use of therapy programs and social services, etc.

Private psychiatric hospitals will require residential treatment centers with minimal housing for patients progressing from an acute inpatient to residential status. As the average acute inpatient length of stay continues to drop, vacated hospital units can be converted to such centers with little or no renovation. Quarterway or halfway housing, however, will require either new construction or the acquisition and renovation of a large house.

Outpatient programs and residential treatment centers are likely to grow tremendously. Intensive outpatient and partial-hospitalization treatment will call for less restrictive settings for patient care. The less stringent engineering or architectural requirements of these settings will make existing facilities that are no longer needed for their original purpose good candidates for such use.

Description of Facilities

A freestanding psychiatric hospital is less costly to build than other specialized medical facilities such as an acute hospital, surgery center, or clinic. Typical per bed building construction costs average $95,000 per bed, compared to $120,000 per bed for acute hospitals of the same type of Class D construction.[13] The physical characteristics of a psychiatric hospital are comparable to a convalescent hospital or skilled nursing facility. They both are typically one-story in height; have building to land ratios of 30% to 40%; have wood frame and masonry, Class C and D type of construction; have similar interior finishes and special health and safety requirements; and have similarly sized patient rooms/wards and common area characteristics. They both generally lack high cost, specialized facilities such as surgical suites, laboratories, imaging units, etc., found in general, acute hospitals. Psychiatric care facilities generally have a higher average building area per bed (usually by a factor of two) than convalescent facilities, due primarily to a greater number of offices, treatment rooms, and recreation areas (indoors and outdoors).

Published cost data for freestanding psychiatric hospitals are rare. Accordingly, replacement cost estimates should be checked against published data for convalescent hospitals and adjusted for differences in characteristics/facilities and converted to units of comparison such as cost per bed or cost per square foot.

In acute general hospitals the psychiatric department typically will encompass an entire floor of a multistory general hospital or at least a wing of one level. Rarely would a separate building for mental patients be developed within a modern community-based hospital campus or medical center. A psychiatric wing will usually have the same construction characteristics as the overall structure. The department may be combined with a substance abuse unit or treatment center. Conversion of unused medical/surgical beds to a psychiatric care unit is relatively uncomplicated and thus has contributed to the excess competition and overbedding problem.

---

[13] The cost estimate for the acute general hospital is from *Marshall Valuation Service*. The estimate for the psychiatric hospital is by the author.

Figure 3.2   Psychiatric Hospital First Floor

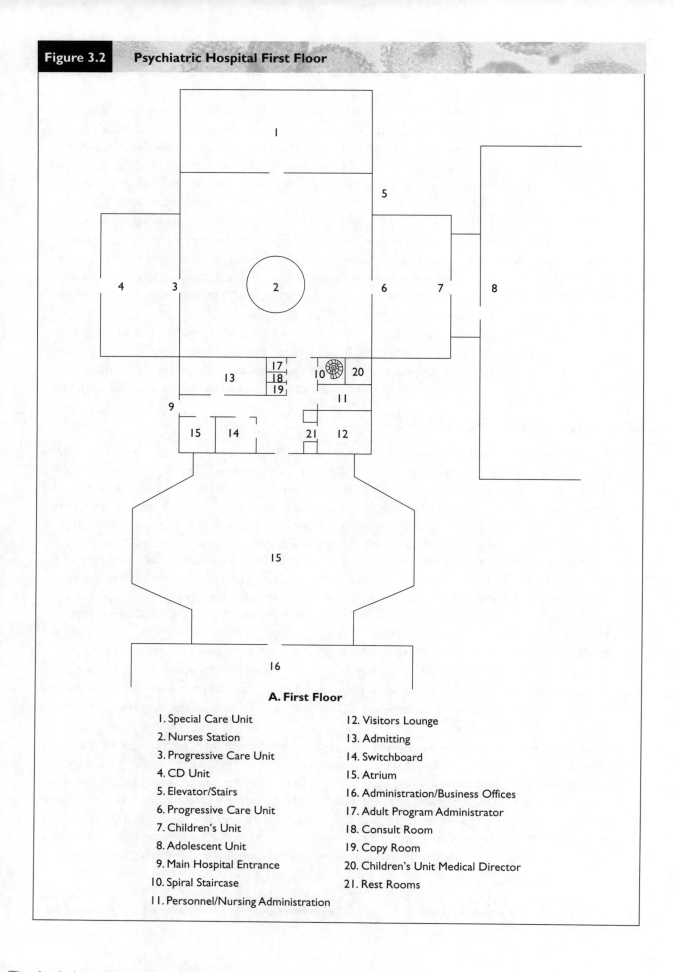

A. First Floor

1. Special Care Unit
2. Nurses Station
3. Progressive Care Unit
4. CD Unit
5. Elevator/Stairs
6. Progressive Care Unit
7. Children's Unit
8. Adolescent Unit
9. Main Hospital Entrance
10. Spiral Staircase
11. Personnel/Nursing Administration

12. Visitors Lounge
13. Admitting
14. Switchboard
15. Atrium
16. Administration/Business Offices
17. Adult Program Administrator
18. Consult Room
19. Copy Room
20. Children's Unit Medical Director
21. Rest Rooms

Figure 3.2   **Psychiatric Hospital Ground Floor (continued)**

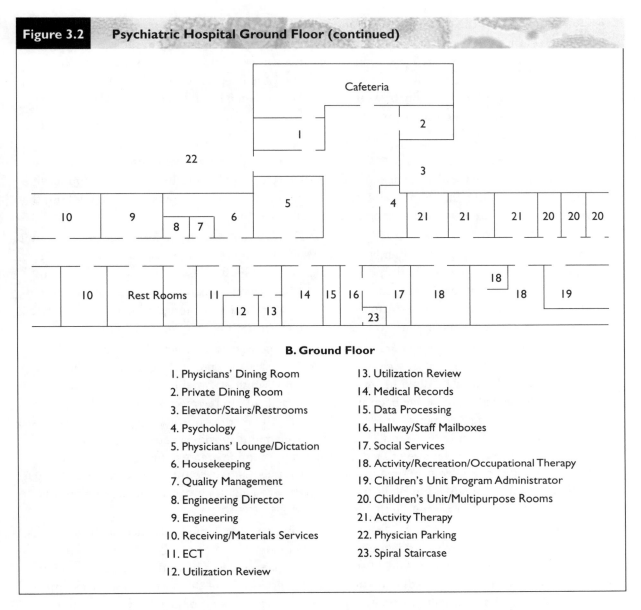

B. Ground Floor

1. Physicians' Dining Room
2. Private Dining Room
3. Elevator/Stairs/Restrooms
4. Psychology
5. Physicians' Lounge/Dictation
6. Housekeeping
7. Quality Management
8. Engineering Director
9. Engineering
10. Receiving/Materials Services
11. ECT
12. Utilization Review

13. Utilization Review
14. Medical Records
15. Data Processing
16. Hallway/Staff Mailboxes
17. Social Services
18. Activity/Recreation/Occupational Therapy
19. Children's Unit Program Administrator
20. Children's Unit/Multipurpose Rooms
21. Activity Therapy
22. Physician Parking
23. Spiral Staircase

A conceptual layout of a contemporary, two-story, freestanding psychiatric hospital (Figure 3.2) shows the various departments and specialized rooms as well as the layout and relationship of the care units to the support facilities. The 94-bed facility illustrated in this figure has a total of about 75,000 sq. ft. of building area (63,000 sq. ft. allocated to the hospital unit and 12,000 sq. ft. to administration/business offices). This is an average of about 800 sq. ft. of building area per bed.

Valuation Considerations

A prime factor for the appraiser to consider is that psychiatric hospitals are special-purpose properties operated as businesses. They have limited alternative uses, mostly ones that are medically related, which means that financial feasibility is a key function in the analysis and valuation of the assets.

In a typical assignment where the report will be used for buy/sell, financing, or securitization purposes, the valuation will encompass land, site improvements, building(s), FF&E, and intangibles. When the facility is a going-concern, all three approaches have applicability. A market analysis is mandatory and a market feasibility study is necessary if the hospital is a proposed project, surplus to the needs of the trade area, or contemplating an addition.

The market for the acquisition of private, psychiatric hospitals can be considered as national in scope because of the numbers and sizes of hospital systems operating in the U.S. Comparable sales from distant cities may have applicability in a variety of circumstances, but they should be thoughtfully analyzed. An allowance or allocation for the business enterprise component is appropriate, but when the industry is in a downward financial trend, the component for intangibles may be shrinking or nonexistent.

Financial Ratios

The following data, derived from *The Sourcebook,* provide some guidelines for analyzing individual properties. Although specific data will vary depending on the date of the appraisal and trends prevailing in the marketplace at the time, the items mentioned are among those that should be considered when analyzing this type of property.

Gross Patient Revenue per Adjusted Discharge. This is a measure of the inpatient price per unit (per case) in a hospital, although it is not equivalent to the unit revenue actually received. "It serves as a measure of a hospital's pricing policies, although it is less revealing in markets in which few third-party payers are charge-based."[14] This amount decreased in the median psychiatric hospital from $13,392 in 1990 to $12,003 in 1994, which represented a decrease of 10.4%. At the 25th percentile the amount was $9,700 and at the 75th percentile it was $14,675 in 1994.

Deductions from Gross Patient Revenue. Deductions consist of contractual allowances and discounts, bad debts, and charity care. They are expressed as a percentage of gross patient revenue and calculated by dividing by gross patient revenue. Favorable values are below the median. These deductions have been increasing drastically in recent years for psychiatric hospitals, increasing 72% between 1990 and 1994 for the median hospital. "The steady increases in deductions are mainly the result of reduced government subsidies and increasing payer differentials, growth in the size of Medicaid shortfalls, and the greater prevalence of HMOs, PPOs, and other managed care organizations which negotiate discounts from charges."[15] In 1994 deductions for the median hospital came to 45.33%; at the 25th percentile the deduction was 35.29% and at the 75th percentile the deduction was 52.87%.

Operating Revenue per Adjusted Discharge. Total operating revenue is defined as the sum of net patient revenue (payments actually received or expected to be received by the hospital) plus other operating revenue. An adjusted discharge is calculated by multiplying the number of acute care discharges by the adjustment factor. It expresses all of the hospital's services, inpatient and outpatient, as acute care discharge equivalence. This ratio measures the amount of operating revenue the hospital collects per unit of output (per case) and thus is an indicator of a hospital's ability to generate revenues from its patient care operations. The median amount has declined in recent years, dropping from $9,046 in 1988 to $6,736 in 1994. In 1994 the 25th percentile was at $5,301 and the 75th percentile was at $8,452.

Operating Expense per Adjusted Discharge. Operating expense per adjusted discharge is a measure of the hospital's average cost of delivering inpatient care per unit (per case). Favorable values are below the median. A typical hospital has had significant decreases in recent years, following the same trend in operating revenue, going from $8,937 in 1988 to $10,073 in 1991, and down to $7,158 in 1993. At the 25th percentile in 1993 the amount was $5,439 and at the 75th percentile it was $8,777.

Outpatient Revenue as a Percentage of Gross Revenue. This measure approximates the portion of a hospital's revenue that is attributable to services provided to outpatients. Management of

---

[14] Op. cit., *The Comparative Performance of U.S. Hospitals: The Sourcebook,* 1996.

[15] Ibid.

psychiatric hospitals is attempting to diversify the hospital's sources of revenue. The median hospital in 1988 secured only 0.44% of its gross revenue from outpatient sources. In 1990 this ratio increased to 1.41%; it then jumped to 4.02% in 1992 and 7.91% in 1994.

Operating Profit Margin. This is a measure of a hospital's profitability with respect to its patient care services and operations. It is the difference between total operating revenue and total operating expense (which includes depreciation and interest), expressed as a percentage of total operating revenue. Due to the problems of the industry, the typical hospital has fallen into the red since 1990, with a negative -1.65% return in 1994. At the 25th percentile the return was -9.90%, while at the 75th percentile there was profitability, but only at 4.17%.

Net Investment per Bed. This ratio measures the degree of a hospital's investment in capital assets in relation to its size. It calculates total plant, property, and equipment less accumulated depreciation, divided by the total number of beds in service in a facility. The median psychiatric hospital had an investment of $50,559 per bed in 1994. At the 25th percentile the investment was $24,584 per bed and at the 75th percentile the investment was $75,430 per bed. These figures have dropped significantly due to recent sales of psychiatric hospitals at highly discounted prices.

Return on Assets. Net income divided by total assets is another measure of overall profitability. It compares the amount of total revenue over total expense generated in relation to the amount of assets controlled by the hospital. The median hospital in 1994 had a negative return of -2.12%, with the 25th percentile hospital at -11.64% and the 75th percentile hospital at a positive 6.48%. The last profitable year for the typical hospital was around 1990.

Debt per Bed. This measures of the amount of a hospital's debt in relation to its size. It is the ratio of total liabilities (both long-term and short-term) to the total number of beds in service at a facility. The average amount of debt per bed for the median psychiatric hospital increased from $47,136 in 1988 to $71,149 per bed in 1992, and then declined to $47,676 in 1994. It is interesting to note that the debt per bed is only slightly less than the net investment per bed shown above, which is another indication of the declining values in the business and the uncertain equity position of owners.

Cash Flow per Bed. Total cash flow is equal to the sum of net income, depreciation, and interest. Cash flow per bed indicates the amount of cash available that a hospital can use for debt-service payments as well as other purposes. This factor has drastically declined in recent years, going from $12,258 per bed for the median psychiatric hospital in 1989 to $5,528 in 1994. Hospitals at the 25th percentile were in a loss position at $-1,177 per bed, while those at the 75th percentile performed at a positive $13,022 per bed in 1994.

Cash Flow to Total Debt. This ratio is one measure of a hospital's creditworthiness. It measures the proportion of a hospital's total debt obligations that could be met with available cash flow if demanded by creditors within one year. It is the sum of net income and current depreciation expense, divided by total liabilities. In 1994 the median psychiatric hospital had a ratio of 0.10, which means that it would take 10 years for the hospital's available cash flow to meet its total debt obligations. This ratio is down 55% from 1988 when it was at 0.22. At the 25th percentile, cash flow to total debt ratio was -05; for the 75th percentile (favorable values are above the median), the ratio was 0.32.

Debt Service Coverage Ratio. Debt service coverage measures the ratio of funds available for payment of debt service to the same year's principal and interest payments. It is an important measure of creditworthiness. It is the sum of cash flow (net income and current depreciation expense) and interest expense, divided by the same year's debt service. Debt service ratios for the median psychiatric hospital have been declining rapidly in recent years, from 2.23 in 1988 to 0.95 in 1994. At the 25th percentile the debt coverage ratio in 1993 was negative at -.59. For the 75th percentile, the debt service coverage ratio was quite favorable at 3.44.

Income Approach

The income approach is typically applied to the entire revenue stream and operational expenses of a psychiatric hospital, which is similar to the methodology commonly applied in the appraisal of nursing homes (see Figure 3.3 for an illustration of a conventional direct capitalization technique).

Figure 3.3	Income Approach Summary of a Successful Psychiatric Hospital			
Number of beds	98			
Available patient days	35,770			
Adult patient days	5,956	$482.79	45.00%	
Adolescent patient days	4,632	$494.92	35.00%	
C.D. patient days	2,647	$458.43	20.00%	
Total patient days	13,235			
Inpatient occupancy	37.00%			
Average prof fee/psych PD	$0			
Average hospital visit charge	$242.31			
Number of hospital visits	6,562			
Net Revenues	**1994 (est.)**	**$/Patient Day**	**$/Bed**	**% Total**
Adult psych revenue	$2,875,467	$482.79	$29,342	35.25%
Adolescent psych revenue	$2,292,446	$494.92	$23,392	28.11%
C.D. revenue	$1,213,464	$458.43	$12,382	13.88%
Hospital visit revenue	$1,590,005	$120.14	$16,225	19.49%
Other net revenue	$0	$0.00	$0	0.00%
Ancillary revenue	$185,290	$14.00	$1,891	2.27%
Total routine revenue	**$8,156,673**	**$616.30**	**$83,231**	**100.00%**
Less Expenses				
Salaries & wages	($3,904,101)	($294.99)	($39,838)	-47.86%
Employee benefits	($1,370,740)	($103.57)	($13,987)	-16.81%
Professional fees	($257,994)	($19.49)	($2,633)	-3.16%
Purchased services	($643,527)	($48.62)	($6,567)	-7.89%
Supplies	($453,390)	($34.26)	($4,626)	-5.56%
General & admin.	($540,740)	($40.86)	($5,518)	-6.63%
Other expenses	($64,818)	($4.90)	($661)	-0.79%
Management expense	($163,133)	($12.33)	($1,665)	-2.00%
Replacement reserve	($81,567)	($6.16)	($832)	-1.00%
Total expenses	**($7,480,010)**	**($565.17)**	**($76,327)**	**-91.70%**
Net operating income	$676,663	$51.13	$6,905	8.30%
Add real estate taxes	$52,718			
R.E. tax adjusted NOI	$729,381			
Capitalization rate	15.00%			
Add R.E. tax rate	1.03%			
R.E. tax adjusted cap rate	16.03%			
Indicated value	**$4,550,101**	**(per bed: $46,430)**		

When vast changes are taking place, as they have been in the health care industry, historical financial performance may not be a guide to the future. The expectancy regarding future operations (and therefore revenues) may be drastically altered. Under current conditions a well-managed and successful hospital cannot expect to maintain market share unless it lowers its rate structure. Introduction of a "gatekeeper" program could have a major impact on occupancy rates, ALOS, and number of discharges. In these circumstances the appraiser should analyze the subject's operating history combined with national and regional data to make future estimates of revenue, expenses, and net income. An example of the projected performance of an actual hospital under two possible scenarios is presented in Figure 3.4. In this example the appraiser has effectively considered industry trends to estimate net income before management and revenues.

Figure 3.4	A. Comparisons between Subject Hospital Operating Results and National Statistics			
	1991	1992	1993	Projection
ALOS (in days)				
50th Percentile	19.2	16.7	14.8	
75th Percentile	23.2	20.4	18.4	
Subject	16.6	18.1	16.2	13.0
Number of Discharges				
50th Percentile	873	960	1,041	
75th Percentile	1,331	1,332	1,508	
Subject	1,605	1,451	1,723	1,750-1,860
Operating Revenue Per Discharge Day				
50th Percentile	$494	$536	$531	
75th Percentile	$554	$560	$537	
Subject	$418	$477	$465	$420-$450
Operating Expense Per Discharge Day				
50th Percentile	$531	$560	$542	
25th Percentile	$484	$538	$537	
Subject	$340	$353	$347	$350-$375

(continued)

| Figure 3.4 | B. Summary of Income Approach (continued) |

Scenario No. 1

Assumptions:

a.   ALOS of 13 days

b.   Same discharges as 1993 or about 1,750

c.   Revenue of $450 per discharge day (3.2% lower than 1993)

d.   Expenses of $375 per discharge day (71.1% higher than 1992-93 mean of $350)

e.   5% for management and reserves

f.   Capitalization rate of 15%

Total operating revenue (13 x 1,750 x $450)		$10,237,500
Operating expenses (13 x 1,750 x $375)	$8,531,250	
Fixed expenses (5% x $10,237,500)	511,875	
Total expenses		$9,043,125
Net operating income		$1,194,375
Capitalized at 15%		$7,962,500
Called		$7,960,000

Scenario No. 2

Assumptions:

1.   Same as above for items a, e and f above

2.   Discharges of 1,860 or an increase of 8% over 1993

3.   Revenue of $420 per discharge day or about 10% less than 1993

4.   Expenses of $350 per discharge day or same as mean of 1992 and 1993

Total operating revenue (13 x 1,860 x $420)		$10,155,600
Operating expenses (13 x 1,860 x $350)	$8,463,000	
Fixed expenses (5% x $10,155,600)	$507,780	
Total expenses		$8,970,000
Net operating income		$1,184,820
Capitalized at 15%		$7,898,800
Called		$7,900,000

Fixed Expenses

Fixed expenses include management and reserves. In the psychiatric hospital business (as well as in other health care businesses) costs for outside management include compensation for the functions of staffing (hiring, firing, training, motivation and supervision), marketing and promotion, accounting, maintenance, and minor capital improvements. As a general rule, the fixed portion of management compensation ranges between 3% to 5% of defined gross revenues, and incentive compensation usually represents an equivalent or larger portion of defined net income.

Reserves, typically ranging from 2% to 4% of total revenues, are necessary to replace short-lived components of hospital improvements and FF&E. They may be estimated sometimes by reference to replacement costs. In a hypothetical example, the short-lived portions of the property amount to about 20% of the estimated replacement cost of the buildings or $1,590,000, while FF&E has a replacement cost of about $658,000. A reasonable replacement rate to be applied to these two figures would be 10% per year, which amounts to about $225,000. This figure is also equivalent to 2.25% of the estimated total operating revenue of $10,000,000.

Capitalization Rate

Although hospitals (including psychiatric facilities) are commonly described as local businesses dependent on a population within, say, a 20-mile radius, market values are not largely a function of a consumer base but rather an investor/owner base and, indirectly, a payer base. The investor/owner base is best characterized by multistate and national companies that stand ready to bid on available facilities largely on the basis of yield potential and expected profit margins. These goals directly affect market value and are based on capitalization rates that tend to be national rather than local due to the nature of the competition, its financing and its investors. The payer base includes various insurance companies (typically on a national basis), the federal government, and state governments disbursing federal Medicaid funds. The payer group tends to merge practices and policies with a high degree of commonality. Even regional differences in labor costs, prices, and building codes tend towards similarity in this industry. These differences can be ignored in the income approach since yields, profit margins, and capitalization rates are a flexible guide to maximum return on capital regardless of local differences and other factors.

Overall capitalization rates or component rates for various categories of assets are difficult to derive from hospital transactions. Every facility tends to have unique characteristics and relationships, and each accounting period tends to include unusual and so-called "nonrecurring" events that make the appraisal concept of normalized income difficult to apply. Also, sales of productive facilities are rare compared to sales of "troubled" properties that often have a negative cash flow. Therefore, cap rates must be supported by other financial studies, investment yield surveys, and individual interviews. Except for financial services that report publicly traded, individual corporation and industry performance, there is little, if any, aggregation of such data.

It should be noted that most purchasers of psychiatric hospitals are owner/users (operators) who typically give less weight to the facility's past performance than to their opinion of the amount of income a facility will generate under their ownership and operation. That this is the case is supported by comments from officials of a chain of psychiatric centers during the sale of a number of its facilities. When questioned about the range of capitalization rates that would be reflected by on-going sales price negotiations, the response was "you cannot derive a capitalization rate from a negative NOI." Based on this statement, it is reasonable to assume that if these negotiations are consummated, the resulting capitalization rates, derived from the "at time of sale" NOI, will be negative. The same officials also reported that they were unaware of rate-of-return levels being projected by the potential buyers. The appraisers involved were also unable to obtain any rate-of-return projections from the major proposed purchaser. Therefore, the appraisers were unable to make any verified projections as to the proposed buyers' anticipated or subsequent capitalization rates, which would be calculated from the net income generated under their ownership and operation.

In attempts to determine market supported capitalization rates, appraisers may have discussions with lenders, buyers, sellers, and other professionals knowledgeable about psychiatric hospital facilities. Capitalization rates can be highly variable when tremendous changes are occurring in the industry. A current consensus is that a broad range of 13% to 20% is appropriate given the risk of these facilities, their specialized nature (lack of alternative uses), unique management requirements, and the general lack of knowledge or interest about them among lenders and investors.

Appraisers could also research and review capitalization rates applicable to other specialty health care property types that are considered to have similar risk, specialization, and management factors. The most appropriate of these alternative capitalization rates would appear to be from the sales of general acute care hospitals, particularly those that emphasize psychiatric care. However, appraisers probably will not be able to identify any such transactions from which market-supported capitalization rates could be derived. The next most appropriate of these alternative capitalization rates would appear to be from the sales of either general acute care hospitals or skilled nursing facilities. Appraisers should be aware that the use of market-derived capitalization rates from the sales of a different property type is not considered to be typical. However, given the lack of psychiatric hospital transactions from which capitalization rates can be derived, it may be considered to be the most accurate method available. A recent survey indicated a range of 13% to 20% for hospital facilities and 11% to 17% for skilled nursing facilities. The lower to mid-range capitalization rates are representative of historically profitable and better located facilities. The higher rates usually reflect distressed or more specialized properties. In comparison the capitalization rates derived from skilled nursing facilities tend to be lower due to their greater marketability and more secure future outlook.

Sales Comparison Approach

Appraisers need to acquire in-depth data about transactions to make appropriate adjustments. Since local sales transactions of psychiatric hospitals may be limited or nonexistent, comparables on a regional and national basis should be considered. The appraiser should watch for sales activity involving on-going disposition programs of chains and other providers. Reliable and accurate comparisons are difficult to make and financial data tends to be minimal. At best the sales comparison approach should be expected to yield only a range in value on a price-per-bed basis.

Adjusting a money-losing comparable to a successful enterprise is extremely difficult unless data on all of the assumptions are available so that the appraiser can quantify the *NPV* of future revenue shortfalls to the point of profitable financial performance. Typical adjustment factors dealing with age, condition, capacity, efficiency, land/building ratios, etc., may be revealing and helpful as far as physical differences are concerned, but they cannot account for economic differentials and buyers' calculations. In a falling market where prices are a "moving target," transactional values for comparable facilities tend to be at the bottom of the range.

Acquisition of "street knowledge" through interviews with major players, whether buyers or sellers, can be the best resource for making adjustments. Overall, adjustments that quantify a large amount of information about facility and enterprise differentials may be the best technique for application of the sales comparison approach. An example of a sales comparison grid and the type of key information that should be considered is shown in Figure 3.5.

Figure 3.5   Summary Grid: Hospital Improved Sales Comparables

Name/ Location/ APN	Sales Date	# Of Beds	Sales Price	Price per Bed	Bldg. Size (SF)	Price per SF	NOI	OAR	Occ. at Sale	1991-92 OSHPD Stated Occ.	Year Built	Gross Avg. Bed Size	Land Area (AC)/Land to Bldg. Ratio	Remarks
Hospital AA	Escrow	80	$5,500,000	$68,750	53,000	$103.77	N/A	N/A	N/A	49.39%	1991	663 sf	6.84 / 17.79%	Cost $12-13 mil. to construct in 1991; scheduled closing 5/31/94
Hospital BB	6/90	151	$10,150,000	$67,219	96,000	$105.73	N/A	N/A	N/A	21.78%	1990	636 sf	5.72 / 38.53%	Purchased just prior to completion; cost $15,150,000 to construct
Hospital CC	Listing	74	$4,000,000	$54,054	32,240	$124.07	N/A	N/A	N/A	N/A	1970	436 sf	1.68 / 44.06%	Former psych. hospital closed for over 2 yrs; recent $300,000 renovation for chemical dependency use; anticipated price $2,500,000
High		151		$68,7850	96,000	$124.07					1991	663 sf	44.06%	
Low		74		$54,054	32,240	$103.77					1970	436 sf	17.79%	
Average		102		$63,341	60,413	$111.19					1984	578 sf	33.46%	
Subject Property Hospital X	N/A	96	NA	N/A	53,297	N/A	$676,663	N/A	37.00%	49.71%	1914 to 1962	544 sf	14.6 / 8.38%	Subject property est. 1994 NOI & occupancy; site is 14.60 acres, with addl. 10.22 acres of excess land

Cost Approach

Since valuation approaches for psychiatric hospitals are similar in concept to nursing homes and medical-surgical (acute) hospitals, an example of the cost approach is not included here. Futhermore, it is not used by buyers or sellers. Nevertheless, the appraiser should have the knowledge and capability to accurately estimate replacement costs for improvements and FF&E and apply various depreciation measurements. External obsolescence is a primary consideration and the appraiser must look beyond local conditions to make an accurate estimate. When buyers and sellers are operating on a national basis and industry-wide trends are prevail, depreciation deductions should be derived from analysis of the types of financial ratios discussed in this chapter. For example, the difference in cash flow per bed between a 75th percentile hospital and a 25th percentile hospital could be capitalized to show why costs must be heavily depreciated. Another similar technique would be to capitalize the differential between actual or projected net income and a pro forma net income necessary to support the value of a facility after physical depreciation factors have been considered. In rare situations where there is significant intangible value to the enterprise, the appraiser will find the cost approach of valuable assistance in accounting for the various categories of physical assets and identifying a value for the business.

C H A P T E R
F O U R

Ambulatory Care (Surgery) Centers

Ambulatory care centers (ACCs) provide a cost-effective substitute for more expensive medical procedures that are performed in acute general hospitals. Many ACCs are focused on the provision of ambulatory or short-term surgeries, but the category also includes dialysis centers, emergency or urgent care centers, fertility clinics, imaging and radiation treatment centers, and birthing centers. This chapter focuses entirely on surgery centers (SCs) and the expanded concept of surgery recovery centers (SRCs). They are a major presence in the medical market and by the year 2000 are expected to account for a growing majority of all surgical procedures performed in the United States. Also, unlike other alternative care facilities, many of which are found in storefront locations or traditional medical office buildings, ambulatory care centers are a unique building type, given their high-cost surgical and imaging suites.

Background

The concept of a freestanding, outpatient surgery center is about 25 years old. The first center opened in 1970 in Phoenix, Arizona, and real growth began to occur about five years later. With the endorsement of the American Medical Association and the American College of Surgeons as well as the demonstrated success of early projects, surgery centers became a strong reality. By 1983 about 240 surgery centers had opened, and currently more than 2,000 such facilities exist in the United States. In one year alone (1986) as many as 190 were added.

Recovery centers focus on medical procedures that require a one- to three-day inpatient hospitalization. Procedures involving ear/nose/throat, orthopedic, plastic surgery, urological, and gynecological specialties, among others, are typical of this type of facility. The addition of patient recovery to surgery centers started in the mid-1980s when the state of California approved the establishment of pilot SRC projects. These projects were allowed a maximum of 20 beds each, and the length of stay could not exceed 72 hours. Currently, there are about 10 existing or proposed projects in California, and at least 20 other states have approved or are considering legislation to establish recovery centers.

Rationale for SCs and SCRs

While large institutional hospitals may tend to be inefficient and unfriendly, surgery centers are generally thought of as efficient and friendly. Physicians prefer to operate in an SC because it saves them time and allows them to perform more procedures. Patients prefer SCs because the facilities provide more amenities and personal attention and because they are less expensive and more convenient than hospitals. Insurance companies, HMOs, and other providers favor SCs because of their substantially lower costs for certain medical procedures. Typically, costs at SCs are 20% to 25% less than they are at general hospitals, which generally have higher overhead, occupancy, and management costs than SCs. Independent SCs have the lowest charge per case, followed by corporate chain facilities, and those that are hospital owned.

A less publicized reason for developing SCs is the profit motive. Physicians and other investors have made very attractive returns on their investments in SCs. Operating profit ratios exceed those of general hospitals by several hundred percent. Internal rates of return (*IRRs*) have reached 20% and more. (A discussion of financial feasibility is included later in this chapter.)

Surgery recovery centers have expanded the concept of ambulatory care into mini-hospitals. About 2,500 different types of procedures are now possible in an outpatient setting. Again, this innovation is driven by large cost efficiencies as well as the better use of physicians' time. Because the desire to control the costs of health delivery ranks high in the United States, SCs will likely continue to grow in numbers and SCRs could have impressive growth. However, competition and government regulation could limit the future growth of both types of facilities. According to the SMG Marketing Group, Inc., many competitive factors may speed or slow the growth projected through 1995 for surgery centers. Any of these events could rapidly change the surgery center market. For instance:

- Hospitals may respond strongly to the establishment of surgicenters in their service areas, using their political and marketing clout to defend their mainstay business of surgery.

- Changes in medical technologies could unexpectedly increase the number of procedures conducted in surgery centers.

- Legislative changes could further encourage the use of surgery centers in both the hospital and freestanding settings. The relationship between hospital and surgery center fees deserves careful attention. Currently, facilities encourage doctors to use surgery centers when possible.

- Cost containment efforts could drastically change the current use patterns of outpatient facilities. Payers such as HMOs and insurers and the federal government could lead this effort. For example, the Inspector General's Office within the Department of Health and Human Services has made repeated efforts to crack down on unnecessary cataract surgery.

- The degree of physician specialization could allow many more types of surgery centers through the advancements of surgical technologies.

- Restrictions placed on Medicare reimbursement to surgery centers through the Ethics in Patient Referrals Act. This bill would disallow payment for patients referred to a facility in which the referring physician has a financial interest. Although several lawmakers will try to insist on stiff regulation of patient referrals, any actual legislation is unlikely to completely ban physician participation in these ventures.

- Impact of the "safe harbor" regulations on physician joint ventures in surgery centers.[1]

Statistics

SMG Marketing Group, Inc., located in Chicago, is the primary source of health care statistics and trend analyses for ambulatory and other care facilities. Their publications, database, and software are available for purchase. Most of the statistical data included in this chapter are

---

[1] SMG Marketing Group, Inc., *Market Letter*, June 1994.

derived from SMG publications such as the *Market Letter* and *Freestanding Outpatient Surgery Centers Report and Directory.*

Surgery centers increased by over 700% in one decade, going from 239 facilities in 1983 to about 2,100 in 1995. At the same time the number of surgeries increased over nine-fold, from approximately 377,000 in 1983 to over 3.75 million in 1995 (see Table 4.1). During 1994, completed ambulatory care center projects or those in the pipeline accounted for over $8.8 billion in construction, or about 20% of all health care projects under construction in the United States (see Table 4.2).

Table 4.1	Growth of Surgery Centers		
Year	**Number of Facilities***	**Total Procedures**	**Per Facility**
1983	239	377,266	1,578
1984	330	517,851	1,569
1985	459	783,864	1,708
1986	592	1,033,604	1,746
1987	865	1,383,540	1,712
1988	964	1,722,367	1,787
1989	1,221	2,162,391	1,771
1990	1,383	2,317,741	1,676
1991	1,515	2,583,147	1,705
1992	1,660	2,870,792	1,729
1993	1,826	3,197,956	1,751
1994	1,986	3,495,000	1,760
1995	2,115	3,750,000	1,773

* Open as of December 31
Source: SMG Marketing Group, Inc.

Table 4.2	Projects by Construction Phase, 1994					
		Completed		**Broke Ground**		**Designed**	
Type		**Projects**	**Cost ($000)**	**Projects**	**Cost ($000)**	**Projects**	**Cost ($000)**
Freestanding outpatient facilities		419	$2,171.5	239	$1,722.4	370	$3,267.7
Freestanding outpatient facility expansions or renovations		454	$746.1	160	$355.0	233	$582.1
Percentage of all health care projects		26.2%	24.4%	25.1%	16.7%	19.7%	17.8%

Source: "Healthcare by Design," *Modern Healthcare,* March 27, 1995, p. 38.

The typical surgery center has two to three surgical suites. About 1,700 procedures per year are performed in the average SC, which works out to 6.8 procedures per working day per facility or 2.27 procedures per day per surgical suite. The most common surgical procedures are set forth in Table 4.3.

Table 4.3	Surgical Procedures by Type, 1994
Procedure	**Percent Performed***
Ophthalmology	30.8%
Gynecological surgery	9.1%
Gastroenterology	11.9%
Ear, nose and throat	6.1%
Orthopedic	6.1%
General	6.2%
Plastic	14.8%
Urology	3.4%
Podiatry	7.3%
Pain block	3.0%
Dental	1.1%
Neurology	0.2%
Total	100%

* "Percent Performed" refers to the percentage of total surgeries represented by each procedure.
Source: SMG Marketing Group, Inc.

Independently owned surgery centers dominate the industry. In terms of market share by percentage of surgeries, through early 1994 independents accounted for 58.3%, hospital-owned SCs accounted for 10.4%, and corporate chains had 3.13%. In terms of numbers of facilities, independents have an even higher percentage with 74%, followed by corporate chains (20%), and hospital-owned (6%). Corporate chains are increasing their market share on a consistent basis in recent years, due in large part to their ability to attract more managed care contracts from HMOs and PPOs. A breakdown of the volume of surgeries by type of facility is summarized in Table 4.4.

Geographically, California leads the nation with 356 SCs and 511,000 surgical procedures in 1994, followed by Florida with 174 SCs and 356,000 surgical procedures. Surgery centers appear to enjoy both a more favorable regulatory climate and greater consumer acceptance in the Sun Belt states than other geographical regions.[2] A complete state-by-state summary of surgery centers is shown in Table 4.5.

---

[2] SMG Marketing Group, Inc., *Market Letter*, January 1995, 4.

Table 4.4	Number of Facilities* by Volume of Surgeries, 1994								
	Corporate Chain		Independent		Hospital-Owned		Total	
Number of surgeries	No.	%	No.	%	No.	%	No.	%
Fewer than 1,000	60	16%	729	50%	17	14%	806	41%
1,000 to 1,999	88	23%	408	28%	27	23%	523	26%
2,000 to 2,999	91	24%	169	12%	16	14%	276	14%
3,000 to 4,999	94	25%	116	7%	41	36%	251	13%
5,000 or more	48	12%	48	3%	16	13%	112	6%
Total	381	100%	1,470	100%	106	100%	1,968	100%

*Data based on facilities open one year or more.
Source: SMG Marketing Group, Inc., Chicago, 1995

Physical Characteristics

Freestanding outpatient surgery centers are located in specially designed, single-use buildings while other surgery centers are located within medical office buildings. A center may focus on one medical specialty, such as oral surgery, or provide numerous medical specialties. They vary significantly in size, ranging from 3,000 sq. ft. up to 35,000 sq. ft. The typical SC has about 8,000-10,000 sq. ft. of floor area. The larger facilities often house surgery recovery centers.

Generally, surgery centers are constructed to hospital standards and often have specialized HVAC systems, customized plumbing components, and specially insulated walls, for example. On a unit basis building costs are higher for SCs than general hospitals because the costly surgical suites represent a greater portion of the building area than they do in hospitals (see Table 4.6).

Typically an SC has the appearance of an upscale professional building. Interior finishes are of good quality, with vinyl and tile wall coverings and ceramic, quarry, or vinyl tile or carpeted floors. Other features include indirect and specialized lighting, interior communication systems, conveying and piping systems, and complete HVAC systems. Facilities may include a laboratory. Group I equipment is permanently attached to the building and is part of the general contract. A typical floor plan is shown in Figure 4.1.

Many smaller SCs are found within medical office buildings, which provide office space for independently operating physicians as well as group practices whose medical specialists actively use the SC. In many cases these specialists are the owners of the SC facility. In such an appraisal situation the cost estimator must allow for special tenant improvements in the SC space; this allowance can easily amount to a unit cost equivalent of the Class D, average cost per square foot, shown in Table 4.6. A key variable as far as cost of development is concerned is the number of surgical suites, which number is a function of the size of the entire SC.

Market Analysis

Surgery centers account for only about one sixth of the inpatient and outpatient surgeries in the United States, even though outpatient or ambulatory surgeries comprise over 50% of all surgeries (see Table 4.7). Thus, it would appear that there is no limit to the number of SC facilities that

Table 4.5   Summary of Surgery Centers* by State, 1994

State	No. of Surgery Centers	No. of Surgeries Performed[†]	No. of Operating Suites[†]	State	No. of Surgery Centers	No. of Surgeries Performed[†]	No. of Operating Suites[†]
Alabama	25	90,250	90	Montana	8	11,612	13
Alaska	3	7,557	10	Nebraska	11	14,997	22
Arizona	76	107,536	140	Nevada	22	40,197	43
Arkansas	26	46,583	48	New Hampshire	12	13,307	20
California	356	511,343	735	New Jersey	48	101,252	90
Colorado	30	42,884	72	New Mexico	8	12,669	17
Connecticut	17	35,932	41	New York	32	92,071	102
Dist. of Columbia	10	23,331	27	North Carolina	52	130,125	142
Delaware	2	'3,901	6	North Dakota	6	11,853	15
Florida	174	356,330	434	Ohio	57	109,218	135
Georgia	72	95,148	135	Oklahoma	25	35,692	55
Hawaii	12	13,129	21	Oregon	18	34,816	33
Idaho	16	16,648	32	Pennsylvania	40	97,030	104
Illinois	74	160,450	193	Puerto Rico	8	12,764	12
Indiana	45	89,612	111	Rhode Island	5	14,516	10
Iowa	9	16,560	24	South Carolina	25	37,709	54
Kansas	23	52,872	52	South Dakota	7	10,580	21
Kentucky	18	42,506	47	Tennessee	64	118,176	143
Louisiana	54	83,232	120	Texas	115	196,851	295
Maine	9	8,455	13	Utah	16	45,036	47
Maryland	76	91,497	122	Vermont	2	1,694	4
Massachusetts	17	25,566	42	Virginia	39	80,599	84
Michigan	39	78,953	107	Washington	75	97,580	133
Minnesota	12	29,473	31	West Virginia	8	9,108	14
Mississippi	12	29,481'	36	Wisconsin	23	53,071	72
Missouri	31	67,066	81	Wyoming	4	4,521	8
				Total	1,968	3,513,432	4,458

* Data based on facilities open one year or more
† Includes estimated data
Source: SMG Marketing Group Inc., Chicago, May 1995.

Table 4.6	Comparison of Base Construction Costs per Square Foot for Freestanding Surgery Center	
Type	**Surgery Centers**	**General Hospitals**
Class A-B, Average	$138.61	$120.90
Class C, Good	$151.86	$123.55
Class C, Average	$107.88	$97.21
Class D, Good	$147.31	$115.13
Class D, Average	$104.68	$91.85

Source: *Marshall Valuation Service,* March 1995, Section 15, p. 22-23.

could be added, given their superior patient costs and amenities and the trend toward less intrusive medical procedures, which reduce the need for hospitalization. New development, however, is based not necessarily on supply and demand but such limiting factors as the availability of financing, medical politics, government regulation, and the increasingly competitive posture of general hospitals.

Government factors that have had a negative impact on the recent development of SCs include greater scrutiny of costs by Congress due to charges that expensive procedures are used in an excessive manner; a 1993 economic plan approved by Congress that put a reimbursement freeze on some procedures and reductions on others; and a $50 reduction in the amount Medicare will pay for intraocular lenses in cataract surgery.

Developing a market analysis for a surgery center may follow these steps:

- determining the service or trade area boundaries;
- collecting demographic data on the service or trade area population;
- collecting inventory, market share, and other performance data for outpatient surgery providers;
- making projections of outpatient surgery procedures for the service or trade area; and
- arriving at conclusions as to projected market share for an existing or proposed facility and the influence of a recovery center.

Service or Trade Area Analysis

Hospital service area boundaries may be used for the existing or proposed location of an SC or SRC. A vast array of pertinent statistical data is available relative to established service areas. In large urban areas hospital service areas may be too big and a smaller delineation may be needed to accurately reflect the trade area of the SC. This delineation should be based primarily on patient travel time, developed from historical data of the surgeons involved in the project, combined with local statistical area or government jurisdiction boundaries.

Socioeconomic Characteristics and Trends

Overall population trends of the facility's service area are an important consideration. The statistics should include historical data as well as forecasts into the future. Most frequently, these data focus on a five- to 10-year period dating back from the most recent decennial census to estimates for the present and projections for a five-year period into the future. Several

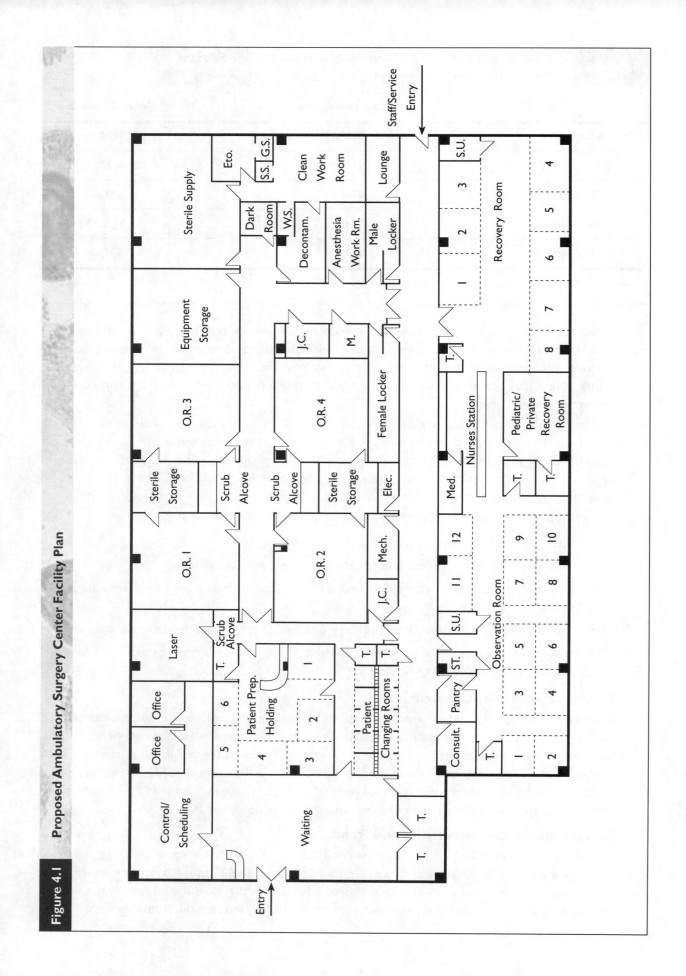

Table 4.7	Outpatient Surgery Performed in Hospitals: 1980 to 1993									
Type of Hospital	1980	1985	1986	1987	1988	1989	1990	1991	1992	1993
Outpatient Surgeries (1,000)										
All hospitals	3,198	7,309	8,705	9,758	10,586	10,953	11,678	12,209	12,849	13,098
Ownership:										
Non-federal hospitals	3,063	6,984	8,272	9,145	10,038	10,362	11,085	11,724	12,316	12,641
Community hospitals[1]	3,054	6,951	8,247	9,126	10,028	10,351	11,070	11,712	12,308	12,624
Nongovernmental nonprofit	2,416	5,392	6,265	6,903	7,577	7,834	8,389	8,989	9,500	9,685
Federal hospitals	135	325	434	612	548	591	593	486	533	457
Size of hospital:										
6 to 99 beds	354	752	966	1,146	1,229	1,241	1,303	1,366	1,464	1,473
100 to 199 beds	571	1,502	1,811	2,030	2,252	2,360	2,498	2,636	2,824	2,927
200 to 299 beds	630	1,521	1,836	2,023	2,297	2,383	2,543	2,695	2,790	2,906
300 to 499 beds	977	2,069	2,368	2,617	2,845	2,920	3,172	3,293	3,340	3,424
500 beds or more	666	1,465	1,725	1,942	1,963	2,049	2,162	2,220	2,431	2,368
Outpatient Surgeries as Percent of Total										
All hospitals	16.4%	34.5%	40.3%	44.2%	47.0%	48.7%	50.6%	52.1%	53.6%	54.9%
Ownership:										
Non-federal hospitals	16.3	34.5	40.3	43.9	46.8	48.5	50.5	52.3	53.8	55.4
Community hospitals[1]	16.3	34.6	40.3	43.8	46.8	48.5	50.5	52.3	53.8	55.4
Nongovernmental nonprofit	17.1	35.5	40.8	44.2	47.0	48.6	50.7	52.5	54.0	55.7
Federal hospitals	18.6	33.9	40.7	49.9	49.7	51.5	51.8	47.8	49.3	45.4
Size of hospital:										
6 to 99 beds	17.9	36.5	44.7	49.4	52.8	54.1	56.2	58.7	61.1	62.5
100 to 199 beds	15.4	36.3	42.9	47.2	50.3	52.3	55.0	56.3	58.3	59.4
200 to 299 beds	16.7	36.4	42.0	45.7	49.2	50.7	52.9	54.6	55.3	57.2
300 to 499 beds	17.2	34.4	40.0	43.1	46.5	48.0	48.8	50.6	51.9	53.2
500 beds or more	15.1	30.4	35.2	39.2	39.6	41.6	43.9	44.4	46.5	46.9

[1] For definition of community hospital, see Table 2.1.

Note: Assuming about 24,000,000 total surgeries (based on 13,000,000 outpatient surgeries representing about 54% of all surgeries), then about 4,000,000 surgeries performed in SCs amounts to a ratio of one in six.

Source: American Hospital Association, *Hospital Statistics*, 1994 edition. Copyright by the American Hospital Association. Reprinted with permission.

companies that can be accessed by computer (e.g., National Planning Data Corporation) provide such forecasts and can tailor the boundaries of the trade area with great flexibility.

Key economic indicators include total population, population by age and income groupings, employment figures and unemployment ratios, retail sales, and housing values. Residential and commercial construction development trends as well as the location of major employers and new shopping centers and malls should also be tracked.

Inventory of Competition

Information on competitors is used in calculating the market penetration required to fill the subject and competitive facilities. Market share measures a center's cases expressed as a percent of the total number of cases in that service area. It is an important measure of the ongoing performance of a facility. Five factors should be considered when analyzing market share. They are:

- Market penetration
- Physician referral patterns
- Patient loyalty
- Patient selectivity
- Price selectivity

Existing surgery centers in a service or trade area can be identified and described by referring to SMG's *Freestanding Surgery Center Directory*. For each SC listed information is provided on location, medical director, telephone, date opened, ownership type, owner, date opened, number of surgeries for the past two years, and a list of medical specialties.

In analyzing the competition it is desirable to obtain operating and financial data as well as performance statistics about the medical staff. Operating data for competitors may be impossible to obtain, but the annual number of cases or procedures is available to determine market share and related trends. Financial data will indicate average revenue per case and provide insights into pricing. A study of the medical staff will provide information about specialties and referral relationships. SCs frequently use patient satisfaction questionnaires to assist management in the analysis of staffing, business operations, and medical services. Physician interviews can document attitudes towards specific SCs; determine willingness to transfer surgical cases from acute general hospitals; and provide insight into future trends, risk factors, and emerging technology. Physician responses relative to medical procedures can be compared to the latest available hospital discharge information to determine market share by specialty.

Geographic relationships involving proximity to primary general hospitals, competitive surgery centers, and the office locations of the SC surgeons should also be explored.

Projections and Pricing

In the analysis and valuation of a proposed SC it is necessary to project annual revenues to the point of stabilization. This may also be true for an existing SC if it is still in the "fill-up" stage. To make such projections separate analyses of categories of surgical procedures as well as unit pricing must be prepared. Average or mean revenues per case should be compared with published data. Table 4.8 shows the average charge per case by ownership for the years 1992, 1993, and 1994. In 1994 the average charge per case at a surgery center was about $1,047, up 6% from 1992.

Larger increases in revenue per case for corporate chain and hospital-owned SCs are indicative of the complexity of surgical cases being transferred from general hospitals, while the smaller increase in revenue for independent SCs was partly due to their higher Medicare caseloads. The overall average charge per case increased only slightly between 1993 and 1994,

Table 4.8

Average Charge per Case by Ownership

Ownership	Charge per Case			Total Centers*		
	1992	1993	1994	1992	1993	1994
Corporate Chain	$1,140.69	$1,256.19	$1,242.58	240	300	327
Independent	$929.35	$968.17	$966.76	970	1,032	1,084
Hospital-Owned	$1,160.96	$1,184.10	$1,280.10	99	99	100
Total	$985.62**	$1,043.49**	$1,047.19**	1,309	1,431	1,511

Data based on facilities open one year or more.
* Total number of centers providing charge-per-case data.
** Total average charge per case.
Source: SMG Marketing Group, Inc., May 1995.

but corporate and independent surgery centers actually reported slightly lower average charges per case in 1994 than in 1993. This reflects the influence of managed care, tight Medicare reimbursement rates, and growing concerns over rising health care costs.[3]

Currently the average number of surgeries per SC is continuing to increase due to shifts of procedures from acute hospitals to SCs, along with greater acceptance of SCs by the general public and the expansion of SCs through the addition of additional surgical suites. Projections through 1995 appear in Figure 4.2. The total market will continue to increase but at a lower annual rate in the near future. The starting point for projecting future caseloads for a proposed SC is to identify the group of surgeons who will support the facility and transfer their caseload. Studies of the growth of similar facilities are helpful in analyzing the annual rate of growth. In

Figure 4.2 **Surgery Center Growth Projections**

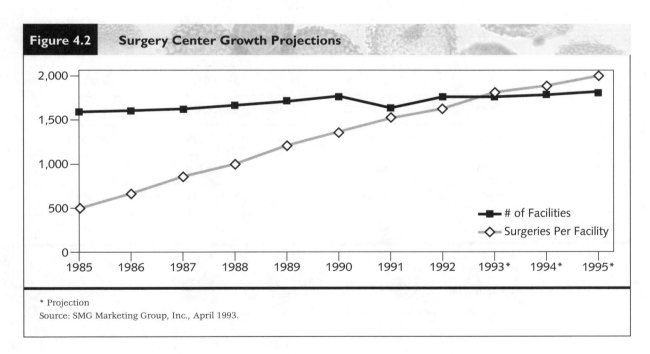

* Projection
Source: SMG Marketing Group, Inc., April 1993.

---

[3] SMG Marketing Group, Inc., *Market Letter*.

some instances an independent SC may be combined with or acquired by a larger and more established SC. The new entity can more efficiently serve a market that will likely become more competitive in the future. Consolidation of facilities will be emphasized in the 1990s.

The addition of recovery units to an existing surgery center can vastly increase the potential surgical caseload —i.e., procedures that normally would require one to three days of inpatient hospitalization. In one of the earliest and most successful SRCs the additional cases amounted to a 40% increase, derived from incremental outpatient surgical cases (10%) and new recovery care center cases (30%).

Financial Data

Nationally, surgery centers accounted for about $3.3 billion in revenue from surgical operations in 1993, which was expected to increase to over $4.6 billion by 1996 (see Table 4.9).

Table 4.9	Revenue Projections for Surgery Centers, 1983-1996			
Year	No. of Facilities	Surgical Operations*	Dollar Volume (000)	Avg. Per Facility
1983	239	377,266	$166,751	$697,703
1984	330	517,851	$329,682	$999,036
1985	459	783,864	$373,479	$813,680
1986	633	1,100,240	$642,540	$1,015,071
1987	853	1,476,236	$847,814	$993,920
1988	984	1,702,397	$1,192,035	$1,211,418
1989	1,227	1,997,856	$1,506,463	$1,227,761
1990	1,364	2,317,741	$1,996,154	$1,463,456
1991	1,556	2,583,147	$2,373,912	$1,525,650
1992	1,690	2,870,792	$2,833,472	$1,676,611
1993	1,862	3,197,956	$3,337,035	$1,792,178
1994**	2,106	3,641,531	$3,813,258	$1,810,664
1995**	2,266	3,970,000	$4,197,084	$1,852,199
1996***	2,386	4,321,000	$4,611,371	$1,932,678

*   Includes estimated data
** Based on centers opened prior to 12/31/94.
*** Projection.
Source: SMG Marketing Group, Inc., May 1995.

Other financial data, such as operating ratios, are not readily available in a detailed format. The analyst should investigate the financial statements of nearby SCs or ones in the same region or state to determine the proper allowances to be made for individual expense categories. Table 4.10 shows actual data on a percentage basis for one of the most successful independent SCs during its early growth period. Operating profit before deduction for management, reserves, depreciation, and interest reached 38%. Typical SCs are much less profitable. The results for a recently completed, hospital-affiliated facility are shown in Table 4.11. Here, operating profit before the same deductions reached 22% but then declined to 17% because of substantial increases in salaries, wages, and purchased services.

Table 4.10	Income & Expense Statement (Unaudited) for Independent Surgery Center			
		Year Ended December 31		
	1990	1991	1992	1993
Cases	1,907	2,931	3,374	3,685
Patient service revenues	99.5%	99%	99%	99%
Other operating revenues	0.5%	1%	1%	1%
Total operating revenues	**100%**	**100%**	**100%**	**100%**
Operating expenses:				
Administrative services:				
Compensation	58%	22%	21%	42%
Rent		16%	14%	13%
Other		9%	7%	8%
Surgery services - supplies	15%	17%	17%	21%
Purchased services	6%	6%	5%	4%
Library	2%	1%	2%	2%
Interest	4%	4%	2%	2%
Depreciation and amortization	9%	9%	6%	5%
Provision for uncollectible accounts		3%	3%	4%
Total operating expenses	**94%**	**87%**	**77%**	**83%**
Net income	6%	13%	23%	17%
Net income before interest and depreciation	19%	25%	31%	25%

Category	6 mos. 1990	%	1991	%	1992	%	5 mos. 1993	%
Operating revenues:								
Gross patient revenues	$3,498.1	116.7	$8,010.6	120.3	$8,809.0	123.5	$3,798	124.3
Less provision for contractual discounts	499.7	16.7	1,350.7	20.3	1,650.2	23.5	734	24.2
Net operating revenues	**$2,998.4**	**100.0**	**$6,659.9**	**100.0**	**$7,158.8**	**100.0**	**$3,034**	**100.0**
Operating expenses:								
Salaries and wages	802.8	26.8	1,741.6	26.2	2,136.4	29.8	937	30.9
Employee benefits	125.8	4.2	276.8	4.1	341.2	4.8	173	5.7
Medical fees	37.5	1.2	91.9	1.4	113.3	1.6	63	1.2
Supplies	710.4	23.7	1,619.5	24.3	1,782.4	24.9	775	25.5
Purchased services, insurance, and other	835.8	27.9	1,172.3	17.6	1,362.3	19.0	579	19.1
Provision for uncollectible accounts	88.2	2.9	238.4	3.6	240.5	3.4	98	3.2
Total	**$2,600.5**	**86.7**	**$5,140.5**	**77.2**	**$5,976.1**	**83.5**	**$2,625**	**86.5**
Net income*	$397.9	13.3	$1,519.4	22.8	$1,182.7	16.5	$409	13.5
Statistics								
Surgery cases	3,346	76.6	7,181	76.6	7,575	76.8	2,987	76.2
GI cases	1,024	23.4	2,195	23.4	2,290	23.2	934	23.8
Total cases	**4,370**	**100.0**	**9,376**	**100.0**	**9,865**	**100.0**	**3,921**	**100.0**
Revenue per case	$686		$710		$726		$774	

Table 4.11 Revenue & Expense Statement (Percentage Basis) for Hospital-Affiliated Surgery Center ($000)

* Before deductions for management, reserves, depreciation and interest

A selection of actual operating ratios from a variety of other sources is set forth in Table 4.12. The reader is cautioned that these data are presented for illustrative purposes only and should not be considered as applicable to any particular SC or proposed project. The data do indicate that SCs can be quite profitable. SCs operate during the workday only and so do not incur the around-the-clock expenses of operating a full-service hospital. Nevertheless, excess profits will attract additional SC competition and this possibility should be considered by analysts and appraisers.

Valuation Methodology

While all three traditional approaches to value may be applicable in valuing a surgery center, only two of them are generally put to use: the cost approach and the income approach. The latter is given the most weight because SCs are considered to be medical enterprises as well as

Table 4.12	Summary of Operating Ratios of Various Surgery Centers		
Year	No. of Cases	Revenue per Case	Operating Ratio*
1988	6,034	$1,083	74.4%
1988	4,120	$785	60.7%
1988	4,052	$780	54.4%
1988	4,946	$894	81.3%
1988	7,574	$621	69.4%
1986	4,072	$650	61.4%
1992	3,374	$861	55.0%
1993	3,685	$825	62.5%

* Before depreciation, interest, income taxes, amortization, management, and reserves.

investment properties, and the income approach measures all components of the business including intangibles or the business value. The sales comparison approach is rarely applicable because sales of surgery centers are few, and those that have taken place usually involve the acquisition of a business and not a freestanding facility or of a chain of health care enterprises.

Cost Approach

The relatively high unit cost of developing an SC plus the provision for a large amount of specialized equipment make the cost approach particularly applicable to valuing an SC. It also accounts for allowances for unique indirect costs such as organizational expenses, inspections, and preopening costs. As noted earlier in this chapter, unit construction costs are very high because the ratio of area for operating suites to the total building area is high. Hospitals have always been the most expensive type of commercial building to construct due to their special functions and regulatory requirements. A traditional cost approach to the valuation of a free-standing surgery center is set forth in Figure 4.3.

In the example in Figure 4.3 a 12,000-square-foot building is divided into the following: a main waiting/reception room, a six-bed patient preparation area, five surgical/operating rooms, an outpatient recovery area, an employee lounge with locker rooms, a decontamination room, sterile work areas, electrical and general storage areas, supply areas, mechanical equipment storage rooms, general offices, and restrooms. Overall cost of all facilities is about $390 per square foot of building area and $940,000 per surgical suite for a very high quality SC.

Income Approach

It is appropriate to base the appraisal of a surgery center on the capitalized value of the total income produced by the enterprise because of a lack of comparable rental data. This is due to the fact that SCs are not typically developed for the purpose of rental to a third party. Many operating entities use related party leases, but these should not be considered unless they are binding and guaranteed to extend for a substantial number of years. Accordingly, an appraiser will investigate past revenues and expenses for the surgery center, operating and published data for other surgery centers, and projected future revenues and expenses. Actual market lease data from a recent appraisal of a surgery center situated within a medical office building is shown in Table 4.13.

Figure 4.3   Cost Approach for a New Surgery Center

Land		$600,000
Improvements		
Building: 12,000 sq. ft. @ $168.61 per sq. ft. (a)	$2,023,320	
Yard construction (b)	400,000	
Total improvements		$2,423,320
Subtotal real estate		$3,023,320
FF&E (c)		1,036,648
Other Costs		
Organization expense (d)	$192,000	
Developer's O & P (e)	400,000	
Contingency (f)	40,000	
Subtotal		632,000
Total Replacement Cost		$4,691,968
	Rounded to	$4,700,000

(a) Base cost of $136.84 for Class C, good-rated building times 1.22 local adjustment and 1.01 times adjustment factors.

(b) Includes paving, landscaping, signage, lighting, and underground lines.

(c) Includes everything from a water softener unit to the most technical surgical instrumentation.

(d) Application cost, partnership materials, legal costs, other consultants.

(e) About 10% of cost of land, improvements, and FF&E.

(f) About 1% of cost of land, improvements, and FF&E.

In this survey, rents for surgery centers average about 20% more than for medical office buildings with similar characteristics.

Using the same facility described in the section on the cost approach, the total projected revenue for valuation purposes is $3,125,000 calculated on the basis of five operating/surgical suites times 2.5 procedures per working day (see Figure 4.4). Direct expenses include salaries and benefits, medical supplies, and food, which in this example come to 47% of gross revenue, or $1,468,750, leaving a gross profit of $1,656,250. General administrative expenses include secretarial, central supply, payroll service computer fees, business office/admitting salaries, office supplies, property insurance, malpractice insurance, utilities, management services, medical director fees, repairs and maintenance, laundry, housekeeping, transcription services, security, legal, tax, accounting, and consulting fees, telephone, postage, and delivery service, marketing, licensing and memberships, interior decorations and miscellaneous. These expenses amount to $703,125, or 22.5% of gross revenue. This leaves a net operating income of $953,125 before depreciation, amortization, income taxes, and debt service, or 30.5% of total revenue. This income stream is attributed to the return on and recapture of the cost of the facility as well as a profit to the business. For appraisal purposes, an additional deduction of 3% for reserves and 2.5% for management is suggested, leaving a net income of $781,250 available to the enterprise.

Table 4.13

Medical Office Rent Comparables

Type	Size	Stories	Yr. Built	Occupancy	Lease Date/ Term	Rent SF/Mo. Escalations	Exp. Basis Expenses/SF/Mo.	NNN Equivalent	Adj. NNN Rent	Comments/Adjustments
Medical Office Bldg.	49,000 sf	4	N/A (older) 1970s	100%	Full for the past 3 years. 5-7 and 10-year terms on last leases.	$1.75 Annual CPI	F.S. gross base year $0.60	$1.15	$1.46 (+27%)	+27% for inferior improvements—the building cost around $130 to $135 PSF to build.
Medical Office Bldg.	70,000 sf	3	1992	82%	3-5 year w/1-5 year option	$2.35-$2.40 flat 5% per year	FS $0.63 to $0.67 (will go up with occupancy)	$1.68 to $1.77	$1.68 to $1.77 (0%)	Similar cost to build. $30 SF TI allowance.
Medical Office Bldg.	25,684 sf	3	1987	96%	Overall rent (effective)	$2.61 N/A	FS $1.00	$1.61	$1.61 (0%)	Very similar building to the subject. 30% of building is leased for dialysis center.
Medical Office Bldg.	55,300 sf	3	1988	100%	Overall rent (effective)	$1.51 5-year term	NNN N/A	$1.51	$1.62	Concrete and steel building. Buyer was former lessee.
Surgery Center	6,500 sf	N/A	1990	100%	1990 26 years	$3.24 (sur.) $2.35 (med off.) $2.69 overall + CPI	Mod. gross FS $0.75 (est.)	$1.94 (overall)	$1.94 (overall) $2.49 (surg.)	Real estate cost $1.6mm or $246.15 to construct; dermatology use; $1.60 adjusted NNN medical office rent.
Surgery Center	6,000 sf	5	1976	N/A	1992 4 years	$2.67 + CPI	Mod. gross	$1.92	$1.92 overall	Steel frame; relet in 1992 after 10 year lease; gynecologist O.R. use; space is leased from separate group. The surg. area is 1,500 SF.
Surgery Center	3,150 sf	multi-	1990	N/A	6/90 15 years w/1-10 yr. option	$3.75 + 5%/year	Mod. gross $0.75 (est.)	$3.00	$2.25 (-$0.75)	Plastic surgeon use; center leases space from third party; $35 TI allowance; one year free rent; 9% load
Medical Office Bldg.	50,000 sf	2	1969	N/A	offer outstanding 5 years	$3.00 annual CPI	FS $0.75	$2.25	$2.25	One month free rent/year; as is; former plastic surgery use.
Medical Office Bldg. & Surgery Center	36,314 sf	3	1985/87	100%	Various	$2.60 (overall)	FS $0.93	$1.67 (overall)	$1.67 (overall)	NNN medical office at $1.00 to $1.75 and surg. center at $2.25.

Figure 4.4   Summary of Income Approach

	$	%
Gross Revenue (net of allowances)		
5 operating suites x 2.5 procedures per day		
x $1,000 x 250 working days =	$3,125,000	100.0
Direct Expenses		
Salaries and Benefits		-29.5
Medical Supplies & Food		-17.5
Total	$1,468,750	-47.0
Gross Profit	$1,656,250	53.0
General and administrative expenses	$ 703,125	-22.5
Net Operating Profit	$ 953,125	30.5
Less fixed costs of reserves and management - estimated at 5.5%	$ 171,875	-5.5
Net Operating Income (NOI)	$ 781,250	25.0
Less return on and recapture of investment in physical plant (12% x $4,700,000)	$ 564,000	18.0
Income attributed to business	$ 217,250	7.0
Capitalized @ 25% =	$ 869,000	
Rounded to	$ 900,000	
Recap		
Physical plant (see Table 4.13)	$4,700,000	
Business	$ 900,000	
Total enterprise	$5,600,000	

In this example, the facility costs $4,700,000. If a capitalization rate of 12% is appropriate ($4,700,000 x .12 = $564,000), a residual of $217,250 is attributable to the business. This amount capitalized at, say, 25% would indicate an additional intangible value of about $900,000, which when combined with the cost approach figure of $4,700,000 would indicate a value for the enterprise of $5,600,000. (The multipliers and capitalization rates referenced here have been reported and analyzed by practitioners in this field. Multiple specialty SCs typically command a lower capitalization rate, say 20%, than do single specialty SCs, which may be 25% to 30%.)

Sales Comparison Approach

If sales of freestanding surgery centers are lacking, it may not be appropriate to attempt to use this approach. If sales are available, they may be compared to the subject property on the basis of price per square foot of floor area, price per number of annual procedures, or price per surgical suite, or on the basis of a gross revenue multiplier. In the above example where the total valuation was $5,600,000 (assumed price for physical plant and the going concern), the price was equivalent to the following:

Price per square foot of floor area	$466.67
Price per annual number of procedures (3,125)	$1,792
(2.5 procedures per day x 250 days x 5 operating units)	
Price per number of operating suites (five)	$1,120,000
Gross revenue multiplier	1.79

When there are no sales of freestanding SCs but an abundance of sales of good quality medical office buildings, it may be possible to use a summation approach through sales comparison. The appraiser would estimate separately the value of the building as a medical office building, adjusted upward for the addition of SC tenant improvements. To this would be added the value of the FF&E and finally the value of the business enterprise. This type of approach, however, probably should be used only as a check on the valuation indicators by the other two approaches. If the assignment involves an appraisal of only the real estate, in such situations the summation approach described above may be quite appropriate.

Analyzing and Appraising Recovery Centers

Recovery centers can increase the number of procedures at a surgery center by tapping an entirely new market in addition to the incremental increase in outpatient surgeries due to physicians having one location for outpatient and recovery care surgical cases. A recovery center will have higher direct expenses than a surgery center, and general administrative expenses will be higher because of additional requirements for staffing, supplies, food, housekeeping, and equipment. Net operating income as a percentage of gross revenue should slightly increase with the successful operation of an SRC due to the fact that the entire business becomes more efficient. Overall, cost savings to users and payers is the primary benefit of an SRC.

Research into the size of the market for a recovery center involves physician questionnaires, published discharge information from area hospitals by DRGs, insurance broker interviews, and the history of market penetration by other recovery centers developed in the United States.

A similar concept to the integrated SRC has been the development of "medical hotels." These are freestanding guest-room facilities, which are separate from medical offices and SCs, designed to keep patients overnight after surgery that does not require admission to a hospital. Tapping a patient base for this new type of facility will depend on overcoming problems of location and physician backing, but the potential apparently is attractive enough that some surgery centers are looking to such link-ups to widen their scope of services and compete with hospitals. That location is a key is apparent in the failure of one such project which had an occupancy level of only 10%. It was located a significant distance from the two nearest community hospitals and physicians were reluctant to drive to another stop to see patients.

C H A P T E R

F I V E

Nursing Homes

Long-term care facilities consist of skilled nursing facilities (SNFs), intermediate care facilities (ICFs), and residential care facilities (RCFs). All three must be licensed, but only SNFs and ICFs may participate in federal Medicaid reimbursement programs. This chapter is concerned with SNFs and ICFs since they are similar in terms of property characteristics and vary only in degree of nursing care. Chapter 6 deals with assisted living or residential care facilities.

Nursing homes, also known as convalescent hospitals, have traditionally served geriatric patients who can generally be characterized as frail and chronically ill. Patients frequently have multiple health problems, including mental illness, which is often referred to as senility among the elderly. Heart disease and arthritis affect one of every three residents. According to a National Center for Health Statistics survey, 32% of nursing home residents could not hear a telephone conversation; 46% could not read ordinary newsprint; 28% had lost bowel and bladder control; 51% had problems with mobility; and 31% were either chair-bound or bedridden. This is in contrast to residents of a residential care facility who may be frail but are usually ambulatory and in fair-to-average general health.

Nursing homes are a multibillion dollar industry (about $60 billion in 1994) but one that is continually facing financial crises and criticism of its practices. It is a highly regulated business, yet it is dominated by private-sector, profit-oriented ownerships. Demographic forces presage a favorable outlook, yet economic factors are placing operators in a risk-oriented environment, including regulated fees, growing costs, proposed cuts in Medicaid, and newer alternatives such as congregate care retirement centers (CCRCs), assisted living facilities (ALFs), and home care.

An Overview

Nursing home markets are measured in terms of number of beds. Currently, there are approximately 1,715,000 beds in the United States in about 16,800 nursing homes. About seven out of ten have a proprietary type of ownership; the balance are operated by nonprofit organizations (23%) or the government (7%). They are not evenly distributed around the country but tend to be located where concentrations of the elderly are found (see Table 5.1). About two-thirds of the nursing home population in the United States are found in the Midwest and South (33% and 30.5%, respectively); the remaining one-third is split between the Northeast and West (18% each). In terms of certification, about two-thirds were SNF beds, 27% were in ICFs, and 6% were uncertified. By size, the typical nursing home has between 90 and 100 beds. The economies of scale generally do not favor operations of less than 50 beds, while facilities in excess of 300 beds tend to be unwieldy and impersonal. Specific state licensing laws dealing with mini-

Table 5.1

Table 5.1   Age of Nursing Home Population by State, 1990

		Number			Percent		
State	**Total, All Ages**	**Under 25 Years**	**25-64 Years**	**65 Years and Over**	**Under 25 Years**	**25-64 Years**	**65 Years and Over**
United States	1,772,032	4,231	177,039	1,590,763	0.0	10.0	89.8
Alabama	24,031	86	1,980	21,965	0.4	8.2	91.4
Alaska	1,202	4	159	1,039	0.3	13.2	86.4
Arizona	14,472	62	1,667	12,743	0.4	11.5	88.1
Arkansas	21,809	43	2,649	19,117	0.2	12.1	87.7
California	148,362	501	16,503	131,358	0.3	11.1	88.5
Colorado	18,506	40	1,770	16,696	0.2	9.6	90.2
Connecticut	30,962	80	3,199	27,683	0.3	10.3	89.4
Delaware	4,596	8	258	4,330	0.2	5.6	94.2
Dist. of Columbia	7,008	118	1,554	5,336	1.7	22.2	76.1
Florida	80,298	305	6,503	73,490	0.4	8.1	91.5
Georgia	36,549	92	3,812	32,645	0.3	10.4	89.3
Hawaii	3,225	23	433	2,769	0.7	13.4	85.9
Idaho	6,318	17	503	5,798	0.3	8.0	91.8
Illinois	93,662	163	11,077	82,422	0.2	11.8	88.0
Indiana	50,845	136	5,334	45,375	0.3	10.5	89.2
Iowa	36,455	64	2,962	33,429	0.2	8.1	91.7
Kansas	26,155	23	2,128	24,004	0.1	8.1	91.8
Kentucky	27,874	85	3,353	24,436	0.3	12.0	87.7
Louisiana	32,072	40	4,098	27,934	0.1	12.8	87.1
Maine	9,855	17	644	9,194	0.2	6.5	93.3
Maryland	26,884	30	2,191	24,663	0.1	8.1	91.7
Massachusetts	55,662	68	4,742	50,852	0.1	8.5	91.4
Michigan	57,622	132	5,885	51,605	0.2	10.2	89.6
Minnesota	47,051	84	3,492	43,475	0.2	7.4	92.4
Mississippi	15,803	48	1,387	14,368	0.3	8.8	90.9

(continued)

Table 5.1	Age of Nursing Home Population by State, 1990 (continued)						
		Number			Percent		
State	Total, All Ages	Under 25 Years	25-64 Years	65 Years and Over	Under 25 Years	25-64 Years	65 Years and Over
Missouri	52,060	119	5,097	46,844	0.2	9.8	90.0
Montana	7,764	20	616	7,128	0.3	7.9	91.8
Nebraska	19,171	29	1,444	17,698	0.2	7.5	92.3
Nevada	3,605	27	516	3,062	0.7	14.3	84.9
New Hampshire	8,202	4	457	7,741	0.0	5.6	94.4
New Jersey	47,054	83	4,088	42,883	0.2	8.7	91.1
New Mexico	6,276	29	602	5,645	0.5	9.6	89.9
New York	126,175	241	14,033	111,901	0.2	11.1	88.7
North Carolina	47,014	138	6,616	40,260	0.3	14.1	85.6
North Dakota	8,159	11	689	7,459	0.1	8.4	91.4
Ohio	93,769	253	9,435	84,081	0.3	10.1	89.7
Oklahoma	29,666	70	3,456	26,140	0.2	11.6	88.1
Oregon	18,200	52	2,072	16,076	0.3	11.4	88.3
Pennsylvania	106,454	144	8,439	97,871	0.1	7.9	91.9
Rhode Island	10,156	3	619	9,534	0.0	6.1	93.9
South Carolina	18,228	38	2,181	16,009	0.2	12.0	87.8
South Dakota	9,356	13	1,065	8,278	0.1	11.4	88.5
Tennessee	35,192	144	3,370	31,678	0.4	9.6	90.0
Texas	101,005	242	8,821	91,942	0.2	8.7	91.0
Utah	6,222	19	762	5,441	0.3	12.2	87.4
Vermont	4,809	9	401	4,399	0.2	8.3	91.5
Virginia	37,762	86	4,729	32,947	0.2	12.5	87.2
Washington	32,840	77	3,028	29,735	0.2	9.2	90.5
West Virginia	12,591	29	1,482	11,080	0.2	11.8	88.0
Wisconsin	50,345	81	4,500	45,764	0.2	8.9	90.9
Wyoming	2,679	0	238	2,441	0.0	8.9	91.1

Note: Column totals may not add due to independent rounding.
Source: U.S. Bureau of the Census, 1990 Census of Population, prepared from the Census Analysis System.

mum nurse staffing requirements have encouraged the development of hospitals of a specific size (e.g., 99, 149, or 199 beds).

The well-promoted boom of the elderly population, also referred to as the graying of America, suggests a significant growth in demand for nursing home beds will occur in the next two to three decades. For example, the group 85 years and older is expected to increase by 39% by the year 2000 from its 1993 level of 3.3 million, and by another 52% by 2025 to 7 million. Table 5.2 shows recent changes in the size and proportions of the elderly age group.

The impact on the real estate market seems obvious. Average occupancy rates should increase, accompanied by a growing demand for new convalescent hospitals. Newly emerging factors, however, have clouded this vision. Reliance on the government in an era of budgetary limitations along with population health trends are raising doubts about generalizations accorded to the elderly. A recent study by the Wisconsin Center of Health Statistics revealed that nursing home utilization decreased by 11% between 1980 and 1990 among individuals aged 75 to 84.[1] At the same time it increased by roughly 20% for the age group 85 and older. These figures would indicate that more elderly are healthier — or at least staying out of nursing homes until a later age.

Dominance of Chains in Market

As of the mid-1990s, chains own, manage, or lease about 41% of the nation's nursing homes. There are about 380 of these chains, controlling over 700,000 beds. The largest chain owns 760 nursing homes with slightly over 81,000 licensed beds, and the second largest owner has 288 facilities with slightly over 36,000 beds. Seven other chains have between 15,000 and 22,000 beds (see Table 5.3). Independent owners accounted for 59% of the facilities and 58% of the beds in 1994.

Government Regulation

The nursing home business is highly regulated. Extensive laws, rules, and regulations dealing with the operation of the industry and provision of facilities have an immediate impact on the value of an enterprise. The federal government is highly involved through funding mechanisms and the setting of minimum standards. Particular programs are mandated in such legislation as the Omnibus Budget Reconciliation Acts (OBRA) of 1987 and 1993 and the Occupational Safety and Health Act (OSHA) of 1992. The individual states implement and enforce federal legislation and set their own requirements. Thus, there are significant differences in funding levels (see Table 5.4), licensing requirements, levels of patient care, and facility standards from one state to another, and these differences are reflected in appraised values.

It is beyond the scope of this text to deal with individual state programs and requirements. Suffice it to say that the appraiser must be familiar with the pertinent laws of the jurisdiction where one is conducting assignments. An experienced nursing home appraiser should have no difficulty in adjusting to varied valuation considerations from one place to another.

Sources of Health Care Revenues

The long-term care industry, which includes nursing homes, home care, assisted living, and CCRCs, had revenues of about $108 billion in 1994. Of this amount, nursing homes accounted for about $57 billion, two-thirds of which were contributed by Medicare, Medicaid, and other government programs (e.g., Veterans Administration). Virtually all of the balance is derived from direct payments (i.e., individuals, families, trusts, etc.) and a very small amount from private health insurance.

---

[1] Victor Jesudason, "Changing Characteristics of Elderly Nursing Home Residents, Wisconsin 1980-90," *Health Data Review*, Wisconsin Department of Health and Social Services, vol. 5, no. 8, August 1991.

Table 5.2

Table 5.2 Elderly Population by Age Group (000s)

Age Group	1985			1988			1990			1995*		
	Elderly Population	As a % of		Elderly Population	As a % of		Elderly Population	As a % of		Elderly Population	As a % of	
		Elderly	U.S. Population		Elderly	U.S. Population		Elderly	U.S. Population		Elderly	U.S. Population
Total Population	28,672	100.0%	12.0%	30,516	100.0%	12.5%	31,798	100.0%	12.7%	34,006	100.0%	13.1%
65-69 Years	9,227	32.2	3.9	9,684	31.7	4.0	10,006	31.5	4.0	9,757	28.7	3.8
70-74 Years	7,635	26.6	3.2	7,896	25.9	3.2	8,048	25.3	3.2	8,766	25.8	3.4
75-79 Years	5,534	19.3	2.3	5,946	19.5	2.4	6,224	19.6	2.5	6,607	19.4	2.5
80-84 Years	3,482	12.1	1.5	3,818	12.5	1.6	4,060	12.8	1.6	4,621	13.6	1.8
85 Years and Over	2,794	9.7	1.2	3,172	10.4	1.3	3,461	10.9	1.4	4,255	12.5	1.6

* Projection
Source: U.S. Bureau of the Census

	1995 Beds	Net patient service revenues (in millions)		Net operating income (in millions)		Assets (in millions)	
		1995	1994	1995	1994	1995	1994
ADS Group	3,720	$64.2	$58.6	$4.6	$3.8	$64.6	$59.1
Advocat	7,324	136.1	99.3	22.8	19.1	57.2	43.7
Alden Management Services	2,934	83.3	63.2	2.2	3.9	51.3	58.8
Allegis Health Services[1]	1,467	59.8	44.2	9.5	6.2	47.2	36.7
American Health Care Centers	1,709	53.5	51.0	—	—	54.1	50.0
Apple Health Care	2,000	96.0	90.5	11.7	12.4	84.4	83.3
Arbor Health Care Co.	3,039	76.9	148.5	13.8	10.8	178.8	136.6
Athena Health Care Systems	3,537	145.4	122.4	25.7	21.5	148.7	135.2
Beverly Enterprises	75,669	3,170.6	2,932.3	276.1	253.7	2,506.5	2,322.6
Britthaven	6,067	154.0	146.0	—	—	—	—
Communicare Health Services	940	55.0	42.0	—	—	—	—
Country Villa Health Services	1,234	57.7	56.7	15.8	15.5	17.6	15.6
Courville Co.	160	7.1	6.7	0.5	0.5	14.8	7.7
Genesis Health Ventures	13,097	458.4	366.0	93.2	69.3	600.3	511.7
Geriatric and Medical Cos.	3,450	192.2	177.9	24.8	18.3	178.2	162.7
GranCare	17,161	811.4	701.8	42.0	30.3	643.0	520.2
Harborside Healthcare	3,008	109.4	86.4	8.0	7.5	99.8	98.0
HCM	3,160	92.4	81.6	—	—	—	—
Healthcare and Retirement Corp.	15,717	713.5	615.1	138.0	122.1	729.2	671.4
Heritage Enterprises	2,067	33.6	32.7	—	—	—	—
Horizon/CMS[2]	17,776	626.6	367.9	—	—	723.8	406.5
Hunter Care Centers	1,497	25.9	22.5	—	—	35.5	26.7
Integrated Health Services	24,700	1,180.0	713.0	91.0	37.0	1,400.0	1,255.0
Lenox Healthcare	1,705	36.3	28.7	—	—	72.5	47.2
Manor Healthcare Corp.	22,527	—	—	246.7	227.1	1,416.3	1,186.5
Mariner Health[3]	6,836	280.9	211.9	263.3	193.0	385.8	273.7
Marrinson Group	322	18.0	16.9	1.8	1.7	12.6	11.4
National HealthCare	18,978	308.0	269.7	21.1	15.9	355.5	396.1
National Health Care Affiliates	4,161	107.3	85.7	15.9	14.5	91.1	80.1
PersonaCare	3,609	—	—	26.4	19.7	185.5	111.0
Quad C Health Care Centers	780	33.3	29.3	2.5	1.7	19.2	22.0
Redwood Care Centers	345	11.0	11.3	0.8	0.9	—	—
Sun Healthcare Group	17,801	1,135.5	673.4	59.8	36.4	—	1,068.8
TNS Nursing Homes	1,099	39.3	38.3	3.5	2.9	63.9	19.0
United Health	16,551	740.9	658.6	—	—	525.6	444.7
Vencor[4]	39,480	2.3	2.0	0.2	0.1	1.9	1.7
White Oak Manor	1,965	57.6	54.2	1.6	0.7	45.5	44.8

All information excludes financials of managed facilities but includes management fees.
[1]Fomerly Global Health Management. [2]Horizon merged with Continental Medical Systems in July 1995. [3]Licensed as skilled-nursing facilities with subacute beds by the Joint Commission on Accreditation of Healthcare Organizations. [4]Financials exclude nonrecurring items.
Source: *Modern Healthcare*, May 20, 1996

Table 5.4	Average Medicaid Per Diem Reimbursement Rates, by State		
	Average 1995 Medicaid Per Diem Rates		**Average 1995 Medicaid Per Diem Rates**
Alabama	$87.15	Montana	$80.15
Alaska	$330.71	Nebraska	$52.30/Urban
Arizona	$211.21/SNF		$46.90/Rural
	$85.30/Urban	Nevada	$79.42
Arkansas	$82.64/Rural	New Hampshire	$105.35
California	$58.02	New Jersy	$135.00
	$59.74/Level A	New Mexico*	$77.69/Low NF
Colorado	$79.71/Level B		$121.32/High NF
Connecticut	$82.37	New York	$132.00
Delaware	N/A	North Carolina	$95.23/SNF
District of Columbia*	$88.18		$71.83/ICF
Florida	$120.00	North Dakota	$79.53
Georgia	$84.22	Ohio	$88.50
Hawaii	$71.11	Oklahoma	$52.50
Idaho	$127.94	Oregon*	$87.98
Illinois	$88.03	Pennsylvania	$93.58/SNF
Indiana*	$70.17		$74.25/ICF
Iowa	$71.72	Rhode Island	$95.00
Kansas	N/A	South Carolina	$70.19
Kentucky	$60.29	South Dakota	$68.89
Louisiana	$69.43	Tennessee	$70.32/Level I
	$73.39/SNF		$108.96/Level II
	$61.50/IC I	Texas	$63.64
Maine	$60.32/IC II	Utah	$74.24
Maryland	$105.96	Vermont	$93.01
Massachusetts	$89.16	Virginia	$68.32
Michigan	N/A	Washington	$98.91
Minnesota	$75.01	West Virginia	$84.00
Mississippi	$92.24	Wisconsin*	$76.32
Missouri	$87.15	Wyoming	$83.71
	$70.26		

* 1994 Data

Source: *The Guide to the Nursing Home Industry, 1995*, Health Care Investment Analysts, Inc., Baltimore MD.

A continual shift in payment responsibility from the individual consumer to third parties has taken place in recent years. Third parties, representing government or public programs and insurance companies, account for about 60% of nursing home revenues. By 1992, when nursing home expenditures reached $67.3 billion, 41.2% came from direct payments, 1.1% from private health insurance, and 57.8% from the government (33.5% federal and 24.3% state).

The government is planning on assuming less of the burden in the future, but this likelihood is uncertain. In theory, expenditures by public programs for nursing home care could decrease because of federal budget cuts. Another factor is the federal government's plan to close loopholes in Medicaid estate planning and to provide financial incentives that encourage the growth of insurance for long-term care. Undoubtedly, responsibility for long-term care will be increasingly shifted to the states since the huge national budget deficit makes it unlikely that the federal government can continue its former role. States are taking steps to deal with the financing problem and to control the situation by limiting reimbursement rates and encouraging programs for alternative financing such as long-term care health insurance, community and home care services, and health care Individual Retirement Accounts (IRAs).

The problems with using individual insurance policies to finance nursing home care are considerable, including high premiums, unequal distribution across demographic groups, unknown impacts from future inflation, and exclusions for or restrictions on coverage for Alzheimer's disease.

Medicaid and Medicare

Medicaid is a federal-state program established by Title XIX of the federal Social Security Act for individuals who meet certain income requirements. Skilled nursing and intermediate care facilities are both eligible for reimbursement through state-operated Medicaid programs.

Medicare is the federal health insurance program established under Title XVIII of the Social Security Act for individuals 65 years of age and older. Available to SNFs but not ICFs, Medicare provides for skilled nursing care for a limited period of time (currently 100 days) after initial hospitalization. Medicare reimbursement for skilled nursing home care was enacted as a cost-saving measure. Its intent was to substitute less expensive nursing home care for inpatient, medical-surgical hospital care, which at that time was reimbursed on a cost-plus basis. Medicare coverage for skilled nursing care continued after the initiation of the hospital DRG system.

Medicare reimbursement for skilled nursing home care is on a retrospective cost basis, i.e., facilities are reimbursed but only up to a specified "routine cost limit." These limits are set separately for urban and rural facilities and for freestanding and hospital-based facilities. Because the definition of "costs" includes an allocation of facility and administrative overhead, well-managed nursing home companies are able to generate relatively high pretax profits from the Medicare program. Medicare regulations provide for certain exceptions and exemptions to the routine cost limits for "atypical services" or new facilities. A provider may request an exemption because its patients require services or equipment that, in aggregate, result in costs exceeding the standard cost limits. In addition, new facilities up to three years old may request an exemption to the routine cost limits.

The government is planning to implement a prospective payment system (PPS) for long-term care services in the near future (October 1, 1997) and a variety of other steps to reduce the levels of reimbursement and promote managed care programs and community based alternatives to hospitalization. These steps are all aimed at balancing the federal budget. Because a PPS provides just one fixed rate per stay, the DRG system has caused hospitals to move patients to subacute and long-term care facilities much faster than before. This has saved the government considerable dollars in acute care costs, but it has resulted in higher subacute and long-term care bills. It has also resulted in occupancy and revenue benefits to some skilled nursing facilities. A prospective payment plan for long-term care will be difficult to estimate because the length of stay is less predictable than in acute care. A PPS may be seen as a way to reduce postacute lengths of stay, but it would have to allow for adjustments after the fact for residents who need extra care.

Medicaid programs, which provide reimbursement for custodial care, are fully administered by the states. Funding for Medicaid is shared between the federal government and individual state governments in a ratio that varies from 50% to 70%, depending upon the state's compliance. Medicaid nursing home policies vary from state to state, which can materially affect the value of an individual facility. (It should be noted that unit values for nursing homes on a per bed basis vary significantly from one state to another, and this factor is primarily a result of varied levels of reimbursement rates.)

The traditional method of Medicaid reimbursement has been a set dollar amount per patient day derived from a retrospective analysis of actual costs for services. Obviously, this system provided little incentive to control costs. The newer prospective payment systems, which set reimbursement rates prior to the delivery of services, provide an incentive to operators to keep their costs within the limits of what is to be received.

Reimbursement rates can vary not only from state to state, but from one hospital service area to another and between individual properties. Several factors determine the amount of the daily rate, including the amount and method of capital valuation, use of case-mix methodology, recognition of the contribution of ancillary income, and performance incentives. Ancillary income is derived from special charges for drugs and medical supplies, special services such as physical therapy, and the use of specialized medical equipment. In the application of a case-mix system a nursing home will group patients into common classifications relating to their physical condition, dietary requirements, and special factors such as incontinence. Consistent reimbursement rates are set for groups of patients with the same overall characteristics. Average per diem reimbursement rates by state are shown in Table 5.4.

Nursing Home Regulations

OBRA 1987 was a reaction to well-publicized complaints about nursing home operations. Scandalous overuse of restraints and tranquilizers in the 1970s gave rise to advocacy groups (e.g., the National Citizens Coalition) for federal reform of nursing homes. Nursing homes are now monitored on a federal level by the Health Care Financing Administration (HCFA), an agency of the U.S. Department of Health and Human Services, and on a state level by agencies called Long-Term Care Ombudsman.

OBRA encompasses new minimum certification standards, detailed regulations, compliance programs, reporting requirements, and enforcement through assessments or more severe sanctions. It aims to eliminate the differentiation of minimum patient nursing requirements between SNFs and ICFs, set higher training standards for nurses' aides, provide readily available statistics on the performance of individual properties, and encourage a higher level of professionalism in the industry.

On July 1, 1995, new HCFA regulations became law. As a result facilities reimbursed by Medicare and Medicaid must contend with important new obligations and enforcement mechanisms. In line with current thinking of hospitals, HMOs, and most other kinds of health care facilities, the HFCA rules attempt to focus nursing home care not only on residents' physical needs but also on their quality of life. In the past the focus was on administrative and procedural detail, documentation was of primary importance, and the sanction for noncompliance was ultimate: a complete withholding of Medicare funds. Not surprisingly, this penalty was so severe that it was rarely used.

The new regulations take a more flexible, quality-oriented approach. The requirement of "perfect compliance" has been replaced by a standard of "substantial compliance." Under this standard, nursing homes reach compliance when deficiencies do not cause actual harm or create the potential for more than minimal harm. In other words, outcomes, not compliance on paper, will determine which facilities will continue to be qualified for Medicare and Medicaid reimbursement. The new rules will be enforced with a range of "graduated" penalties. Examples of severe penalties include fines of up to $10,000 per day for failing an inspection and $2,000 against anyone tipping off a nursing home manager that inspectors are on the way. On the other hand some other violations carry only $50 fines or no sanction at all. Minor oversights will no longer be the basis for denying Medicare certification. If a facility is in substantial compliance, virtually all remedies cease.

HCFA's outcomes-oriented focus, however, will create a larger set of compliance issues for nursing home facilities. The new rules establish more than 100 requirements that facilities must meet to participate in Medicare and Medicaid. Before OBRA '87, there were only about 15 general requirements. The new law also requires nursing homes to conduct initial and annual health assessments of every resident and to develop and update individual plans of care. Assessment of the scope and severity of residents' illnesses and outcomes will become crucial.

The implication of this new law is that nursing homes will place a premium on documented, cost-effective treatments and services. Therefore, products and services that can assist with these "initial and annual" care assessments will be particularly valuable. Although the impacts on valuation will not be immediately apparent, a qualified appraiser/analyst should be aware of these changes.

General Property Categories

Three broad economic classifications are useful for initial valuation planning. At the lowest end of the valuation spectrum are nursing homes that derive all or virtually all of their revenues from Medicaid and Medicare reimbursement programs. Profit margins before rent, depreciation, and interest payments are slim in this category, averaging less than 10%. Operators can partially compensate for this factor by controlling multiple properties, thus taking advantage of the economies of management and centralized purchasing of goods and services.

A mid-value category of nursing homes represents those properties that typically have a weak mix of private pay and a strong mix of Medicaid patients. Many appraisal assignments will involve facilities with a census mix of this type. When one hears about "average" values per bed in a particular area, the reference is usually to such a property.

Top-of-the-line nursing homes focus solely on private-pay patients and market their product by emphasizing a higher level and intensity of personal care and privacy, greater building area per bed, newer and better maintained facilities, established relationships in the medical community, and the exclusivity of the neighborhood. Higher operating costs per patient day reflect these amenities, and daily rates may far exceed and in some cases be as much as double the minimum Medicaid figure amount. On a unit-value-per-bed basis this category may exceed the first category by two to four times.

Private-pay patients (PPPs), who are not eligible for government assistance, occupy a large but decreasing percentage of nursing home beds. They are subject to rate schedules that can range from a small amount over the current Medicaid level to very high rates found in exclusive, upscale facilities. The sources of their payments are generally privately held assets and insurance programs. Private-pay patients are desired by profit-oriented operators because there tends to be a direct relationship between increased percentages of *NOI* and increased percentages of PPPs within the census of any nursing home.

An all private-pay/Medicare facility or one that has only a small number of Medicaid patients will typically be sold at $20,000 to $30,000 per bed more than a typical convalescent hospital with a small mix of private-pay/Medicare patients/residents. It will command an even higher per bed price premium than a hospital entirely occupied with Medicaid patients. The reason for the price advantage is that operating costs will increase at a lower rate than revenues because of the favorable relationship between fixed and variable costs. The following example (Figure 5.1) illustrates how the price differential can be separately estimated.

Figure 5.1	Private Pay/Medicare Valuation Advantage

Assumptions

1. Two 100-bed facilities are alike in size and quality, except that one has a private-pay/Medicare patient ratio of 30% and the other has a ratio of 70%.

2. Private-pay premium over Medicaid is $25 per day.

3. Occupancy level is 95%.

4. Marginal net operating income factor is 75% (i.e., 25% of the excess premium goes to operating expenses).

5. Marginal capitalization rate is 18.75%, representing a premium of 50% over the normal *OAR* of 12.5%. The premium represents an allowance for risk and management reflecting the difficulty of maintaining an advantageous private-pay mix, increasing competition within the market, the long-term trend for the private-pay market to decline, and the future influence of managed care/capitated payment schedules.

Valuation

1.	Beds: 100 x 40% differential =	40
2.	Days	x 365
3.	Price advantage per day	x $25
4.	Occupancy level	x 95%
5.	Marginal profit ratio	x 75%
6.	Total	$260,062.50
7.	Capitalization rate	18.75%
8.	Value premium	$1,387,000
9.	Divided by 40 beds	$34,675
10.	Divided by 100 beds	$13,870

Competitive Strategies

Competing companies in the nursing home industry are currently undergoing a transformation. Once viewed solely as providers of standard geriatric custodial care, they are becoming an increasingly important part of the continuum of care following hospitalization by providing specialty medical services to higher-acuity patients. Some care facilities are seeking to charge higher prices for a product that consumers view as different from that offered by the competition. That is most easily accomplished by constructing a facility with more room and amenities and specializing in private-pay patients, at least for a designated section. Subacute and rehabilitation services are now being emphasized along with provision of designated Alzheimer's units. These services are generally higher margin and serve to differentiate facilities from their competitors.

To raise the acuity level of medical services provided, management has followed one or both of two strategies. They have a) established distinct subacute care units within the nursing facility, or b) treated higher-acuity Medicare and insurance patients in non-distinct Medicare-certified beds. These special care units can typically be provided in existing facilities at capital costs of $10,000 to $15,000 per bed. It must be recognized, however, that it is difficult to recruit and train the administrative and specialized personnel necessary to focus successfully on this market.

The most difficult route to product differentiation appears to be obtaining a "subacute" rate for caring for stabilized patients who might otherwise be in a low-level hospital intensive care unit. Compared to $700-$1,000 per day at an acute care hospital and $850 per day at an acute rehabilitation hospital, average per diem charges range from $300 to $550 for skilled nursing facilities, reflecting both the relative acuity of the patients and the provider's cost structure. Operating margins for subacute patients typically run between 20% and 40%.

Another possible strategy to produce a higher-margin income stream is the integration of ancillary services such as rehabilitation therapy and pharmacy services provided by third parties into existing facilities. Medicare and private-pay patients who require third-party therapy and pharmacy services generate significantly higher operating margins for nursing care operators than custodial geriatric residents. With respect to Medicare patients, this is because an SNF may report both the cost of the therapy provided and an allocation of the overhead required to provide the service.

Another obvious but not necessarily emphasized strategy is for management to improve marketing and to strengthen relationships with referral sources such as physicians, hospital discharge planners, HMOs, and commercial insurers to help increase the flow of higher-margin patients.

A final strategy involves the registration of patients who require the minimum bundle of services provided under a set or capitized rate. Knowledgeable managers recognize that there are high- and low-cost patients, and if a favorable ratio of the latter can be attracted, the profitability of a facility can be enhanced.

The Future of Long-Term Care

Experts in the field have highly varied views of likely developments in long-term care through the year 2000. Payers, patients, and providers have all called for reform of the U.S. health care system, but each group has a different agenda as to who should pay for long-term care and how that should be accomplished. Recent proposals have included the tightening of eligibility rules, moderate restructuring of long-term care insurance, and extending health insurance experiments now in progress. The trend toward the use of case-mix reimbursement systems can be viewed as a reform that offers incentives to nursing home providers.

Medicaid payments, which currently provide about 52% of all nursing home revenues, could increase to about 67% unless the financing system is somehow changed in the next two decades. Many believe that the private sector must be called upon to halt the hemorrhaging of Medicaid spending and help rescue millions of Americans from "impoverishment" due to their long-term care needs.

Managed care has proved that it works and the use of capitated contracts has necessitated long-term care providers to become expense oriented rather than revenue oriented. Managed care places a premium on high-quality and cost-effective alternatives to continued hospitalization. Rate controls on health care providers and health insurance companies have potentially positive implications for the long-term care industry because: 1) further limitations on DRG payments to hospitals would increase the incentive to discharge patients to skilled long-term care facilities; and 2) rate controls on insurance companies would likewise greatly increase the incentive to find the most cost-effective quality alternative to continued hospitalization.

Other recent studies of nursing homes foresee a future of downsized facilities. This is based upon the idea that SNFs will become more specialized and reconfigured to be more consistent with what the consumer wants. Such a facility will be characterized by frequent admissions and shorter lengths of stay. Facilities will have to learn how to define their outcomes, demonstrate quality, and accurately and competitively price their services. Nursing homes are likely to be viewed as one option among many and industry growth will occur in the competitive assisted living facility sector. Lastly, it is likely that hospitals will seek to reclaim the subacute niche, fueling competition in the industry.

Many of these potential trends and other possibilities will not be clear until long after reform of the health care system on a national level has been achieved. However, recent House and Senate budget proposals that have included reductions of several hundred billion dollars in combined Medicare and Medicaid spending over a seven-year period do not bode well for the industry.

Design Considerations

Most of the nursing homes in the United States were built before 1969. The interior design requirements of nursing homes have changed significantly since then due to changes in demographics, service concepts, and government regulatory programs. It is beyond the scope of this chapter to explain the impacts of environmental design. Readers are referred to an excellent text on the subject, *Nursing Home Renovation Designed for Reform,* by Lorraine G. Hiatt,[2] which includes discussions on environmental design, planning a renovation program, converting a nursing home to an assisted living facility, and methodology for estimating the cost for common refurbishments. The book suggests a 12-step technique, which is set forth below, for comparing the cost of renovating an existing facility versus constructing a new one.

1. List the design changes being considered.

2. Calculate the square footage per room, and multiply by the number of rooms affected. Preliminary calculations usually involve inside room dimensions (net square footage). This is the usable space from the consumer's point of view.

3. Add a factor for grossing, which accounts for the thickness of the walls, supporting mechanical spaces, and spaces like stairwells and hallways that are not listed as net areas. These computations vary according to such factors as whether the corridors have nooks, seating niches, or features like recessed doorways. Grossing may range from about 1.6 to 1.74 times the net square footage for resident-use areas along an 8-foot (2.5 meter) corridor, but it may be 1.54 to 1.6 for office areas. An additional 3% may be added where room changes involve expansion of mechanical space. Square foot analyses and costs are not complete without a thorough analysis of the net areas plus the gross areas affected.

4. Add together any special costs related to these changes such as asbestos removal or bringing other systems into compliance and any demolition costs.

5. Add to the subtotal a factor for all the fees involved (design, cost estimation, construction, legal and filing). About 15% to 31% of the subtotal may be appropriate. This may not include planning costs for study of various alternatives.

---

[2] Lorraine G. Hiatt, *Nursing Home Renovation Designed for Reform* (Butterworth Architecture, 1991), 50-51.

6. Add any operational costs associated with lost beds, the purchase of temporary services, moving, filing, and so on.

7. Multiply the total square footage by current costs for nursing home renovations. These might range from $67 to over $140 per square foot ($622 to $1,300 per square meter), depending on local economic and labor situations, the amount of plumbing, and the complexity of the systems involved in the renovation. Some refurbishment projects cost less; they range from $35 to $90 per square foot (or $325 to $835 per square meter).

8. Add together the costs calculated in Steps 6 and 7. This is the cost for renovation.

9. Estimate new construction costs by calculating the total square footage from net and gross areas and multiplying it by the cost per square foot (which may be less than the renovation figure, depending on complexity).

10. Add costs for financing, moving, and lost revenue.

11. Also add land costs, fees, and professional charges for zoning. The result is the cost for new construction.

12. Add a contingency for unexpected discoveries during renovation to the figure in Step 8, and add one for client changes during construction to the figure in Step 11. These contingencies may be as low as 3% to 5%, especially when the client has worked with the design team on a specific design program document, or they may be as high as 10% when the client or board are known for indecisiveness, written documents and decisions are scarce, or work has begun without program consensus. Compare the final figures resulting in Steps 8 and 11 to determine whether renovation or new construction is more economic.

Market Analysis

A study of the current and future supply of nursing home beds; occupancy rates for competitive facilities; private versus public pay rates and ratios for competitive facilities; and demographic trends can provide insight into the future income-producing potential of a subject property, whether it is a proposed project or an existing facility. A market analysis should be performed in every instance, not only because of institutional and regulatory requirements but also the significant information that will be provided to the appraiser before the valuation approaches are performed. In this particular health care specialty a wide range of data is readily available to the analyst on future bed needs (whether positive or negative), but generalized findings need fine tuning. In many states, the department responsible for health planning and statistics will have relatively current estimates of future bed needs by specialized categories for individual health service areas. Such data should be used with caution. Market analysis involves well-defined steps, covering primary research, secondary data sources, and the capability to derive conclusions on a qualitative and quantitative basis. It can be visualized as shown in Figure 5.2.

Defining the Product Capability

A first step is understanding what segment of the elderly population is being targeted by the subject property. This will assist in directing the necessary supply and demand studies and provide for the most efficient use of the appraiser's resources. The general property categories, which have been previously discussed, must be considered as well as the unique capabilities of the subject property. For example, if an SNF has a mix of public and private-pay patients, its competition may range from SNFs whose patient mix is historically limited to Medicaid-funded patients to those SNFs that try to appeal only to private-pay patients.

At the top and low ends of the market the same considerations relative to the competition are at play, except that alternative facilities are probably more readily identifiable. The analyst

Figure 5.2 **Outline of a Market Feasibility Study**

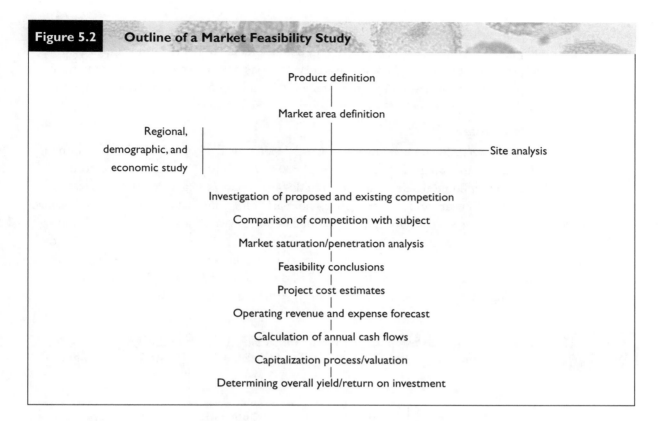

Product definition

Market area definition

Regional, demographic, and economic study ——————————————————————— Site analysis

Investigation of proposed and existing competition

Comparison of competition with subject

Market saturation/penetration analysis

Feasibility conclusions

Project cost estimates

Operating revenue and expense forecast

Calculation of annual cash flows

Capitalization process/valuation

Determining overall yield/return on investment

or appraiser who conducts this aspect of an assignment should first confer with the administrator of the subject property to obtain information about its target patient population as well as hard data on the competition and current developments. At later stages in the market research program, it will be rewarding to interview the administrators of competitive properties to obtain other valuable data and differing views of emerging trends.

Defining the Trade or Service Area

Selection of a specific nursing home for an individual is a complicated process involving proximity to family members, friends, and church or other support groups. In most cases a facility is chosen that is close to a patient's former address. Driving time is probably the most important factor influencing the radius of a facility's service area. Using distance factors and drawing a circle around the subject may be acceptable under certain circumstances, but the following methods may produce more accurate results:

1. Use the boundaries of existing hospital service areas as established by the state's department of health. A single source (usually the state capitol) may yield a wealth of statistical information that may be accessed for a reasonable consideration. Depending on the location of the subject property relative to the boundary and the size of the service area, it may be necessary to use two or more such service areas for proper analysis. Whether or not the established service areas are used for an individual assignment, the statistical information available relative to competitive properties and general trends should not be overlooked.

2. A more precise determination of a trade area can be ascertained from the locational source of a nursing home's patients. The records of every hospital can be summarized in such a way to maintain confidentiality, but also to provide enough information for the analyst to draw a conclusion as to the approximate boundaries of primary and secondary hospital service areas.

With this information, a modem, and computer access to data services such as the Claritas Senior Life Report (see Appendix), it is possible to obtain precise information for individually tailored situations. This technique may involve service areas defined in terms of driving times or distance, zip codes, or governmental units. It should be the preferred method for proposed projects.

Analyzing the Demand

As of 1990 there were 32,200,000 persons in the United States aged 65 or more, and their number is expected to increase to a range of 41,200,000 to 44,600,000 by 2010. Three age groups account for virtually all nursing home residents in the United States: 65 to 74 years old (16%), 75 to 84 years old (39%), and 85 years and higher (45%). The market for potential residents is vast because 4,600,000 persons in these age groups not in nursing homes (or two times the number in nursing homes) have one or more limitations that affect the activities of daily living (ADL). Over 50% of those over 85 are in need of long-term care or assistance with daily living activities compared with 13% of those 65 to 69 years of age. Based on a study of current demographic data, the demand for nursing home beds will be 89% higher in 2010, as shown in Table 5.5.

Table 5.5	Estimates of the Demand for Nursing Home Service with Underlying Demographic and Health Characteristics of the Elderly, 2010 and 2020 (in millions)					
			2010		2020	
Population	1990	Baseline	Optimistic	Baseline	Optimistic
65-74	18.7	21.7	22.4	34.4	36.6
75-84	10.1	12.8	13.8	21.3	23.9
85+	3.3	6.8	8.3	8.7	12.0
Total	32.2	41.2	44.6	64.3	72.5
No. of seniors in community with one or more ADL limitations					
Unmarried	3.1	4.1	4.3	6.4	7.3
Married	1.5	2.1	2.3	3.3	4.1
Total	4.6	6.2	6.6	9.7	11.4
Living arrangements Community-Based					
Married	14.0	17.9	19.9	28.0	33.4
Living alone	10.4	15.1	15.9	25.5	26.9
Living with others	6.0	5.2	5.4	6.5	7.1
Nursing home	1.8	3.0	3.4	4.3	5.3

Source: "The Changing Profile of the Elderly: Effects on Future Long Term Care Needs and Financing." *The Milbank Quarterly* (No. 2), 1992.

More detailed trade area socioeconomic information must be quantified and processed to gain a clear picture of demand over and above gross percentages applied to total population numbers. In particular, factors dealing with ethnicity, income, and overall health rating must be considered. Data on living arrangements prior to admission provide additional material for analyzing the demand side of the equation (see Table 5.6). The appraiser should also keep in mind that not all skilled nursing beds are devoted to the frail elderly. A small but growing portion of patients are treated on a short-term, subacute basis.

Table 5.6	Living Arrangements of Nursing Home Residents Prior to Admission, by Age, Sex, and Race, 1985 (Percent Distribution)								
					Sex		Race		
Living Arrangement	Total	65-74 yrs.	75-84 yrs.	85 yrs. and over	Male	Female	White	Black	Other
Private or semiprivate	40.0%	29.2%	40.5%	43.3%	36.3%	41.2%	40.5%	31.9%	35.6%
Alone	14.7	8.2	14.7	17.0	11.6	15.8	15.2	6.9	15.5*
With family members	18.9	16.0	19.8	19.2	19.3	18.8	18.9	19.0	15.5*
With nonfamily members	3.4	3.1	3.3	3.5	3.2	3.4	3.3	3.9	2.0*
Unknown if with others	3.0	1.8	2.7	3.7	2.2	3.3	3.1	2.1*	2.5*
Another health facility	57.0	67.7	56.5	53.6	60.4	55.9	56.5	65.2	59.0
Another nursing home	12.2	12.9	12.6	11.5	13.1	11.8	12.4	9.2	9.7*
General or short-stay hospital	38.7	39.5	38.2	38.9	35.2	40.0	37.8	49.5	49.4
Mental facility	3.0	7.6	3.2	1.1	5.0	2.3	3.1	1.8*	0.0
Veterans hospital	1.4	4.6	0.9	0.7	5.4	0.0*	1.5	0.9*	0.0
Other facility or unknown	1.9	3.3	1.9	1.4	1.9	1.9	1.8	3.8*	0.0
Unknown or other arrangements	2.9	2.9	2.7	3.0	3.1	2.8	2.9	2.9*	5.4*

* Figure does not meet standard of reliability
Note: Multiple responses resulted in totals exceeding 100%.
Source: National Center for Health Statistics

Statistics for individual nursing homes may reveal important information relative to operational characteristics. Because impairments tend to worsen with age, nursing homes with varied resident age levels could have significantly differing nursing requirements that would impact the cost of labor and benefits.

Conclusion

There are no exact or recommended rules of thumb for estimating demand. A thorough study of the population characteristics of a hospital service area along with an analysis of occupancy data for competitive facilities will reveal important information relative to a projected number of future annual patient days. Many states will have prepared their own estimates, but these may be unreliable. In determining future bed need one state considered the following ratios:[3]

Age brackets	Beds needed per 1,000 population (15-mile radius)
Under 65	1.1
65 to 74	20
75 to 84	70
85 and over	200

Analyzing the Supply

Considerable data are available from state government reports on competitive facilities within defined hospital service or trade areas. Using these data the appraiser can categorize other nursing homes by ratios of private and public-pay patients and analyze their performance including occupancy rates. Nursing home beds can include freestanding SNFs and ICFs, facilities within general hospital medical campuses, special wings within life-care facilities, and other categories such as gero-psychiatric hospitals.

Average occupancy rates are considered to be the key to the future outlook for an area. This information must be confirmed with a quality rating of competitive facilities and data on future additions to the market. Because operating margins are slim in this business, a high rate of occupancy is critical to success. A rate of 90% is considered average. Generally where average occupancy rates in a hospital service area are in the mid-90s, the success of a proposed project is likely. A rate of 85% or less should alert the appraiser to a number of possibilities, including management deficiencies, an overbuilt market, problems of obsolescence, and the likely lack of profitability. Statewide occupancy and other data are found in Table 5.7.

In the past state governments typically controlled nursing home bed supply through a Certificate of Need (CON) process, wherein developers of proposed projects had to demonstrate a sizable bed need to obtain approval. Control was considered a desirable social and fiscal goal because of the restricted nature of Medicaid funds and the marginal profitability of the industry. Excess construction was thought to encourage destructive competition and result in waste. Deregulation of the CON process in the mid-1980s resulted in excess construction in a few states and a drop in average occupancy rates. The CON process, where it still exists, has become somewhat superfluous. Private-pay facilities, which may not require a CON, are being added to the supply in locations with exceedingly attractive demographic characteristics, but these developments will have only a small impact on the overall market. In any event it is recommended that the appraiser make a check of a local hospital service area to determine whether there are any approved, but unbuilt nursing homes and what the requirements are for new construction.

In the 1990s it is expected that some additions to supply will take place despite state and federal government funding crises and uncertain economic conditions in portions of the nation. Indications that construction of new or replacement nursing homes will occur provide a somewhat positive outlook for the industry. In 1994, 45 projects accounting for 4,517 beds in new or replacement nursing homes were completed in the United States at a construction cost of $316,600,000. Expansions and renovations totaling 4,128 beds were also completed, and 367 projects of both types involving 26,408 beds were in the pipeline. Construction costs averaged about $70,000 per bed for new or replacement facilities in 1994.

In addition to the usual considerations of age, condition, and location, a qualitative rating of a facility may also consider such factors as management and appeal, based on a personal visit and inspection. The list in Figure 5.3, compiled by various industry experts, can be an excellent guide.

---

[3] Joe R. Roberts and Eric Roberts, "Nursing Homes: Government Influence," *The Appraisal Journal* (July 1989) 309-316.

Table 5.7   Nursing Home Data by State, 1995

	Nursing Homes (1995)	Beds (1995)	1993 Occupancy Rate (%)	Beds per 1,000 Age 65+	Beds per 1,000 Age 75+
Alabama	229	23,754	98.06	42.50	95.88
Alaska	25	909	88.76	33.60	96.98
Arizona	156	16,895	91.66	30.18	72.26
Arkansas	239	24,714	94.81	65.57	142.77
California	1,248	118,601	92.83	34.47	80.19
Colorado	185	17,808	89.20	46.87	107.95
Connecticut	351	32,708	96.31	72.41	161.88
Delaware	46	5,000	90.91	56.52	138.73
D.C.	21	3,054	98.18	41.67	95.21
Florida	643	75,313	95.36	28.72	65.74
Georgia	341	37,019	97.89	50.92	118.93
Hawaii	42	3,532	95.44	24.51	64.05
Idaho	82	6,024	93.71	41.92	93.27
Illinois	831	106,460	91.64	70.48	156.99
Indiana	589	55,299	87.92	74.21	166.06
Iowa	427	33,864	96.39	76.12	155.91
Kansas	395	29,442	93.14	81.67	169.76
Kentucky	348	31,476	98.21	62.97	140.09
Louisiana	340	37,598	92.98	77.14	178.26
Maine	148	9,920	97.25	58.13	125.41
Maryland	235	27,371	96.57	50.08	121.46
Massachusetts	565	55,186	97.08	65.43	142.09
Michigan	442	48,669	95.23	41.90	97.06
Minnesota	486	45,871	97.83	78.60	162.69
Mississippi	156	15,598	99.08	45.99	100.66
Missouri	622	58,055	89.78	76.64	162.74
Montana	125	8,000	91.43	67.71	150.20

(continued)

Table 5.7   Nursing Home Data by State, 1995 (continued)

	Nursing Homes (1995)	Beds (1995)	1993 Occupancy Rate (%)	Beds per 1,000 Age 65+	Beds per 1,000 Age 75+
Nebraska	242	19,418	92.84	82.63	167.46
Nevada	39	3,690	91.20	22.64	64.22
New Hampshire	75	7,106	96.57	53.33	117.31
New Jersey	343	50,000	94.04	46.59	108.76
New Mexico	84	6,961	97.00	37.36	87.32
New York	652	111,374	97.12	46.26	103.30
North Carolina	356	36,053	96.84	40.76	96.98
North Dakota	86	7,125	98.01	77.29	155.06
Ohio	1,002	99,335	94.65	67.29	154.97
Oklahoma	424	35,129	84.80	78.11	167.46
Oregon	182	14,870	90.32	33.79	75.26
Pennsylvania	710	92,556	94.29	48.94	112.59
Rhode Island	102	10,306	97.19	67.71	149.69
South Carolina	177	16,408	97.91	38.38	96.11
South Dakota	114	8,293	96.53	76.47	156.82
Tennessee	321	37,148	97.59	54.81	123.23
Texas	1,150	124,995	84.76	65.12	147.36
Utah	85	7,356	90.51	41.45	94.24
Vermont	50	3,840	96.71	54.36	116.89
Virginia	257	29,818	95.65	41.59	99.45
Washington	300	29,600	94.07	44.85	102.08
West Virginia	105	9,844	97.77	35.23	79.52
Wisconsin	449	50,489	95.09	72.45	153.65
Wyoming	36	3,112	97.45	60.61	138.37
All states	16,658	1,742,966	91.00	54.61	122.34

Source: *The Guide to the Nursing Home Industry, 1995*, Health Care Investment Analysts, Inc.

Figure 5.3   Selecting a Nursing Home

The criteria that experts recommend to family members in choosing a nursing home can be used by appraisers for comparative and valuation purposes. Among the items to watch for are

1. The number of residents in bed. It is a good sign if people are up, dressed, and groomed.

2. The number of residents involved in activities vs. dozing before the TV. Social programs and amenities should be available seven days a week, days and evenings. Without such programs, a nursing home is little more than a human warehouse. After-dinner activity is a subtle but important quality index. In a poorly managed nursing home, residents may be in bed by 6 p.m. but awake at 3 a.m. needing sleeping pills. Patients who are up until 10 p.m. will sleep better and avoid taking drugs.

3. The quality of meals. Visit during meal time and taste the food yourself.

4. The level of staff responsiveness. Does the staff appear animated or listless with residents? Are call bells promptly answered at night? Ask about family satisfaction surveys and staff turnover rates. Look beyond the "glitz" of the lobby; staff performance matters more than decor.

5. Signs of inadequate care (e.g., patients lying around incontinent)

6. The adequacy of the facility's infection control and immunization plans

7. Special services offered (e.g., rehabilitation programs, "wander guard" bracelets for Alzheimer's patients)

8. Compatibility of roommates, if rooms are shared. A resident who is mentally and socially acute can be unnerved by a roommate who is confused or agitated.

When visiting a nursing home facility, an appraiser should talk to the staff and the residents. All the senses, including those of smell and taste, should be used to determine general quality of care provided.

Source: *The Guide to the Nursing Home Industry, 1995,* Health Care Investment Analysts, Inc.

Example of a Penetration/Saturation Study

The following example represents an actual market saturation analysis for a proposed 99-bed skilled nursing facility (see Table 5.8). The target population for this facility is the group 75 years old and over. In 1993 the population of the market area for this group was 8,843; by 1998 the projected population is estimated to be 10,552 (an increase of 19.3%). Population is primarily female (60%), white (97.5%), and middle-income (median income in 1993 was $22,644 for ages 75 to 79, $22,337 for ages 80 to 84, and $21,079 for ages 85 and over).

In the 75 years and over category, 41.3% are married couple families, 4.6% are single heads of households, and 54.1% are rated as nonfamily (householder living alone or with nonrelations). Ninety-two percent of the total are rated as living above the poverty level. Of the persons who are noninstitutionalized and aged 75 years or more, 43.1% have mobility and/or self-care limitations. Within this category 67.7% have mobility limits, 6.8% self-care limits, and 25.5% both limits.

Thus it can be seen that 832 beds are available to service a potential population of 8,843 persons aged 75 or more, at an absorption or saturation rate of 9.41%, which is considered conservative. With the additional 99 beds the rate is 10.53%, which is highly acceptable. By 1998, assuming no change in the supply, the demand picture improves to rates of 7.9% and 8.8%, respectively.

Table 5.8	Market Saturation Analysis* of a Proposed 99-Bed Hospital				
		Population*	**Saturation Rates for SNFs**		
			W/O Subject (832 Units)	**W/Subject (931 Units)**	**Subject Only (99 Units)**
1993 Estimate					
	75+ all	8,843	9.41%	10.53%	1.1%
	75+@ $15K+	5,872	14.7%	15.8%	1.7%
	@ $25K+	3,861	21.5%	24.1%	2.6%
	@$35K+	2,416	34.0%	38.53%	4.1%
1998 Projection					
	75+ all	10,552	7.9%	8.8%	0.9%
	75+ @ $15K+	8,036	10.3%	11.6%	1.2%
	$25K+	5,966	14.0%	15.6%	1.7%
	$35K+	4,448	18.7%	20.1%	2.2%
Evaluation of Saturation Rates					
Penetration Level			**Estimate of Overall Market Demand**		
0-10%			Conservative		
10-20%			Moderate		
20%+			Aggressive		

* Market saturation rates represent the percentage of total market demand which is necessary to absorb a) existing units not including the subject or b) existing units including the subject.
** Number of income and age qualifying senior households within Central Coast County per Claritas/NPDC.

Highest and Best Use Considerations

Typically, the highest and best use of a nursing home property as improved is continuation of the existing use. However, certain factors must be considered that may have a dramatic effect on depreciation estimates. Among these are market (or supply and demand) conditions, design limitations resulting in functional deficiencies, demographic shifts affecting patient mix, and Medicaid limitations on reimbursement rates that affect revenue production.

Prior periods of rapid expansion of nursing home beds resulted in excess inventory and low occupancy rates. In recent years limited construction of facilities has improved the supply side of the equation. Thus, even older facilities that do not appear to be particularly appealing may perform quite well in terms of occupancy compared to superior nursing homes, but their patient census will be derived mostly from the public or Medicaid sector. Such high occupancy rates (typically in the mid-90s) may be expected to last for many years unless unusual shifts take place in demographics, limitations on government funding, or a preference for home care.

Appraisers need to analyze the physical characteristics of a property to derive indications of design problems. Some properties will require special allowances for future additional investment for remodeling, upgrading to meet code changes, and/or eliminating items of deferred maintenance. Some nursing homes are maintained to an appallingly limited degree. Such properties will have to be either totally upgraded or closed down. The likelihood is that a current operator may fail and the property will be acquired by another entity at a price low enough for the required capital investment to meet current but limited standards. The appraiser can check with the applicable agency to determine if the property meets operational requirements. Constantly changing statutory considerations require these matters to be carefully investigated. The best sources for this information are representatives of the applicable state agency or staff members of the local building or health department.

Demographic shifts occur slowly, but changes in neighborhoods due to these factors may be more apparent to an appraiser. For example, there is a much lower propensity for certain ethnic groups to utilize nursing homes, which could be extremely important in the valuation of a property where racial cohorts are undergoing significant shifts. Due to the aging of the nursing home population in some locations, units that specialize in Alzheimer's patients or those with a related dementia type of illness may be in greater demand. In some respects the increase in the number of such patients represents a business opportunity because of a higher rate structure and the lack of competitive beds. The appraiser can obtain information about such trends in the patient population by researching the types of patients a hospital has had over the years, the relative degrees of their acuity and illness, and changing nursing requirements (see also Chapter 7, where a brief discussion of valuation factors relating to Alzheimer's facilities is provided).

Given the changing environment of publicly supported reimbursement programs, potential factors dealing with DRGs, PPSs, and managed care activities must be factored into revenue projections. These might include appropriate annual inflators as well as higher rates of billings that may not be recovered. Lastly, opportunities in the subacute care market can have a dramatic impact on the bottom line of a skilled nursing facility (see Chapter 7). Ultimately the appraiser must be aware of evolving political, social, and economic factors and their potential effect on the market value of the nursing home facility as well as the entire business enterprise.

Valuation Methodology

Lenders generally require the cost approach, but it rarely has significance as an authentic indicator of total facility value because virtually all assignments involve older facilities that exhibit substantial degrees of various types of physical depreciation as well as external obsolescence. The intangible element of the enterprise is also difficult to quantify separately. These factors will be described in greater detail later in this chapter. Few clients express an interest in the numbers produced by the cost approach except as they support the development cost of a proposed project. However, the cost approach does perform an essential function where the value conclusion must be allocated to its component parts.

Virtually all the appraiser's analytical energy should be focused on the income approach because nursing homes are investment properties first and foremost. Their test of marketability relates to the potential to produce future revenue, whether the facility is operated on a for-profit or nonprofit basis. In the latter situation the appraiser may substitute market rental rates for the subject's subsidized rates if the assignment is to estimate value "in exchange." This situation will be expanded on in a later discussion.

The sales comparison approach is always useful even if it only serves as a check on the result indicated by the income approach. It is entirely appropriate to conclude with a valuation range since sale prices are influenced not only by the usual variances in real estate characteristics but by business judgments involving corporate policies, problems arising from regulatory decisions, the inability or unwillingness to deal with functional inadequacies, and so on. Research into the "sales market" is essential to derive information about investment yields, market activity, and price trends.

Cost Approach

As with most health care facilities, nursing homes comprise the typical group of physical assets, including FF&E, as well as intangibles, the main component of which may be referred to as business value. All of these assets can be estimated by a cost approach methodology, but in most cases the intangible element, where it is positively identified, is derived from an allocation of the total value indicated by the income approach. Following is a discussion of value and cost estimating methods that are uniquely applicable to this type of property. Emphasis will not be on the general theory and principles associated with the cost approach but rather the applications and special appraisal processes that are unique to these properties.

Land Value

A nursing home usually may be found in a location with a residential or commercial zoning designation. Typically, there is no special zoning category for nursing homes, but they normally require use permits whether located in single-family residential, multiple-family residential, or commercial zones. A strict interpretation of the permitted uses within the zone where the subject is sited could mean that the land comparables would all be of the same zoning category. This seems logical, but in many cases the use permit provides for a higher than normal density and the conduct of commercial activities that enhance the value of the land, especially where surrounding parcels are limited to a low or moderate density. Thus, when appraising a nursing home site that is essentially part of a single-family home neighborhood, it can be entirely appropriate to use multiresidential land sales for comparables. This situation is not imperative when the nursing home is located on a commercial site, since it can be assumed that under typical circumstances commercial land unit values reflect a broad spectrum of potential uses that could include a hospital.

Exceptions to these recommendations include a nursing home on a rural site where multiple alternatives for an appropriate location exist, or where the nursing home no longer represents the highest and best use of the land. However, obtaining a use permit may be a time-consuming and costly process, and this factor should be recognized as a unique additive to the land appraisal or possibly as an element of the business enterprise.

Land unit values are usually expressed on the basis of price per square foot or price per bed (bed rather than room since a typical nursing home will vary in the number of beds per patient room). Urban sites are usually cramped, but some sites may have a generous ratio of land area to nursing beds or the appearance of excess land to the needs of the hospital. In such cases an adjustment should be considered to recognize these factors even though they bear no consequence on the economics of the operation, except possibly where the facility is very upscale and exclusive.

Of the four principal elements of the enterprise (land, improvements, FF&E, and business enterprise), land value will typically contribute 15% to 20% of the total. Where the land component represents a high percentage of the total property or facility value, the remaining life of the improvements has been significantly reduced and the future highest and best use may be something else that is more appropriate.

Improvement Value

Convalescent hospitals are typically of one-story frame or masonry construction. Unit costs may range significantly between fair to excellent categories of facilities. (A description of a typical nursing home appears in Table 5.9). Although low-cost facilities in low-income areas

Table 5.9	Component Description of a Nursing Home	
System/Component	**Specifications**	**Unit**
Foundations		
Footings & foundations	Poured concrete; strip and spread footings and 4' foundation wall	S.F. Ground
Excavation & backfill	Site preparation for slab and trench for foundation wall and footing	S.F. Ground
Substructure		
Slab on grade	4" reinforced concrete with vapor barrier and granular base	S.F. Slab
Superstructure		
Elevated floors	Plywood on wood joists	SF Elev. Fl.
Roof	Plywood on wood joists	S.F. Roof
Stairs	Wood	Flight
Exterior Closure		
Walls	Vertical T & G redwood siding (85% of wall)	S.F. Wall
Doors	Double aluminum & glass doors, single leaf hollow metal	Each
Windows & glazed walls	Wood double hung (15% of wall)	Each
Roofing		
Roof coverings	Built-up tar and gravel with flashing	S.F. Roof
Insulation	Perlite/urethane composite	S.F. Roof
Openings & specialties	Gravel stop, hatches, gutters and downspouts	S.F. Roof
Interior Construction		
Partitions	Gypsum board on wood studs (8 S.F. Floor/L.F. Partition)	S.F. Partition
Interior doors	Single leaf wood (80 S.F. Floor/Door)	Each
Wall finishes	50% vinyl wall coverings, 45% paint, 5% ceramic tile	S.F. Surface
Floor finishes	50% carpet, 45% vinyl tile, 5% ceramic tile	S.F. Floor
Ceiling finishes	Painted gypsum board on wood furring	S.F. Ceiling
Interior surface/exterior wall	Painted gypsum board on wood furring (8% of wall)	S.F. Wall
Conveying		
Elevators	One passenger elevator	Each
Mechanical		
Plumbing	Kitchen, toilet and service fixtures, supply and drainage (1 fix./230 S.F.)	Each
Fire protection	Sprinkler, light hazard	S.F. Floor
Heating	Oil fired hot water, wall fin radiation	S.F. Floor
Electrical		
Service & distribution	600 ampere service, panel board and feeders	S.F. Floor
Lighting & power	Incandescent fixtures, receptacles, switches and misc. power	S.F. Floor
Special electrical	Alarm systems and emergency lighting	S.F. Floor

Source: R.S. Means

exist, they generally will not meet today's regulatory requirements and are candidates for replacement or extensive renovation in the near future.

By definition a nursing home should have a higher unit construction cost than a structure of equivalent room density because of safety, handicap, communication, and medical care requirements. In actual practice many existing nursing homes were constructed on a highly competitive/minimal basis in the 1950s and 1960s using standardized plans and specifications where the total floor area per bed was 200 square feet or less. Superior facilities should have much more square feet per bed. The floor area indicator can be one test of the general quality and capability of a facility.

Nursing homes with 200 square feet of gross floor area per bed are generally cramped facilities. In such homes many residents are in wards, recreation and common dining areas are minimal, and space for therapy, management, and maintenance functions is limited. The design may allow for only one nursing station. A rule of thumb is that there should be one nursing station per 50 beds and no more than 55 feet between the nursing station and the farthest room. Repair and maintenance department needs have usually resulted in the addition of a shop or storage building. Tight space situations are common, but, nevertheless, the nursing quality can still be above average and the enterprise can be a resounding success due to good management combined with a high occupancy ratio.

A functionally desirable design for a nursing home will provide for ample resident bed, therapy, recreation, and dining space as well as room for management, nursing, dietary, employee support, and repair/maintenance departments. Ratios of gross floor area per bed of 250 square feet or more are usually indicative of such situations. However, when a nursing home occupies space originally designed for another purpose, such as acute hospital beds, this ratio may not be appropriate because it may include space of marginal utility.

As of this writing an average quality convalescent hospital building of frame construction will cost $66 per square foot to build in an average American city.[4] Good quality buildings can go as high as $87 per square foot and still be economically viable. Very costly convalescent hospitals may not be financially viable investments unless they have a constantly high occupancy rate with private patients paying an average rate of over $120 per day.

As a convenient basis for analysis, construction or development costs may be commonly referred to on a per bed basis. In fact, rules of thumb such as a room rate multiplier used in hotel valuation can be developed for quick "takes" on the value of a facility. Although readers should not place much weight on the following example, it illustrates the direct relationship between cost and the average daily hospitalization rate required to satisfy typical yield and amortization requirements. In the hotel business the "rule of 1,000" has gained some notoriety. In the nursing home business a similar test for proposed facilities may be referred to as the "rule of 500." A convalescent hospital that cost $60,000 per bed to develop would have to produce an average daily revenue per bed of $120 to be an economically viable investment. The rationale for this cost/revenue relationship will be described in the income approach section which follows. Obviously, the relationship can be reversed to produce a transaction-derived multiplier that can be used in the sales comparison approach.

It is beyond the scope of this chapter to present all of the replacement cost possibilities of nursing home improvements. The reader is referred to such publications as the *Marshall Valuation Service,* which provides detailed replacement cost data on a square foot and per bed basis as well as more detailed component cost and price data. Considering the value limitations

---

[4] *Marshall Valuation Service,* Marshall and Swift, Los Angeles, 1996.

of the cost approach, it is not recommended that the appraiser spend the time and effort involved in preparing such estimates unless they are necessary for insurance, litigation, or development financing purposes.

In addition to building improvements a nursing home will have a significant investment in yard construction for landscaping, fencing, paving, enclosures, and underground utilities. These items are commonly estimated on an average per square foot of site area basis but can also be individually detailed.

Depreciation

The typical nursing home is about 30 years old and thus suffers from a significant degree of depreciation, most of which is due to a combination of physical deterioration and external obsolescence. Functional problems are common, but their effect on total value is usually small and curable. Effective age and life expectancy tables can be employed to estimate depreciation. Appropriate allowance should be made for the fact that older facilities may still be in use for a long time because it isn't generally financially feasible to develop new ones, except those which serve the higher paying, private-pay market. Revenues from facilities with extremely high ratios of Medicaid-supported residents cannot come close to supporting the costs of replacement. This is another reason for not employing a cost approach.

Because most nursing homes serve Medicaid-supported residents, which means that the reimbursement rate is controlled by a political agenda, the major depreciation factor is related to economic considerations or the capitalized difference between the rate normally needed to provide an appropriate return on cost and what the government actually provides.

It is not recommended that the appraiser employ sophisticated techniques to separately estimate various factors of depreciation. Textbook depreciation calculations should be applied only where they are significant to the function of the appraisal. Rather, the appraiser should use easily understood general estimating techniques based on age-life-condition considerations and present the depreciated replacement cost only as an approximate method for valuing this type of enterprise.

FF&E Value

Real estate appraisers have always had problems in estimating the value of FF&E (fixtures, furnishings, and equipment) for any type of property since it represents a large number of relatively low-valued items for which readily usable market data are not available. The problem with FF&E is that many of the individual items are old (and probably fully depreciated on the books) and do not represent "state-of-the-art" capabilities but still have considerable utility. They could be replaced with equally equivalent used items from the secondhand market (and frequently are), but would never be purchased new unless there was a dramatic event such as a fire. Because they perform a significant function, they have market value "in place" but only "in exchange" when part of an overall enterprise.

Several techniques are usually applied where an "estimate" of value is required and a high degree of accuracy for FF&E is not essential to the function of the appraisal. Typically, the process is referred to as an allocation of the total appraised value. This is an attempt by the appraiser to indicate that the manner in which the total value of this component is derived is not an appraisal (and therefore the appraiser should not be liable for an exact estimate). It also is an attempt to minimize the time and cost required since the client also minimizes this aspect of the assignment and allocates little if any of the appraisal fee to it. It is suggested that some type of formula technique should be acceptable to those clients who require a breakout of the components of the enterprise and that detailed information be provided only in cases involving loans where securitization of the assets is contemplated.

Marshall and Swift publish broad estimates of ranges in FF&E value or FF&E cost per bed or square foot. There are also generally accepted ratios that FF&E may represent of the total cost or value. Combining this information with some knowledge of the original or book cost can assist the appraiser in developing a conclusion for this component that will satisfy reviewers and be reasonably accurate.

Other Costs

An allowance for entrepreneurial risk or developer's overhead and profit is typically applied by appraisers and is justified except possibly in circumstances where a project is of minimal profitability or is losing money. An allowance of 5% to 15% may be reasonable under appropriate circumstances. An additional factor that may overlap the allowance for entrepreneurial performance is the absorption cost factor or cost to fill the project when the appraisal involves an existing entity. These costs may range from $3,000 to $5,000 per bed, and much more for a highly profitable operation. For example, if a 99-bed hospital has a depreciated cost of $30,000 per bed, an allowance of 10% for developer's profit, *or* a $3,000 per bed absorption allowance to fill the hospital, the result will be an identical amount of $297,000.

Business Value

The true measure of the value of the intangible component of a nursing home business is the enhancement in value over and above the physical assets created by the ability of typical but enlightened management to produce "excess" earnings. Since business opportunities are rarely transferred, except as part of a sale of a leasehold interest, little or no data from transfers exist to provide independent valuation indicators.

The simplest technique for isolating a business value is to attribute any intangible value to the difference between the value indicated by the cost approach for physical assets only with the concluded total enterprise value developed from the income and sales comparison approaches, both of which should reflect all contributory components, sometimes referred to as the agents of production. Management and staff-in-place, which is one of the key agents, is just another term for part of the business value component when its unique contribution to profits is separately capitalized.

Separate methodologies for estimating a business value component were presented in Chapter 3. While acute general hospitals are much more complicated than skilled nursing facilities, the basic techniques for estimating business value are comparable and do not have to be repeated here.

Some basic principles, however, should be considered in addressing the subject of business value. One is that only a moderate percentage of nursing homes are truly successful in that they produce "excess profits." It is our position that most operations that are heavily oriented to Medicaid residents have low profit margins and cannot be considered to have a major business value component. This leaves the field of intangible value to those nursing homes that successfully serve the private-patient market. Of course, it is recognized that private patients are essentially subsidizing the public sector. Some type of monumental reversal could take place if Medicaid rates were adjusted to reflect true operating costs (which will never happen) and the price differential between the public and private sector was narrowed (see the discussion of cost shifting under the income approach). Thus, few buyers will pay significant consideration for intangibles in a single property unless it is uniquely positioned or managed in a tightly controlled market. More likely significant allowances for intangibles will be allocated where a large system or block of properties is being acquired, due to efficiencies of management and economies of scale that can be realized.

This does not mean that buyers will not attempt to allocate a significant portion of the purchase price to various categories of businesses or intangible value. The motivation for such an action can be to minimize the value of real estate assets for tax assessment reasons (significant allocation scenario), or to maximize the value of real estate assets for mortgage loan purposes (insignificant allocation scenario). Within these strategies can be scenarios involving physical asset valuation allocations to reflect depreciation advantages for income tax purposes.

Where a separate estimate of business value is indicated and appropriate, consideration of two or three techniques may be preferred to provide a well-supported conclusion. The combination of the residual method with excess profits as a check, or excess profits with the capitalized net management fee as a check, is recommended. The cost to replace personnel and management systems is another methodology that recognizes the value of a successful "going concern."

When the appraiser researches transactions, it may be revealed that a significant portion of the total price paid has been mutually allocated to intangibles by the buyer and seller. The appraiser should recognize that there are special tax benefits to an allocation of this type if it can be shown that there is a definite life for the particular category of intangibles and that the rate of write-off is much higher than the average percentage allowed by the Internal Revenue Service for depreciation of other assets. In another situation the business value component may purposely not be recognized even where it exists, since for financing purposes the buyer may want to show the highest possible cost for the physical assets. These two unique investment factors should be carefully explored when analyzing sales.

Conclusion

A full example of a cost approach summary is shown in Figure 5.4. The example represents a 15-year-old, well-maintained, financially successful skilled nursing facility with 99 beds. It has a 25% ratio of private patients and a consistent occupancy rate of 96%, and it is situated in a market with a good demographic outlook as far as the elderly population is concerned. Such a facility is reasonably worth a value in the range of $30,000 to $35,000 per bed. The conclusion in the example is $3,300,000.

Income Approach

Virtually all appraisals of nursing homes employ a business valuation/capitalization process rather than a capitalization of estimated or actual rental income, which is traditional for most investment properties. The operational characteristics of a nursing home are similar to that of a hotel and so are the appraisal procedures and techniques.

In the past it was common for contractors to develop nursing homes for investment purposes and to lease the real estate to an operator. Where such arrangements are common and sufficient lease and transactional data exist to estimate a current rental value and an appropriate capitalization rate for the subject, it is entirely appropriate to appraise the real estate or physical assets portion of the enterprise as one would with a single tenant valuation assignment.

Direct Rental Capitalization

In the 1960s and 1970s, builders who knew little about the operation and management of nursing homes were responsible for developing a major portion of the current inventory. In those days it was common to enter into a 20-year lease with options. Typical terms were absolute net with the rent adjusted for Consumer Price Index changes or some other periodic escalation. Many of these leases are still in existence, but for the most part this practice is not followed anymore. With the decline in third-party rental arrangements came a decline in the valuation of nursing homes by net rental income capitalization. When such data are found, however, the comparison to the subject can be on the basis of rent per bed or rent as a percentage of total revenue. Today, when an assignment calls for a rental estimate for the physical facilities, the appraiser generally has difficulty in obtaining current rental comparables. When rental data are found, the appraiser

Figure 5.4   **Cost Approach Example**

			Totals	Per Bed
Land:				
By price per sq. ft. - 50,000 sq. ft. @ $9 =	$450,000			
By price per room - 50 rooms @ $10,000 =	$500,000			
Conclusion			$475,000	$4,798
Improvements (direct and soft costs)				
Building:				
25,000 sq. ft. @ $85 =	$2,125,000			
99 beds @ $23,000 =	$2,277,000			
Conclusion		$2,200,000		
Yard:				
50,000 sq. ft. @ $4 =	$200,000			
99 beds @ $2,000 =	$198,000			
Conclusion		$200,000		
Subtotal			$2,400,000	$24,242
FF&E				
25,000 sq. ft. @ $20 =	$500,000			
99 beds @ $5,500 =	$544,500			
Conclusion			$525,000	$5,303
Subtotal replacement cost			$3,400,000	$34,343
Developer's overhead and profit (15%)			$510,000	
Total replacement cost (empty project)			$3,910,000	$39,495
Less depreciation (improvements)				
By separate estimates:				
Deferred maintenance	$150,000			
Incurable deterioration	$200,000			
External obsolescence	$350,000			
Subtotal	$700,000			
Age-life-condition (as a check)				
$(15 \div 50 = 30\% \times \$2,400,000)$	$720,000			
Conclusion		$700,000		
Less depreciation (FF&E)				
By observed condition				
$(50\% \times \$525,000)$	$262,000			
By age life				
$(10 \div 15 = .33$ left $\times \$525,000)$	$175,000			
Conclusion		$200,000		$2,020
Total depreciation			$900,000	
Depreciated value			$3,010,000	$30,404
Business value				
By excess profits	$310,000			
By capitalized management fee	$320,000			
By cost to replace in-place personnel and systems	$278,000			
By cost to reach stabilized occupancy	$250,000			
Conclusion			$290,000	$2,929
Total value estimate			$3,300,000	$33,333

should examine the relationship between the lessor and lessee to be sure of an arm's-length transaction and the fairness of the terms. Because rental income has a higher priority (and thus a lower risk) than business-derived revenues from commercial activity, the capitalization rate will be significantly lower. An example of a rental survey is shown in Table 5.10.

There are two basic methodologies for appraising a rental ownership. One is to capitalize the net rental income into perpetuity by the following formula:

$$\frac{\text{Net Rental Income}}{\text{Overall Capitalization Rate}} = \text{Value of Leased Fee}$$

The other is to capitalize the rental income and reversion components of the owner's rights separately. The factors controlling the selection of the appropriate method are the length of the lease and the market support for the capitalization and discount rates.

This is the extent of the discussion on rental valuation. There are no rules of thumb or commonly accepted ratios to determine the relationship between net business income and fair

Table 5.10	Summary of Nursing Home Leases					
No./Name Location	Lease Date/ Term/Options	Expense Terms	No. of Beds	Rent per Bed	Rent as % of Revenue	Comments
A	12/94 20 years no option	NNN	190	$264	9.63%	Annual CPI increase (3%-6%); FF&E included; built 1969
B	12/94 20 years no options	NNN	151	$281	11.32%	Annual CPI increase; FF&E included; built 1968
C	1/95 3 years six 3-year options	NNN	144	$235	7.49%	Annual CPI rent increase; FF&E included; built 1967
D	10/94 15 years one 10-year option	NNN	59	$225	8.83%	Annual rate increase based on Medi-Cal rates; FF&E included; built 1960
E	4/95 10 years 1 - 10 year options	NNN	56	$225	9.51%	Annual rate increase based on Medi-Cal rates; FF&E included; built 1960
F	8/93 20 years options - N/A	NNN	205	$210	10.59%	Built late 70s, early 80s
G	2/95 10 years one 10-year option	NNN	124	$250	11.43%	Annual CPI rent increases; verification not complete; FF&E included; built 1954 and 1970
Subject	1995	NNN	112	—	—	FF&E not included; built 1968

Source: Arthur Gimmy International

rental value. The emphasis in the following section will be on the traditional analysis and capitalization of the income produced by the enterprise.

Business Enterprise Capitalization

This valuation alternative involves an estimate of actual or effective gross revenues, a deduction for operating expenses and fixed charges, and a capitalization of the resultant net income or cash flow figure into a valuation conclusion. It can be on a one-year basis or a series of projected cash flows that are discounted and capitalized. The estimate of value covers all of the physical assets of the enterprise as well as intangibles if there are any. It is not necessary to repeat the step-by-step process of analyzing all of the components of revenues and expenses, but it is beneficial to understand the relationships between revenues and individual expense/cost categories and how sensitive the impact is of small adjustments in occupancy and expenses/costs on profitability.

Certain basic or minimum costs are necessary to operate a nursing home on an acceptable basis. Beyond this point the individual categories can vary significantly from property to property due to quantitative differences in services and facilities, the amount of ancillary income, management capabilities, and the ratio of private patients to the total census.

Total Revenues

Virtually all of the revenues of a typical nursing home are derived from the basic daily rate. Ancillary income can be quite significant for those facilities that have a specialized market niche, offer rehabilitation or subacute services, or have a highly affluent resident population. Ancillary charges include items such as physical therapy, extra nursing care, and medical treatment items. Extensive lists of a la carte charges, sometimes representing hundreds of items, exist in private facilities, but most of these charges are small in price and beyond the scope of this chapter.

Potential revenue for a nursing home that is totally occupied by Medicaid-supported residents is much less compared with one that has a strong ratio of private patients to the total census. Because Medicaid reimbursement rates vary extensively from state to state, and within states by hospital service area and property, the following example does not represent any geographic location. Assume that the Medicaid rate is $77 per day and the private-pay rate is $120 per day, or a difference of 56%. If one SNF has a census of 90% Medicaid and 10% private-pay patients and the other SNF has a census of 80% private pay and 20% Medicaid, the revenue differential for the two properties at the same occupancy rate is 37%.

Revenues are typically reported as gross billings less contractual adjustments. An example of this procedure is for management to bill all patients at the current market (or private) rate and then adjust this figure to the actual amount collected or estimated to be received.

Cost Shifting

The differential between Medicaid rates and those charged to private patients can typically vary by 35% or more in the same facility. Many industry specialists feel that those who have the means to pay are being significantly overcharged throughout the country. About one-third of private nursing home residents who are not eligible for Medicaid are actually paying for 20% to 30% of the long-term care received by Medicaid-supported residents. Jane Sneddon Little of the Federal Reserve Bank of Boston argues that: "Such cost-shifting is inherently unfair and counterproductive. By increasing the already heavy burdens of those private payers who are unfortunate enough to require such care themselves, the practice hastens the painful day when they exhaust their savings and move onto Medicaid. It also tends to encourage families to hide assets to avoid depleting their savings. And by muddying the cost picture, it impedes efforts to control Medicaid costs. A better policy would be for states to require nursing homes to charge public and private payers the same rates 'within the same facility' [as Minnesota already does]. Fees that reflect the true costs of services would be fairer to private patients. They would also make it easier for regulators to spot inefficiencies and curb the explosive rise in Medicaid spending."[5] The author of this text is not challenging the rationale for rate differentials or attempting to explain how Medicaid reimbursement rates are derived, except to note that the concept of cost shifting is accepted and corrections to it could have a significant impact on *NOI*s and, therefore, value.

Competitive Rate Survey

The appraisal assignment should also include a survey of competitive facilities. This information is necessary to compare the performance of the subject to alternate properties and to determine the correctness of the rate structure. The results of a typical survey are summarized in Table 5.11. Key data from competitive projects include distance from subject; age; number of licensed beds; occupancy rates for recent years; current census breakdown of private-pay, Medicare, and Medicaid patients; and current private-pay rates for various sized rooms.

After the market rates are determined for the subject property and applied to the appropriate bed classifications, the only calculation left is the average occupancy rate (est.). In most cases there is little movement in average occupancy rates because the competitive supply rarely changes. Currently in many markets it is uneconomic to develop new facilities, and those that are developed are generally oriented to a private patient market. The market could become less competitive in the future as older, noncode–conforming facilities are closed in light of Medicaid revenue restrictions, which make the cost of conformity uneconomic.

Operating Expenses/Costs

This category includes estimates of all the varied expenses of operating a nursing home including

- general and administrative
- management
- advertising/marketing
- accommodations/housekeeping
- utilities
- maintenance/repairs
- social activities/recreation
- dietary
- real estate taxes/licenses
- insurance
- staff education
- reserves
- miscellaneous

Expenses are typically analyzed on a per-patient-day basis, but they can also be compared on the basis of the percentage of actual or effective gross revenue. Operating ratios of 80% to 85% for all of these expenses usually indicate a well-managed operation, assuming that all other ratings for the facility are positive. Operating ratios closer to 90% or more are more typical of the general performance of the overall market, where management tends to be less effective.

---

[5] Jane Sneddon Little, *New England Economic Review*, August 1992.

Table 5.11 Competitive Rate Survey

#	Miles From Subj.	Name/Location	Age (Yrs)	# of Lic. Beds	% Occ 1993	% Occ 1992	% Occ 1991	% Occ 1990	1993 Census Breakdowns % Prvt Pay	% Medi-care	% Medi-cal	1991 Census Breakdowns % Prvt Pay	% Medi-care	% Medi-cal	1993 Private Pay Rates Prvt Room Rate	Semi Private Room Rate	Ward Rate	Primary Or Secondary Comp
1	1.00	Alpha C.H. 6000 Vista, City D	30	71	77.50%	70.00%	64.30%	77.40%	90.00%	2.00%	8.00%	95.40%	3.80%	0.80%	$140.00	$102.00	$100.00	P
2	1.50	Beta C.H. 3000 Ralston St, City D	4	188	53.00%		17.60%					93.15%	6.85%	0.00%	$135.00	$93.50		P
3	5.00	Delta C.H. 2000 "C" St, City E	24	99	77.27%	75.00%	61.70%	64.10%	90.00%	5.00%	5.00%	95.80%	4.20%	0.00%	$125.00	$100.00		P
4	12.50	City Care Center 35 Main St, City F	+30	50	96.00%		97.50%	96.10%	49.00%	1.00%	50.00%	47.80%	1.40%	50.80%	$112.00	$97.00	$85.00	P/S
5	15.00	Quail C.H. 1500 Quail Ave, City G	40	28	98.00%	98.00%	98.70%	97.90%	77.60%	1.00%	21.40%	82.90%	0.00%	17.10%		$115.00		P/S
6	11.00	Dove C.H. 1200 Dove St, City H	+20	115	93.00%	83.00%	84.00%	84.60%	45.00%	10.00%	45.00%	39.10%	0.20%	60.70%	$127.00	$98.00	$94.00	P/S
		Total/Avg (Excluding Subject)		551	82.46%	81.50%	70.63%	84.02%	70.32%	3.80%	25.88%	75.69%	2.74%	21.57%	$127.80	$100.92	$93.00	
		Avg OCC (Excluding Subject & #2)			88.35%	81.50%	81.24%	84.02%										
		High (Excluding Subject)		188	98.00%	98.00%	98.70%	97.90%	90.00%	10.00%	50.00%	95.80%	6.85%	60.70%	$140.00	$115.00	$100.00	
		Low (Excluding Subject)		28	53.00%	70.00%	17.60%	64.10%	45.00%	1.00%	5.00%	39.10%	0.00%	0.00%	$112.00	$93.50	$85.00	
S	N/A	Subject Property Seaview C.H. 5400 Sea Pine Rd, City D	32	71	67.72%	68.72%	74.42%	77.85%	86.61%	3.43%	9.96%	84.30%	3.31%	12.39%	$135.00	$97.00	$93.00	N/A
		Total # of Licensed Beds		622														

An example of a survey of operating expenses for average facilities within a defined hospital service area is shown in Table 5.12. Published information is generally available from state regulatory agencies, but there may be a one-year lag in the data.

Table 5.12 Income and Expenses, 1992										
Skilled Nursing Facility	1	2	3	4	5	6	7	8	9	Mean
Net revenue per patient day	$77.52	$80.31	$84.09	$76.28	$73.52	$88.47	$86.34	$78.96	$93.59	$82.12
Expenses:										
Nursing services	$33.29	$35.56	$34.20	$30.85	$30.88	$41.20	$34.81	$29.46	$37.52	$35.38
Plant operations & maintenance	$3.35	$4.06	$4.57	$4.15	$4.74	$3.65	$4.88	$7.00	$4.37	$4.27
Housekeeping	$2.77	$2.89	$3.67	$4.71	$4.23	$2.74	$1.85	$2.84	$4.03	$3.11
Laundry & linen	$1.60	$3.33	$1.61	$2.95	$1.98	$2.20	$1.92	$2.32	$1.70	$2.20
Dietary	$8.85	$8.73	$7.11	$10.10	$9.25	$7.96	$9.38	$11.26	$9.58	$8.83
Social services	$2.03	$1.61	$2.32	$1.28	$2.22	$1.69	$1.55	$4.18	$1.50	$1.83
Administration	$15.60	$12.52	$13.94	$8.92	$8.23	$11.84	$9.78	$19.20	$14.22	$12.34
Other property expenses	$0.78	$0.74	$1.87	$5.29	$3.35	$1.30	$0.96	$1.66	$1.40	$1.58
Other expenses	$0.09	$0.33	$0.19	$0.18	$0.01	$4.06	$2.00	$0.65	($0.05)	$1.13
Ancillary expenses	$0.87	$2.06	$0.06	$0.25	$0.54	$8.92	$5.20	$0	$10.31	$3.13
Total expenses:	**$69.23**	**$71.83**	**$69.56**	**$68.68**	**$65.43**	**$85.56**	**$72.34**	**$78.57**	**$84.58**	**$73.80**
Net income	$8.29	$8.48	$14.53	$7.60	$8.09	$2.91	$14.00	$0.39	$9.01	$8.32
Operating ratio	0.89	0.89	0.83	0.90	0.89	0.97	0.84	0.99	0.90	0.90

Source: OSHPD

Statewide Statistics

Financial operating data provided by *The Guide to the Nursing Home Industry,* published by HCIA, are shown in Table 5.13. Median values are shown for revenue and expense items for each state, concluding with total profit per patient day and as a percentage of net patient revenue. *The Guide to the Nursing Home Industry* also provides a breakdown by state of median values of for-profit units and all other facilities. These data are helpful to the appraiser in comparing a subject property with an "average" facility. More specific information relative to facilities in individual hospital service or planning areas should be acquired from the pertinent agencies in each state.

Table 5.13   Income and Expense Statistics per Patient Day Basis, 1993

State	Net Patient Revenue	Expenses					Total Profit	
		Operating	Direct Care	Indirect Care	Admin. & General	Ancillary	PPD	%
Alabama	$71.38	$60.70	$26.31	$12.37	$19.50	$2.52	$10.68	15.0
Alaska	211.18	181.29	66.50	37.04	63.37	14.38	29.89	14.2
Arizona	93.52	81.18	31.62	14.04	25.63	9.89	12.34	13.2
Arkansas	55.19	45.78	17.43	10.51	16.64	1.20	9.41	17.0
California	81.87	81.37	28.37	16.27	30.97	5.76	0.50	0.6
Colorado	79.41	67.41	33.87	13.47	15.66	4.41	12.00	15.1
Connecticut	128.14	98.37	41.68	17.30	35.92	3.47	29.77	23.2
Delaware	98.62	92.25	37.85	21.64	26.94	5.82	6.37	6.5
District of Columbia	141.20	122.45	54.62	31.27	33.14	3.42	18.75	13.3
Florida	91.67	79.85	30.45	15.07	24.49	9.84	11.82	12.9
Georgia	65.85	54.91	22.43	10.94	19.65	1.89	10.94	16.6
Hawaii	122.64	103.15	41.25	21.72	35.79	4.39	19.49	15.9
Idaho	79.92	71.30	32.74	11.71	26.23	0.62	8.62	10.8
Illinois	71.17	57.90	23.61	12.15	19.62	2.52	13.27	18.6
Indiana	77.74	62.97	27.32	13.48	22.17	N/A	14.77	19.0
Iowa	57.35	50.73	20.12	11.28	14.97	4.36	6.62	11.5
Kansas	57.46	50.12	19.44	11.97	18.16	0.55	7.34	12.8
Kentucky	68.43	52.55	23.84	10.43	14.30	3.98	15.88	23.2
Louisiana	59.32	42.56	17.98	8.69	15.62	0.27	16.76	28.2
Maine	94.81	69.73	36.22	14.77	16.42	2.32	25.08	26.5
Maryland	92.16	74.46	30.22	15.61	26.69	1.94	17.70	19.2
Massachusetts	110.65	89.97	41.76	17.85	27.18	3.18	20.68	18.7
Michigan	78.07	62.43	31.26	13.97	14.39	2.81	15.64	20.0
Minnesota	75.90	70.12	32.33	16.15	19.54	2.10	5.78	7.6
Mississippi	61.57	51.09	19.53	10.12	19.04	2.40	10.48	17.0
Missouri	66.42	61.12	23.38	10.93	25.65	1.16	5.30	8.0
Montana	72.72	67.76	27.29	13.95	24.79	1.73	4.96	6.8
Nebraska	62.11	56.13	26.25	14.13	14.55	1.20	5.98	9.6
Nevada	96.60	74.22	33.24	13.17	23.54	4.27	22.38	23.2
New Hampshire	104.53	91.37	36.51	19.78	31.05	4.03	13.16	12.6
New Jersey	107.61	85.12	35.50	19.31	26.71	3.60	22.49	20.9
New Mexico	79.42	62.48	22.85	11.10	25.90	2.63	16.94	21.3

(continued)

State	Net Patient Revenue	Expenses					Total Profit	
		Operating	Direct Care	Indirect Care	Admin. & General	Ancillary	PPD	%
New York	$133.28	$114.15	$48.22	$25.79	$36.24	$3.90	$19.13	14.4
North Carolina	77.26	65.72	30.02	13.52	19.61	2.57	11.54	14.9
North Dakota	79.24	67.73	30.37	15.99	19.79	1.58	11.51	14.5
Ohio	86.37	69.92	34.77	15.50	15.73	3.92	16.45	19.0
Oklahoma	N/A	39.26	15.19	10.15	15.67	0.86	N/A	N/A
Oregon	82.90	72.13	32.51	12.21	23.57	4.14	10.77	13.0
Pennsylvania	96.35	77.47	31.77	15.38	26.55	3.77	18.88	19.6
Rhode Island	105.49	80.46	35.14	15.77	26.82	2.73	24.98	23.7
South Carolina	82.21	60.31	25.04	14.07	18.20	3.00	21.90	26.6
South Dakota	69.16	55.31	23.48	12.74	15.68	3.41	13.85	20.0
Tennessee	67.12	55.26	21.76	12.40	18.95	2.15	11.86	17.7
Texas	57.66	47.73	20.28	10.47	15.77	1.21	9.93	17.2
Utah	73.60	60.91	26.37	10.95	23.59	N/A	12.69	17.2
Vermont	75.40	62.66	24.01	15.56	17.52	5.57	12.74	16.9
Virginia	91.66	71.22	35.87	12.72	18.43	4.20	20.44	22.3
Washington	103.05	78.58	36.05	12.99	26.18	3.36	24.47	23.7
West Virginia	77.83	53.52	23.60	11.75	15.97	2.20	24.31	31.2
Wisconsin	86.69	73.78	32.22	15.19	24.49	1.88	12.91	14.9
Wyoming	75.82	73.15	33.06	16.69	22.84	0.56	2.67	3.5
All States	73.50	61.09	25.61	13.16	20.41	1.91	12.41	16.9

Legend:
All of the above revenue, expense and profit categories represent the sum of the individual items in each category divided by the number of resident days in a nursing home. Net patient revenue is a measure of the patient care revenue per day received by a nursing home. Total operating expenses include salaries, supplies, etc. but do not include extraordinary items or charges against income. Direct care expense represents nursing costs and the related expenses attributed to patient care. Indirect care expense includes categories such as laundry and linen service, housekeeping, dietary, cafeteria, central services and supply, pharmacy and social services. Administrative and general expense include non-patient telephone bills, cashiering, patient billing, maintenance and repairs, operation of plant, maintenance of personnel, employee benefits and medical records. Ancillary costs include all services incurred during a patient's stay except for room and board, nursing, dietary, physician services and blood. Total profit is a measure of the overall profitability of a nursing home without the inclusion of philanthropic contributions, endowment revenue, government grants, investment income and other revenues and expenses not related to patient care operations, and also exclusive of those expenses that are associated with the maintenance of long-term assets and liabilities, including capital lease payments, depreciation and interest expense.

Source: *The Guide to the Nursing Home Industry,* Health Care Investment Analysts, Inc.

Capitalization Rates

Because a nursing home is a business, the capitalization rates reflect a risk or entrepreneurial component that typically is about 300 basis points over an average commercial real estate investment. The sources of capitalization rates include publications such as the *Nursing Home Acquisition Report,* published by Irving Levin & Associates, Inc., and the individual analyses of comparable nursing home sales. The appraiser should also attempt to obtain opinions of capitalization rates from specialists in the industry such as those involved in financing skilled nursing facilities or brokerage firms such as Marcus & Millichap, which has a senior housing division. Irving Levin Associates, Inc., reported that the average capitalization rate based on a large number of transactions was 13.8% in 1992.[6]

Valuation

An example of the application of an income approach is shown in Figure 5.5. The subject has 71 beds and a patient mixture as follows:

Private	(83%)
Medicaid (or MediCal in California)	(8%)
Medicare	(2%)
Other or VA	(1%)
HMO	(6%)

HMO patients are also considered to be private but at a higher reimbursement rate due to greater health care requirements.

Total gross care revenue amounts to $103.74 per patient day (PPD). Ancillary revenue from therapy and related services amounts to a net of $1.44 PPD, while miscellaneous revenue provides $0.66 PPD. After deductions for collection loss, total effective revenue is $2,509,334. Operating expenses, including management and reserves, of 86.73%, or $2,176,269, are deducted, providing a net operating income of $333,066. This example also solves for real estate taxes since the subject is underassessed and will undergo a sharp increase in taxes subsequent to sale. Thus, the real estate tax rate (1.03%) is added to the property capitalization rate (12.00%). The value estimate comes in at $2,700,000, or $38,028 per bed for the entire enterprise.

Sales Comparison Approach

The sales comparison approach is a popular indicator of value, but it is difficult to apply accurately in nursing home situations because of the large variations in physical and performance characteristics among properties. The common unit of comparison is price per bed, but if properly derived other indicators such as a gross revenue multiplier or price per square foot of building area can be equally accurate. Since there can be a significant intangible value attributed to an SNF, it would appear that comparisons and adjustments made only on the basis of physical and locational characteristics can be inaccurate. It is sometimes recommended that the sales comparison approach be used to show a range in potential value for a property rather than a precise measure unless sale properties are exceedingly comparable to the subject in overall characteristics and performance.

In addition to sales of nursing homes, knowledge of nursing home acquisitions can provide the appraiser with an understanding of market forces that are at work in the industry. For example the pace of mergers in the industry appears to have intensified in recent years, which has been motivated partially by the potential profitability of operating subacute care facilities. Table 5.14 lists 10 major long-term care acquisitions made in 1993 and 1994.

Critical data necessary to analyze sales transactions include age of the facility, occupancy at time of sale, private pay ratio, Medicare ratio, Medicaid ratio, operating expense ratio, gross revenue per patient day, and net income per patient day. Information on all of the expense categories to be analyzed is also critical because usually there is a significant variance from performance averages for these categories within a service area, larger region, or entire state.

---

[6] *The Nursing Home Acquisition Report,* 2nd edition (New Canaan, CT: Irving Levin Associates, Inc., 1993).

Number of beds	71		
Available patient days	25,915		
Medicare patient days	492	$116.59	2.00%
Medi-Cal patient days	1,970	$77.41	8.00%
Private patient days	20,434	$101.50	83.00%
VA/other patient days	246	$86.00	1.00%
HMO patient days	1,477	$168.50	6.00%
Total patient days	24,619		
Occupancy	95.00%		

Revenues	Est. 1994	$/PD	% Total
Medicare rate revenue	$57,362	$116.59	2.25%
Medi-Cal rate revenue	$152,498	$77.41	5.97%
Private rate revenue	$2,074,051	$101.50	81.21%
VA/Other rate revenue	$21,156	$86.00	0.83%
HMO revenue	$248,875	$168.50	9.74%
Total routine revenue	$2,553,941	$103.74	100.00%
Ancillary revenue	$78,145	$3.17	100.00%
Ancillary expense	($113,654)	($4.62)	-145.44%
Net ancillary revenue	($35,509)	($1.44)	-45.44%
Misc. revenue	$25,850	$1.05	100.00%
Misc. expense	($9,602)	($0.39)	-37.14%
Net other revenue	$16,249	$0.66	62.86%
Total revenue	$2,534,681	$102.66	100.00%
Less: deductions	($25,347)	($1.03)	-1.00%
Effective gross income	$2,509,334	$101.93	99.00%
Less: Expenses			
Nursing services	($965,382)	($39.21)	-38.47%
Plant operations	($155,354)	($6.31)	-6.19%
Housekeeping	($103,401)	($4.20)	-4.12%
Laundry/Linen	($100,000)	($4.06)	-3.99%
Dietary services	($321,770)	($13.07)	-12.82%
Social services	($62,999)	($2.56)	-2.51%
General & admin.	($248,797)	($15.50)	-9.91%
Management	($125,467)	($5.10)	-5.00%
Property & other	($17,819)	($0.72)	-0.71%
Replacement reserve	($75,280)	($3.06)	-3.00%
Total expenses	($2,176,269)	($88.40)	-86.73%
Net operating income	$333,066	$13.53	13.27%
Add: R.E. taxes	$14,423		
R.E. tax adjusted NOI	$347,489		
Capitalization rate	12.00%		
Add: R.E. tax rate	1.03%		
RE tax adjusted dap rate	13.03%		
Indicated value	$2,666,836		
Rounded to:	$2,700,000	$38,028 per bed	

Table 5.14

Table 5.14   Nursing Home Acquisitions, 1993-1994 (Purchase Price and Revenues in Millions)

Closing Date	Buyer	Acquisition	Purchase Price	Revenues Acquired	Bed Capacity Acquired	Price Per Bed[1]
Oct 1993	Living Centers of America	Vari-Care, Inc.	$71	$65[4]	2,541	$27,942
Nov 1993	Regency Health Services	Braswell Enterprises	$14	NA	777	$17,600
Nov 1993	Welsh, Carson	The Cardinal Group	NA	$82[5]	2,814	NA
Dec 1993	Genesis Health Ventures	Meridian Healthcare	$205	NA	5,465	$37,511
Dec 1993	GranCare, Inc.	CompuPharm, Inc.	$63	$70	NA	NA
Dec 1993	Integrated Health Services	Central Park Lodges	$182	$137[6]	5,050	$36,040
Feb 1994	Horizon Healthcare	Greenery Rehabilitation	$85	$175[7]	2,803	$30,325
Mar 1994	Multicare Companies	Providence Health Care	$30	$33[7]	1,245	$24,096
Apr 1994	Regency Health Services	Care Enterprises, Inc.	$120[2]	$197[2]	5,040	$23,810
May 1994	Sun Healthcare Group	Mediplex Group, Inc.	$320[3]	$398	5,729	$55,856

1. Price per bed may reflect revenues generated by pharmacy, home health, and rehab services included in purchase. Does not reflect any adjustments for leased facilities.
2. Estimated value when deal was announced (12/93). Given Regency's 3/17/94 stock price of $17.38, transaction is now worth approximately $165 million.
3. Estimated value when deal was announced (1/94). Given Sun Healthcare's 3/17/94 stock price of $25.50, transaction is now valued at approximately $430 million.
4. Trailing four quarters.
5. Estimated first year's revenues.
6. Previous year's U.S. revenues.
7. Annualized revenues.

Source: *The Genesis Report/MCx: Managed Care Strategic Planning* (November 1994).

Since general and administrative expenses may be reported (or juggled) to affect the reimbursement rate positively, the appraiser should study what is a fair allowance for these functions.

Certain principles should be kept in mind by the health care appraiser or analyst. They are

1) keep current on all transactions or have a network where information can be provided in an efficient, timely manner;

2) utilize transactions on a statewide basis;

3) confirm and analyze transactions in depth; and

4) compare facilities and make adjustments based on financial performance.

Other variables are generally difficult to quantify but should be considered.

An example of the application of a sales comparison approach grid is shown in Figure 5.6.

Conclusion

Nursing homes are probably the most common health care facilities that are appraised by real estate appraisers. Due to regulations and financing or reimbursement rates that vary from state to state, property values also vary extensively. Analysts must be familiar with the pertinent information and codes to properly study and appraise individual projects. Considerable research is required for a typical SNF whether it is small or large.

Figure 5.6	Sales Adjustment Grid					

Number		#1	#2	#3	#4	Subject
Name/Location		Pacific View 5200 Ocean Avenue City A	Valley C.H. 1800 Valley Avenue City B	Mountain C.H. 2300 Mountain Rd. City C	Tri-City C.H. 4000 Midway Rd. City C	Ocean View C.H. 5400 Sea Pine Road City D
Sales price		$2,600,000	$2,000,000	$2,047,500	$4,900,000	N/A
Size (gross S.F.)		28,065	19,527	14,976	60,000	22,856
Price per S.F.		$92.64	$102.42	$136.72	$81.67	N/A
# of Beds		99	99	64	176	71
Price Per Bed		$26,263	$20,202	$31,992	$27,841	N/A
Year Built		1959	1964	1961	1971	1961
Construction Type		WF/Stucco	WF/Stucco	WF/Stucco	WF/Stucco	WF/Stucco
Average bed size (S.F.)		283	197	234	341	322
Percent of private pay		16.12%	3.50%	35.00%	15.00%	89.00%
Occupancy at sale		N/A	95.17%	95.80%	79.55%	95.00%
Sales date		2/92	7/93	5/92	9/93	N/A
1.	Financing terms	($181,000)	$0	($154,000)	($320,000)	N/A
2.	Other terms	$0	$0	$0	$0	N/A
	Normal sales price	$2,419,000	$2,000,000	$1,893,500	$4,580,000	N/A
3.	Market trend	0.00%	0.00%	0.00%	0.00%	N/A
	Time adj. normal sales price	$2,419,000	$2,000,000	$1,893,500	$4,580,000	N/A
	Time adj. normal price/unit	$24,434	$20,202	$29,586	$26,023	N/A
4.	Location	0.00%	20.00%	0.00%	0.00%	N/A
5.	Facility size	0.00%	0.00%	0.00%	5.00%	N/A
6.	Age/condition	10.00%	10.00%	0.00%	-5.00%	N/A
7.	Quality	0.00%	0.00%	0.00%	0.00%	N/A
8.	Unit type/mix/size	0.00%	5.00%	5.00%	5.00%	N/A
9.	Project/unit amenities	0.00%	0.00%	0.00%	0.00%	N/A
10.	Income characteristics	25.00%	25.00%	10.00%	25.00%	N/A
	Sub-total adjustment	35.00%	60.00%	15.00%	30.00%	N/A
	Indicated value per/bed	$32,986	$32,323	$34,024	$33,830	N/A
	Total subject indicated value	$2,342,032	$2,294,949	$2,415,692	$2,401,898	N/A

Appraisers should also have the capability of analyzing the business component of the property because many assignments require a separate allocation for the real and personal property as well as the intangibles.

Future Medicaid cuts can have a major impact on the SNFs that serve the public pay market sector. The likelihood is that future government spending will be capped at growth rates of 8% in 1996, 7% in 1997, 6% in 1998, and 5% in 1999 and at 4% per year thereafter. Without these caps federal Medicaid spending was projected to increase from about $90 billion in 1995 to nearly $150 billion in 2000, an average growth of over 10% per year. Further, the funds are likely to be distributed to the states on a block-grant basis, effectively giving the states more control over their Medicaid programs. The negative impact on value from the spending cap is obvious. The implications of greater state control (regulations and funding) are unknown.

CHAPTER

SIX

Assisted Living Facilities

Assisted living facilities are designed to provide a level of personal care within a residential environment to residents who are generally frail and/or elderly. Typically such residents require assistance in one or more activities of daily living (ADLs) including housework, shopping, and meal preparation as well as with personal care.

The real estate projects are variously known as residential care facilities (RCFs), residential care facilities for the elderly (RCFEs), personal care facilities (PCFs), assisted living facilities (ALFs), residential care homes, board and care facilities, senior hotels, adult homes, domiciliary care homes, homes for the aged, foster care homes, adult foster care homes, catered living facilities, retirement homes, and community residences.

Resident characteristics can vary significantly from one project to another based on the objectives for which a project has been developed. Residents typically are in the middle of the continuum of care, between independent or congregate living and a nursing home residence. Varied emphasis on residents' age ranges and health status and the levels of assistance to be provided result in differing requirements for unit mix, unit size, services (e.g., health care, personal care or both), size of project, and other design features. Some assisted living facilities are specialized to serve unique health care markets such as Alzheimer's disease patients.

An assisted living facility is not a hospital, and its appearance should offer a home-like atmosphere that emphasizes the individual requirements of each resident. Assisted living units can be found in freestanding facilities and as wings or separate floors within congregate/independent living projects or nursing homes. Life care projects typically will have a separate personal care component as part of the continuum of care concept. Independent living projects are able to broaden their market appeal by providing a separate residential care section, which allows residents to stay in their existing surroundings even when their health starts to fail.

Assisted living is an economically attractive alternative to other living and care arrangements because of its favorable cost. A recent study[1] found that in one state assisted living saved up to 67% compared to home health care and up to 54% compared to skilled nursing care (see Table 6.1).

---

[1] JoAnn Clipp, "Pursuing the Frail Elderly," *Assisted Living Today*, 1995.

Table 6.1		Monthly Cost of Service to the Customer in Three States									

	Monthly Cost of Service ($)									
	Assisted Living			Home Health			Nursing		
Service/Expense[1]	MI	PA	NY	MI	PA	NY	MI	PA	NY
Basic Service[2]	1,909	2,340	2,085-2,700[3]	5,323	3,600	2,760[4]	3,534	4,125	5,170
Property Tax	NA	NA	NA	193	446	218	NA	NA	NA
Utilities	NA	NA	NA	60	170	110	NA	NA	NA
Property Insurance	NA	NA	NA	25	30	30	NA	NA	NA
Maintenance[5]	NA	NA	NA	100	100	100	NA	NA	NA
Total Cost	1,909	2,340	2,085-2,700	5,701	4,346	3,218	3,534	4,125	5,170

[1] For purposes of this study it is assumed that home appreciation will offset the interest income one would earn from the sale of their primary residence.
[2] Includes: Three meals per day; weekly housekeeping, weekly linens change; emergency response; seven hours of personal care; transportation (two times per week); activities (three per week); medication; care management; and overnight companion service.
[3] This fee ranges from $2,085 for an efficiency apartment to $2,700 for a two-bedroom, one and one-half bath apartment.
[4] Only two meals per day (main meal and sandwich).
[5] Assumes home maintenance to average $100 per month.
Source: Jo Ann Clipp, "Pursuing the Frail Elderly," *Assisted Living Today*.

Defining the Market

The market for assisted living facilities is larger than most people realize. Functional impairment is the measure by which a resident qualifies for occupancy in an assisted living facility. It is defined as a partial or complete inability to carry out activities of daily living (ADLs) such as bathing, dressing, toileting, eating, and ambulation, and instrumental activities of daily living (IADLs) such as doing housework, preparing meals, shopping, and performing other tasks considered essential to living alone. Obviously, assisted living facilities primarily serve the so-called "old-old" age market, which is exceedingly large and expected to grow rapidly in the future. For example, the age cohort of 85 and over, which currently numbers about 3,500,000 persons, is projected to increase 42% during the 1990s and 32% between the years 2000 and 2010 (see Table 6.2).

The large increases in the elderly population are due not only to the natural forward progression of larger-sized age groups but also to major increases in life expectancy. For example, life expectancy at age 85 has increased 24% since 1960 and is projected to increase another 44% by 2040. These enormous increases in life expectancy over a relatively short period of time are due to improved health, preventive care, and medical care. Nevertheless, older people will eventually get frail and need assistance with activities of daily living.

According to the U.S. General Accounting Office approximately 7 million older people need assistance with ADLs or IADLs at the present time and this figure could double by the year 2020. The National Health Interview Survey estimates that currently 56.8% of the population 85 and over need help with at least one ADL or IADL (see Figure 6.1).

Many older persons are often placed in institutional-like nursing homes because they or their families could not find or did not know of other, more appropriate residential care settings where 24-hour personal care is provided. Recent studies of nursing homes have found that some residents could have been placed in residential care settings. Providers have only begun

Table 6.2	Growth of Older U.S. Population: 1960 to 2050 (population numbers in thousands)								
		65 to 74 Years		75 to 79 Years		80 to 84 Years		85 Years & Over	
Year	All ages	Number	Percent*	Number	Percent*	Number	Percent*	Number	Percent*
Total Population									
1960	179,323	10,997	6.1	3,054	1.7	1,580	0.9	929	0.5
1970	203,302	12,447	6.1	3,838	1.9	2,286	1.1	1,409	0.7
1980	226,546	15,581	6.9	4,794	2.1	2,935	1.3	2,240	1.0
1990	248,710	18,045	7.3	6,103	2.5	3,909	1.6	3,201	1.2
Projected: Middle Series**									
2000	268,266	18,243	6.8	7,282	2.7	4,735	1.8	4,622	1.7
2010	282,575	21,039	7.4	6,913	2.4	5,295	1.9	6,115	2.2
2020	294,364	30,973	10.5	8,981	3.1	5,462	1.9	6,651	2.3
2030	300,629	35,988	12.0	13,023	4.3	8,464	2.8	8,129	2.7
2040	301,807	30,808	10.2	14,260	4.7	10,790	3.6	12,251	4.1
2050	299,849	31,590	10.5	12,042	4.0	9,613	3.2	15,287	5.1

* Percentage of total U.S. population
** Middle Series Projections: Middle Fertility, Mortality, and Immigration Assumptions
Source: U.S. Bureau of the Census, "Sixty-Five Plus in America," Current Population Reports, P23-178

Figure 6.1	Need for Assistance Among the 85 Year and Older Population

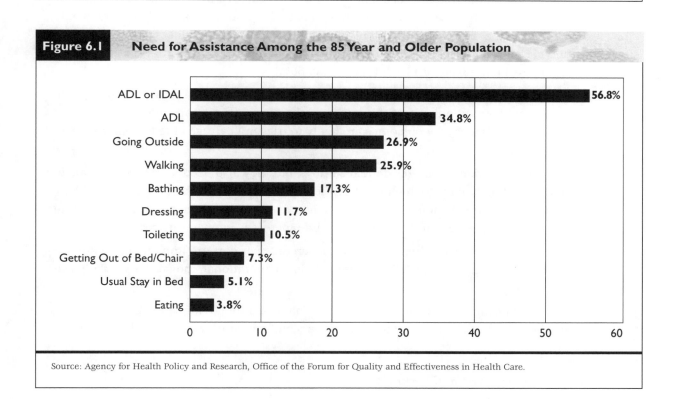

ADL or IDAL — 56.8%
ADL — 34.8%
Going Outside — 26.9%
Walking — 25.9%
Bathing — 17.3%
Dressing — 11.7%
Toileting — 10.5%
Getting Out of Bed/Chair — 7.3%
Usual Stay in Bed — 5.1%
Eating — 3.8%

Source: Agency for Health Policy and Research, Office of the Forum for Quality and Effectiveness in Health Care.

to recognize this market. In the past, the tendency was to move the slightly impaired group into nursing homes (intermediate or skilled). Now there is the fine recognition that many elderly persons can thrive in an assisted living facility designed to meet the needs of those with limited impairments at a lower cost.

There is no question that the size of the market needing assistance with ADL or IADL is much larger than most analysts have projected. However, some demographic factors that revolve around affordability could negatively impact the demand for future facilities, as could family and social traditions. Considerations include the financial impact of a move when one spouse requires personal care and another spouse must remain at home or that of financial support from family members. Ethnically, there are differences in family care provided to the aged. Lastly, the impact of home care, which serves many who can be marginally classified as potential residents of assisted care facilities, must be considered. Furthermore, the influence on future resources of national and other health plans, insurance, and other types of assistance programs is expected to be significant but cannot be accurately gauged on a macro-basis at this time.

Emerging Market Trends

While assisted living is recognized as the most cost-effective method for housing a frail, elderly population and is well positioned for future growth, there are uncertainties relative to resident turnover, future regulation, control of operating costs, pricing, and potential overconstruction. According to Jim Moore, a national seniors housing and health care consultant and president of the National Association for Senior Living Industries and of Moore Diversified Services, Inc., these five trends could change the assumptions about assisted living[2]:

1. *High acuity levels and high resident turnover.* Many operators have had visions that the residential or social model of assisted living would attract the frail elderly, who could be cared for with relative ease and at moderate cost. However, changing entitlement systems and managed care market forces are bringing high-acuity patients into nursing homes, and the effect is filtering through the levels of long-term care to assisted living. Add to that the natural effects of aging and it is not surprising that assisted living facilities are finding themselves with an unexpectedly high number of residents who need complex and expensive care. As a result, facilities are losing residents to institutions that provide more intensive care. A number of assisted living sponsors are experiencing annual resident turnover rates of more than 50%.

2. *Threat of regulation.* As acuity levels rise, assisted living may well cross the line into the domain of licensed nursing. If this happens, the types of assistance offered, staffing levels, and resident care outcomes are likely to trigger a barrage of federal and state regulations.

3. *Cost creep.* Residents want residential settings, but they also need increased assistance in activities of daily living, which must be met through a strong, albeit largely invisible, medical structure. Although this phenomenon does not entail the obvious large expense of high-acuity services, it does result in subtle increases in operating costs.

4. *Complex pricing systems.* In response to cost creep, operators are implementing tiered, multilevel pricing policies. While these policies seem rational, they cause marketplace confusion.

5. *Market proliferation.* The consumer demand that is assisted living's greatest strength may also be a weakness. Inexperienced developers and operators, eager to cash in on that

---

[2] Jim Moore, "Senior Housing," *Long Term Care*, March 1995.

demand, may overbuild. This could result in a glut of poorly planned facilities and a tarnished reputation for the industry, as people unfamiliar with assisted living underestimate the complexities of resident care.

A recent article in the *Wall Street Journal*[3] points out the attractiveness of ALFs to investors in terms of the rapid gains in stock prices for companies that have recently gone public and the large financial commitments that are being received for new facilities. Analysts are quoted as being unconcerned about the possibility of overcapacity, pointing out that many companies have pre-rented 80% of their units. Experts emphasize the advantages of an ALF over an SNF in terms of quality of life and also that most ALFs have the benefit of dealing only with privately paying residents. They point out that there is a strong move towards consolidation among ALFs, similar to that occurring in the SNF industry, and also point to the importance of strong management. One portfolio manager stated that "The industry is so new right now that any well-capitalized company could come in and steal the market. Assisted living is sure to take off, and once bigger companies focus on it, the whole industry could change."

Demand Factors

In analyzing the market for a proposed or existing facility, it is first necessary to establish a territory, service, or planning area for the subject project. Maximum driving time is a key factor and a 20- to 30-minute distance that allows for varied traffic conditions is generally considered acceptable to family members and friends.

Once the proposed market territory has been established, demographic data can be procured by computer from sources such as the Claritas Senior Life Report (see Appendix B), which supplies information by state, metropolitan statistical area (MSA), county, census tract, and numerous other breakdowns. Among demographic data that are available, in addition to standard information on population by age, household income by age of householder, and monthly owner cost as a percent of household income, etc., are estimates of the aged population with mobility and disability limitations. This latter type of information will be of interest to analysts because it provides counts of those individuals with a health condition (mental and/or physical) that has lasted for six or more months that makes it difficult for them to go outside the home alone.

As indicated earlier in this chapter, documentation of demand indicates a dramatic increase of the "old-old" in the coming decades (see Table 6.2). Affordability issues can dramatically affect the market potential of the project. If the size of the market of individuals who are 80 years or more and who need assistance with more than one ADL is 4,000,000 without consideration of income, the target market is reduced to 1,200,000 persons if 30% have incomes of $15,000 or more. Other variables influence the size of the market at any particular location.

As of 1995 basic fees of for-profit facilities range from approximately $38 (lower quartile) to $66 (upper quartile) per day and average about $53, compared to nursing homes which generally range from a low of about $70 to a high of about $150 per day and average about $90.[4]

Residents or their families generally pay the cost of care from their own financial resources. Only about 5% of those over the age of 65 have long-term care insurance; therefore, the source of reimbursement is limited. Government payments for assisted living mostly involve double-occupancy conditions and residency in older, "hotel-sized" projects. Some states provide subsidies in the form of additional payments to those who receive Supplemental Security Income

---

[3] "Assisted Living Health Centers Are Making Investors Feel Better," *Wall Street Journal*, February 26, 1996.

[4] See *The State of Seniors Housing 1995* (Washington, D.C.: American Seniors Housing Association) for assisted living costs; estimates for nursing homes are by the author.

(SSI). Oregon has pioneered a plan that uses Medicaid funds, SSI payments and state resources to make assisted living residences available to anyone in the state who needs this level of care. Under the Federal Medicaid Home and Community Care Options Act of 1990, states have the option to use Medicaid funds to support services for low-income, frail older persons in assisted living facilities.

The Health Care Financing Administration encourages continued government financing to assisted living through the Medicaid waiver program. Funds shifted from skilled nursing facilities to assisted living allow states to trade in institutional bed capacity for noninstitutional bed capacity. About 14 states have waivers permitting Medicaid funding for care and assisted living and other alternative facilities, although some states have been slow to take advantage of the program because they fear that it will be a cumbersome process.

In Oregon a client can choose a nursing home, assisted living facility, home care, adult foster care, or daycare. In this type of arrangement the money follows the individual and can be used wherever it is most appropriate. (See Appendix C for a state-by-state summary of regulations pertaining to assisted living, prepared by the American Health Care Association.)

Supply Factors

Considerations of supply are subject to exact measurement but are complicated by the terminology first discussed in this chapter. The Assisted Living Facilities Association of America estimates that there are 30,000 to 40,000 facilities housing an estimated 1,000,000 individuals in the United States. These facilities may be freestanding or combined with other residential options, such as independent living or nursing care; many are in older-type "rest homes." The analyst/appraiser is concerned primarily with larger facilities, typically 60 beds or more in size that are recently built (within the past 10 years) or are proposed.

The analyst is also concerned with estimating and analyzing "competitive" facilities. They are easily identified by management personnel, regulatory agencies, local senior center activists or organizations, and possibly by the local chamber of commerce. Typical assisted living facilities house between 25 and 120 individuals, but projects can range as high as 250 beds. Existing facilities range from converted hotels, schools, dormitories, convents, or single-family homes to specially constructed and designed residential care facilities. It should be noted that individual states vary in the level of care allowed in assisted living facilities; a number of states are currently considering revisions to their regulations. States have been encouraged to limit regulatory oversight to basic safety concerns and to avoid attempts to create quality through over-regulation.

Often confused, the number of living units and beds are both used to define the capacity of assisted living facilities. Beds are the most accurate measure because revenues are measured on an occupant basis and licenses are issued by states on the same basis. In most projects some units are designed for double occupancy. All residents typically require a varied level of care or assistance. It is rare to find an instance where couples reside in an assisted living unit and only one spouse requires assistance. Rate schedules typically provide for a variety of occupancy arrangements to maximize market penetration. Unrelated individuals may share a two-bed unit.

In determining the supply of competitive beds, it is imperative to properly determine what is appropriately competitive and which facilities serve alternate markets, as defined by income levels and quality of facilities. Most assisted living facilities charge month-to-month rates.

An example of a supply and demand analysis is shown in Table 6.3. In this study it might appear that the market is oversaturated with competitive ALF projects. Within a seven-miles trade area, over 40% of all persons over 75 years with an annual income of $15,000 or more are accounted for by existing beds, including the 82-bed subject. However, after classifying and categorizing the "competitive" beds to compare more properly to the subject, the saturation measure was cut in half to slightly more than 19% of the current $15,000-plus population. This particular project turned out to be highly successful. All units in the subject property were absorbed within a year, illustrating that well-managed and designed ALFs can succeed in what would otherwise appear to be an overdeveloped market.

Table 6.3	Market Saturation Analysis (within seven-mile radius)			
	Head of Household*	Without Subject 1,345 Beds	With Subject 1,427 Beds	Primary Competition With Subject 639 Beds
1994 Estimate				
75+, All Income	18,379	7.32%	7.76%	3.48%
75+, $15,000+ Income	3,353	40.11%	42.56%	19.06%
75+, $25,000+ Income	2,589	51.95%	55.12%	24.68%
75+, $35,000+ Income	2,160	62.27%	66.06%	29.58%
1999 Projection				
75+, All Income	20,720	6.49%	6.89%	3.08%
75+, $15,000+ Income	3,761	35.76%	37.94%	16.99%
75+, $25,000+ Income	2,936	45.81%	48.60%	21.76%
75+, $35,000+ Income	2,529	53.10%	56.43%	25.27%

Market saturation rates represent the percentage of total market demand necessary to absorb a) existing beds not including the subject, b) existing beds including the subject and c) subject and existing primary competitive beds. As of the date of appraisal, there are no new license applications for residential care beds in the subject property's primary market.

Evaluation of saturation rates:

Penetration Level	Estimate of Overall Market Demand
0-10%	Conservative
10-20%	Moderate
20%+	Aggressive

* Number of income and age qualifying senior households within seven miles of the subject site, as per National Planning Corporation.

Size and Age Data

Recent studies undertaken by an accounting firm for the American Seniors Housing Association surveyed various types of living facilities for seniors, including assisted living facilities.[5] From those statistics the following data dealing with ALFs have been extracted. The mean unit mix by age of facility is shown in Table 6.4. The total for all units surveyed shows 51.4% as studios, 26.6% as one-bedroom units, 7% as two-bedroom units, and 12.3% as other (an example of "other" could be a combination of two studios or a combination studio/one-bedroom or a junior one-bedroom).

Table 6.4	Mean Unit Mix by Age of Facility				
Type Unit	**Built 1970-79**	**Built 1980-85**	**Built 1986-90**	**Built 1991-93**	**Overall**
Studio	57.1%	77.3%	23.6%	94.4%	54.1%
1-Bedroom	42.9%	3.1%	43.1%	5.6%	26.6%
2-Bedroom	0	0	16.1%	0	7.0%
Other	0	19.6%	17.2%	0	12.3%

Source: American Seniors Housing Association

The mean unit size in square feet by age of facility is shown in Table 6.5. Studios average 348 square feet; one-bedroom units, 499 square feet; two-bedroom units, 836 square feet; and "other" units, 414 square feet. The gross building area per unit is typically 50% higher than the average rentable area.

Table 6.5	Mean Unit Size in Square Feet by Age of Facility		
Type Unit	**Built 1980-85**	**Built 1986-90**	**Built 1991-93**	**Overall**
Studio	288	366	391	348
1-Bedroom	374	519	605	499
2-Bedroom	None	836	None	836
Other	288	540	None	414

Source: American Seniors Housing Association

The median project age was six years (as of 1994), with 14% built before 1980, 59% between 1980-1989, and 27% after 1989. Median costs were $45,536 per unit for development and $47,244 for acquisition.

---

[5] *The State of Seniors Housing,* 1993 and 1995 reports prepared for the American Seniors Housing Association using survey data compiled by Coopers & Lybrand LLP.

Monthly Fees and Resident Turnover

Monthly fees by unit and age are set forth in Table 6.6. The most recently built facilities showed a mean monthly rent of $1,454 for studios, $1,650 for one-bedrooms, and $2,140 for two-bedroom units. Table 6.7 sets forth the same monthly fees by unit and region on a minimum, maximum, and mean basis. The 1995 survey reported monthly revenues per typical unit of $1,132 for the lower quartile, $1,575 for the median, and $1,978 for the upper quartile.

Table 6.6	Monthly Fees by Unit and Age		
Type	**Built 1970-79**	**Built 1980-85**	**Built 1986-90**
Studio	$936	$1,565	$1,454
1-Bedroom	$1,467	$2,430	$1,650
2-Bedroom	–	–	$2,140
Other	$1,059	$1,700	$1,704

Source: *The State of Seniors Housing 1993,* American Seniors Housing Association.

Table 6.7	Monthly Fees by Unit and Region								
	Southeast			**North Central**			**West**		
Type	**Minimum**	**Mean**	**Maximum**	**Minimum**	**Mean**	**Maximum**	**Minimum**	**Mean**	**Maximum**
Studio	$1,350	$1,522	$1,650	$575	$753	$855	$705	$1,439	$1,950
1-Bedroom	$1,350	$1,959	$2,430	$870	$900	$929	$748	$1,681	$2,225
2-Bedroom	$2,195	$2,198	$2,200	$1,183	$1,206	$1,229	$1,015	$2,152	$2,871
Other	$1,000	$1,763	$2,650	$829	$829	$829	$405	$1,701	$2,385

Source: *The State of Seniors Housing 1993,* American Seniors Housing Association (insufficient data reported for Northeast and South Central regions).

Annual resident turnover is probably the biggest headache for administrators because it means that the marketing program never ends. Median project turnover in the 1995 survey was 55%, which means that the typical resident only stays for 22 months. Most operators report a turnover range of two to three years per resident.

The biggest reason for turnover is the need for more care (42%). Other turnover factors include residents' moving in with family (10%) or to a competing facility (6%), financial hardships (7%), being a seasonal guest/snowbird (6%), and death (16%). These data show that price competition is not a significant problem but that management should focus its resident selection process on those who are most healthy and likely to stay for an extended period.

Financial Data

The financial performance results from the 1995 survey of 67 ALF projects are set forth in Table 6.8. This is exceedingly valuable information from which comparisons can be made with properties that are being appraised. The ALF projects in the survey show a high degree of profitability with a mean return on equity of 17.19% on a leveraged basis and 12.6% on an unleveraged basis. These figures exceed the return on investment of all senior housing investments.

Table 6.8	Assisted Living National Profile		
Description	**Lower Quartile**	**Assisted #/Mean/Median**	**Upper Quartile**
Property Profile			
Total number of properties		67	
Total number of units		5,948	
Total gross building area (SF)		3,137,154	
*Total cost per unit/bed	$35,635	$45,640	$58,482
*Total debt per unit/bed	$25,328	$32,785	$45,003
*Property age	1985	1988	1991
*Occupancy	90.0%	97.0%	100.0%
*Project size (units)	66	92	115
Revenue Profile			
Total annual revenues		$115,455,493	
*Revenues per unit/bed per year	$14,341	$18,824	$23,246
*Revenues per resident per month	$1,132	$1,575	$1,978
Expense Profile			
Total annual operating expenses		$83,655,078	
*Expenses per unit/bed per year	$10,652	$13,253	$16,370
*Expenses per resident per month	$813	$1,120	$1,579
Net Operating Income (NOI) Profile			
Total annual NOI		$31,434,759	
*NOI per unit/bed per year	$3,084	$5,105	$7,080
*NOI per resident per month	$247	$407	$537

(continued)

Table 6.8	Assisted Living National Profile (continued)		
Description	Lower Quartile	Assisted #/Mean/Median	Upper Quartile
Departmental Annual Expense/Resident			
*Wages and benefits	$760	$1,179	$1,918
*Property taxes and insurance	$522	$739	$1,039
*Raw food	$1,107	$1,299	$1,487
*Utilities	$675	$803	$1,152
*Management fees	$653	$933	$1,337
*All other departmental expenses	$949	$1,234	$2,011
Operating Highlights			
*Gross margin (NOI/revenue)	19.0%	28.0%	35.0%
*Raw food per resident day	$3.03	$3.56	$4.07
*Annual resident turnover	42.0%	55.0%	71.0%
*FTE's per resident	0.31	0.43	0.53
% Annual change in occupancy		8.0%	
*Annual % change - in-house rents	3.0%	4.0%	4.0%
*Annual % change - street rents	3.0%	4.0%	5.3%
*Capital expenditures per unit/bed	$204	$297	$468
Financial Highlights			
*Debt coverage ratio	1.1	1.6	1.9
*Debt to equity ratio	2.9	4.0	7.8
% Properties covering debt service		76.8%	
*Return on equity (leveraged)	3.6%	17.1%	35.1%
*Return on investment (unleveraged)	8.3%	12.6%	15.9%

*Denotes median statistics

Source: *The State of Seniors Housing 1995,* American Seniors Housing Association and Coopers & Lybrand LLP. Reprinted with permission.

Other key statistics are summarized below:

	Lower Quartile	Median	Upper Quartile
Management fees (% of revenue)	4.9%	5.0%	6.0%
Property taxes & insurance (% of revenue)	3.8%	3.9%	4.4%
Capital expenditures or reserves (% of revenue)	1.5%	1.6%	2.0%

Design and Construction

The architecture of assisted living facilities should respond to residents' needs and enhance the quality of their lives. Among the unique design elements that must be considered are the placement and location of doors, electric switches, lighting, cabinets, faucets and handles, call pulls, and thermostats. Other considerations include access to cooking facilities, circulation for walkers or wheelchairs, the height of closet shelves, rods, grab-bars, and towel racks, open shelving, color coding, and so on. Many projects do not provide cooking facilities in the unit, and others are limited to "mini-kitchens." (Figure 6.2 shows a typical studio/alcove unit.) Residents typically provide their own furniture and other furnishings, but many residents do not.

Private occupancy units are most responsive to the residents' need for privacy, dignity, and autonomy, which may mean that double-occupancy units will be harder to market if the supply of private units increases. Nevertheless, double-occupancy units are required at certain income levels; the percentage of need for such units would be revealed by market analysis and a financial feasibility study.

Other than specific design features that are necessary for this market, the common facilities in an assisted living project are comparable and typical of those in congregate types of senior living facilities. These include a dining room, meeting/activity area(s), reception area, and beauty salon, along with areas for management offices, service facilities, kitchen, storage, and maintenance. An example of a simplified floor plan of typical common facilities is shown in Figure 6.3.

Unit sizes vary greatly depending on the economics of the targeted market. Not counting low-income boarding homes, the units in most assisted living projects in urban areas fall into two broad categories: hotel-sized or apartment-sized units.

- *Hotel-Sized Units.* Sized to reach maximum market penetration, these projects will typically range from 300 to 600 square feet per bed. Individual units will range in size from 220 to 380 square feet and double-occupancy units as small as 250 square feet. These units typically have no kitchen. Bathroom arrangements range from two-fixture, half bath (with common bathing rooms) to shared baths (with a connecting unit) to full baths with walk-in shower. Shared baths are not recommended and should be considered as an item of functional obsolescence.

- *Apartment-Sized Units.* The total square footage per bed for these more upscale assisted living facilities ranges from 600 to 950 square feet and averages 800 square feet. Individual units range in size from 380 to 610 square feet, with double occupancies typically in the larger units. A kitchen is generally included, but some units will be limited to a mini-kitchen and others may not have ovens and ranges for special residents. All units will have at least one full bathroom, and larger units may have one-and-one-half baths.

Circulation Features
All circulation space dimensions for ease of circulation in walkers and wheelchairs
Pocket or folding doors wherever possible to eliminate door clearance requirements
Provide built-in night light on path to bedroom
All passage doors to be 3' wide for ease of passage in wheelchairs
Bath situated for easy direct circulation from sleeping area and convenient to living area.
Open plan area with no corridors for ease of movement through unit and direct access by nurse's aide.

Fixtures
Thermostat with large numerals mounted at 48"
Mount electrical outlets at 18" to 24" above floor
Mount switches 36" to 40" above floor for easy reach for wheelchair and walker residents
Adjustable height closet shelf and rod between 46" and 60"
Pull u-shaped handles on doors (no knobs) for persons with limited dexterity
Wall mounted task lighting at sink area to eliminate shadows

Special Features
Lockset to prevent accidental lockout
Emergency call pulls in bedroom and bathroom areas.
Wall mounted sconce light for front door image and identity
Tenant identity feature and entrance for orientation and easy recognition of the resident's unit.
Overhead light in closet for better visibility
Open shelving for ease of access. Bottom shelf at 18" to reduce stooping.
Beverage bar with outlet for microwave, sink, and refrigerator on 18" high platform

Materiality and layout
Utilize wood cabinets for residential character
Recessed entry for identity and to break the corridor (institution image)
Unit configuration includes turret for residential character and expanded space.
Drop down sprinkler heads for residential appearance

Bathroom amenities
Grab bar towel rack for safety. Vinalized (colored) grab bars with contrast to wall color for residential character and visibility.
Continuous grab bar from shower to water closet for movement between fixtures
Counter hung lavatory with removable front panel for residential character
Large floor area in bath for wheelchair/walker refuge and ambulation, and to accommodate assisted bathing.
Shower controls mounted on entry side of shower for temperature adjustment prior to entry or by nurse's aide
Slip resistant shower with built-in or fold-down seat, anti-scald device and detachable spray head.

Plan reprinted with permission from *Assisted Living Housing For the Elderly*, by Victor Regnier, Van Nostrand Reinhold, New York, 1994.

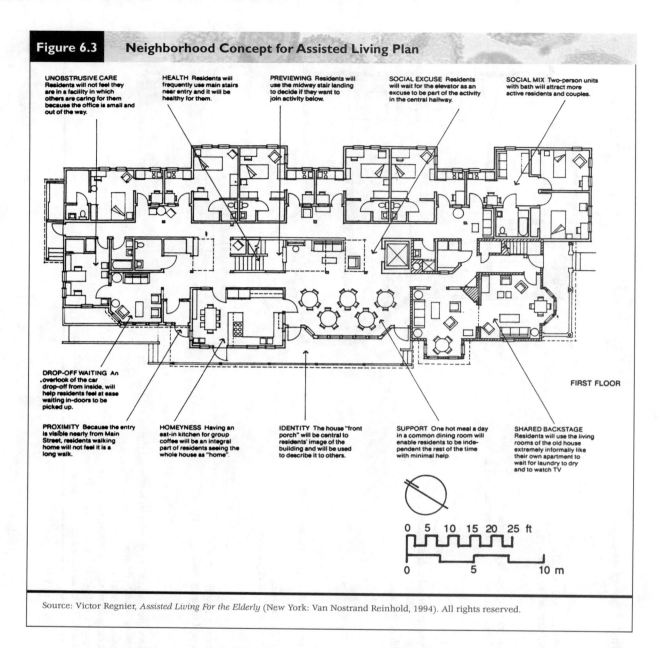

Figure 6.3   **Neighborhood Concept for Assisted Living Plan**

UNOBSTRUSIVE CARE Residents will not feel they are in a facility in which others are caring for them because the office is small and out of the way.

HEALTH Residents will frequently use main stairs near entry and it will be healthy for them.

PREVIEWING Residents will use the midway stair landing to decide if they want to join activity below.

SOCIAL EXCUSE Residents will wait for the elevator as an excuse to be part of the activity in the central hallway.

SOCIAL MIX Two-person units with bath will attract more active residents and couples.

DROP-OFF WAITING An overlook of the car drop-off from inside, will help residents feel at ease waiting in-doors to be picked up.

PROXIMITY Because the entry is visible nearly from Main Street, residents walking home will not feel it is a long walk.

HOMEYNESS Having an eat-in kitchen for group coffee will be an integral part of residents seeing the whole house as "home".

IDENTITY The house "front porch" will be central to residents' image of the building and will be used to describe it to others.

SUPPORT One hot meal a day in a common dining room will enable residents to be independent the rest of the time with minimal help.

SHARED BACKSTAGE Residents will use the living rooms of the old house extremely informally like their own apartment to wait for laundry to dry and to watch TV

FIRST FLOOR

0 5 10 15 20 25 ft

0   5   10 m

Development costs of assisted living facilities are similar to typical congregate/elderly projects, and both are similar in development costs to hotels. Based on Marshall Valuation Service, a good quality, Class C (insurance rating) home for the elderly has a base cost of $75.57 per square foot (before adjustments for sprinklers, elevators, balconies, canopies, basements, time, and location). This compares with a good Class C hotel with a base cost of $70.19 per square foot. Homes for the elderly are slightly higher in unit cost due to the higher degree of life safety requirements and special designs for elderly residents.

- *Other Projects (Conversions).* A variety of development models exist in the ALF market, ranging from converted buildings to state-of-the-art European models. Some developers and operators have acquired vacant hotels and motels in overbuilt lodging markets such as Florida for the purpose of conversion to an ALF. These projects may be cost effective and appropriate for certain income/rental levels, but design inefficiencies and institutional appearance may present marketing disadvantages. Some conversion projects have been successful and others have failed. The appraiser needs to apply an extra amount of effort in the analysis and valuation of such projects to make sure that the developer is not attempting to place a round peg into a square hole.

Management and Operations

While physical design and amenities are very important considerations in creating a successful facility, the programs, staffing levels, and other aspects of resident care and services are equally important. A management plan that addresses the needs profiles of the targeted resident group is a critical factor to a successful operation. The residents' individual and collective needs, skills, interests, and preferences should control the day-to-day implementation of carefully prepared policies, objectives, and standards.

The management plan should be centered on four critical areas: resident care and service, staff organization, staff development, and physical environment. A key factor involves the interaction of staff and residents. Anticipated benefits for the residents of this organizational structure include increased ADL functioning and reduction of confusion, memory loss, and social withdrawal as well as a reduction in medication use. Anticipated benefits for the staff include improved morale and attitude, increased accountability, and reductions of staff turnover and absenteeism. The development of personal relationships between staff and residents can increase the expectations of the staff regarding resident capabilities and potential and increased personal satisfaction.

Documented standards for the care, services, amenities, and benefits available at the facility are communicated through residency agreements, residents' handbook, and written procedures for handling grievances and suggestions. A residents' council is also important. It is important to recognize that an assisted living facility is an operating business enterprise with special departments and functions including administration, accounting, health and food services, housekeeping, laundry, maintenance, and security. The *Assisted Living Manual* published by the Assisted Living Facilities Association of America is recommended reading for appraisers and other analysts who are or hope to be specializing in this unique property type.

Lastly, it should be noted that assisted living facilities operate within a carefully defined regulatory climate that involves detailed licensure requirements and rules and regulations that vary from state to state. It is critical that the operator provide only those services that are clearly within the scope of the facility's license.

Highest and Best Use Considerations

The appraiser may be confronted with a situation wherein a developer proposes to initiate a new elderly housing project based on a congregate type of housing. This was typical in the 1980s, and an extraordinary number of projects were completed. Unfortunately an excessive number of independent and congregate housing developments were developed primarily because of the ease with which projects could be financed along with a misunderstanding of the requirements of the market. Many developers failed to realize that the true need was for more assisted living beds. Most seniors prefer to stay in their existing arrangement and won't consider moving until their care needs require or necessitate a change. Thus, it is incumbent upon the analyst/appraiser to recognize that the demand factor is primarily influenced by those with care needs and that a proposed elderly housing project should at worst have a mix of assisted living beds and congregate type of housing.

Recognition of these market elements early in the development stage is imperative because of the special design considerations that are required by assisted living facilities. In a number of cases projects have been reconfigured from all or part congregate housing to assisted living beds. In such situations, the actual capacity of the housing component of the project may be increased, but this is not a critical element as far as market feasibility is concerned.

The important thing about the highest and best use analysis is that it brings together the various aspects of supply and demand, costs, revenues, and expenses in a way that can reveal the financial feasibility of a venture as well as comparative yields for various alternatives involving the mix of level of care, beds, and housing units.

Relative to highest and best use, the notion of critical mass is recognized but there is no consensus as to the optimal size of a facility except that a range of 50 to 100 units is preferred. Also, the most efficient size is not only a function of operational staffing and organization but the length of time it takes to reach normalized occupancy whether it be 97%, 95%, or 90%. Up to a point larger facilities are the most efficient, but that assumes an equally large, continuous, and stable market of new residents to maximize the occupancy level.

For these reasons as well as risk management, most new projects are sized from 80 to 120 beds. This is not to say that an upscale 50-bed project is not feasible. There are many such developments in niche markets that are highly successful, but the key to efficiency may be operation of a group of these facilities under a single management organization.

Valuation Methodology

All three approaches are applicable to the appraisal of assisted living facilities. The biggest problem is application of the sales comparison approach since, in any market area, there is generally a paucity of improved sales. Of those that are available, some will likely have been consummated as a result of the excesses of the 1980s, the inability of an owner to refinance a loan, or poor management.

Cost Approach

Newer projects are good candidates for a valuation estimate by the cost approach. The estimate of depreciation for older assisted living projects, especially rest homes, is difficult due to a high degree of obsolescence or the fact that the improvements represent a conversion from some other type of residential or institutional use. Many design inadequacies may be present.

In the valuation of land, the appraiser may be faced with a problem typical of all health care facilities: the site may be surrounded by a neighborhood zoned for low-density residential uses that are not appropriate indicators of the unique locational aspects of the subject. They also may not reflect the value of development entitlements such as a use permit, zoning variance, or planned unit development (PUD). Therefore, if the subject site is clearly not in a commercial zone, it is recommended that the appropriate land comparables should be those with a similar housing density. Obviously, the best comparables are sites acquired for the same purpose. The appraiser is justified in going out of the immediate area to use such comparables.

As far as the replacement cost estimate is concerned, actual or trended cost estimates are preferred, followed by comparable cost data for similar assisted living facilities. Average cost data (e.g., those reported previously in this chapter) or square foot cost data from a published cost manual are least preferred. Where heavy reliance is placed on the cost approach estimate, the greatest possible degree of accuracy should be applied to the replacement cost estimate.

Assisted living facilities are quite expensive to develop because of the small unit size and the density of costly components such as HVAC, plumbing, and electrical installations. Assisted living facilities are more costly than hotels with a similar quality rating or type of construction. Unit cost breakdowns for assisted living facilities from the *Marshall Valuation Service* "Homes for the Elderly" category appear in Table 6.9. These unit costs must be adjusted for additional factors such as time, locale, sprinklers, elevators, decks/balconies, and height.

Table 6.9 Homes for the Elderly (Calculator Method)

CLASS	TYPE	EXTERIOR WALLS	INTERIOR FINISH	LIGHTING, PLUMBING AND MECHANICAL	HEAT	COST Sq. M.	Cu. Ft.	Sq. Ft.
A	Good	Face brick, metal and glass, architectural concrete	Plaster or drywall, carpeting, vinyl composition, ceramic tile	*Good lighting, alarm system, some special plumbing fixtures	Hot & chilled water (zoned)	$981.14	$9.12	$91.15
A	Average	Brick, concrete or metal and glass, little ornamentation	Plaster or drywall, carpet, vinyl composition	*Adequate lighting/plumbing, some extras	Warm & cool air (zoned)	765.86	7.12	71.15
A	Low cost	Concrete block or panels, little trim	Plaster or drywall, painted block, low cost carpet, vinyl composition	*Minimum lighting/plumbing	Hot water	606.44	5.63	56.34
B	Good	Face brick, metal and glass, architectural concrete	Plaster or drywall, carpeting, vinyl composition, ceramic tile	*Good lighting, alarm system, some special plumbing fixtures	Hot & chilled water (zoned)	956.38	8.89	88.85
B	Average	Brick, concrete or metal and glass, some ornamentation	Plaster or drywall, some exposed block, carpeting, vinyl composition	*Adequate lighting/plumbing, some extras	Warm & cool air (zoned)	744.65	6.92	69.18
B	Low cost	Concrete block or panels, little trim	Exposed block, acoustic tile, drywall, vinyl composition	*Minimum lighting/plumbing	Hot water	588.36	5.47	54.66
C	Good	Face brick, metal or concrete and glass, good design	Plaster or drywall, vinyl composition, some carpeting and ceramic tile	*Good lighting, alarm system, some special plumbing fixtures	Warm & cool air (zoned)	813.44	7.56	75.57
C	Average	Brick or block, concrete panels, little ornamentation	Plaster or drywall, some exposed block, carpeting, vinyl composition	*Adequate lighting/plumbing, few extras	Hot water	614.19	5.71	57.06
C	Low cost	Brick, block, concrete panels, very plain	Exposed block, drywall, vinyl composition	*Minimum lighting/plumbing	Forced air	463.93	4.31	43.10
D	Good	Brick veneer, best stucco or siding, good trim	Plaster or drywall, vinyl composition, some carpeting and ceramic tile	*Good lighting, alarm system, some special plumbing fixtures	Warm & cool air (zoned)	774.79	7.20	71.98
D	Average	Brick veneer, good stucco or siding, some trim	Plaster or drywall, acoustic tile, vinyl composition	*Adequate lighting/plumbing, few extras	Hot water	582.98	5.42	54.16
D	Low cost	Stucco or siding	Drywall, vinyl composition	*Minimum lighting/plumbing	Forced air	438.74	4.08	40.76
S	Good	Best sandwich panels, good fenestration and ornamentation	Drywall, good finish, good carpet and vinyl composition	*Good lighting, alarm system, some special plumbing fixtures	Warm & cool air (zoned)	782.22	7.27	72.67
S	Average	Sandwich panels, little trim	Drywall, carpet, vinyl composition	*Adequate lighting/plumbing	Hot water	577.49	5.37	53.65

BASEMENTS

CLASS	TYPE	EXTERIOR WALLS	INTERIOR FINISH	LIGHTING, PLUMBING AND MECHANICAL	HEAT	Sq. M.	Cu. Ft.	Sq. Ft.
A-B	Finished basement	Finished interior	Plaster or drywall, vinyl composition, therapy and housekeeping rooms	Adequate lighting/plumbing, high voltage outlets	Hot water	$461.67	$4.29	$42.89
CDS	Finished basement	Finished interior	Plaster or drywall, asphalt tile, therapy and housekeeping rooms	Adequate lighting/plumbing high voltage outlets	Forced air	336.05	3.12	31.22

Fireplaces, balconies, and built-in appliances are not included.

BASEMENT UNITS – Use 80% of comparable above ground units. For semi-basement living units, use 90%.

MULTISTORY BUILDINGS – Add .5% (1/2%) for each story, over three, above ground, to all base costs, excluding mezzanines, up to 30 stories; over 30 add .4% (4/10%) for each additional story.

CANOPIES – Large entrance marquees or carport canopies generally cost 1/4 to 2/5 of the final base cost per square foot of the building, or they may be computed from the Segregated Costs, Section 41, or from Unit-in-Place Costs.

BALCONIES – Exterior balconies generally cost 1/5 to 1/3 of the final base cost per square foot of the building, or they may be computed from the Segregated Costs, Section 41, or from the Unit-in-Place Costs.

*ELEVATORS (Homes for the Elderly) – Buildings marked with an asterisk (*) include elevator costs. If elevators are not included in your subject property, deduct the following from the base costs on this page which are so marked. For buildings not marked, or for basement or mezzanine stops, add costs from Page 21.

	Sq. M.	Sq. Ft.		Sq. M.	Sq. Ft.		Sq. M.	Sq. Ft.
CLASS A & B								
Good	$28.52	$2.65	Average	$20.99	$1.95	Low cost	$15.61	$1.45
CLASS C, D & S								
Good	$18.30	$1.70	Average	$13.46	$1.25	Low cost	$10.23	$.95

SPRINKLERS – Systems are not included. Costs should be added from Page 21.

MEZZANINES – Do not use story height or area-perimeter multipliers with mezzanine costs.

Source: *Marshall Valuation Service*, Marshall & Swift, March 1996, Section 11, p. 16.

In addition to building construction, assisted living facilities will have additional costs for yard improvements, landscaping, paving, parking, underground utilities, etc. The replacement costs for these items can be measured on a unit basis based on the appropriate measure of quantity (i.e., square feet, lineal feet, number of items, etc.). Due to the shorter useful lives of these components, the percentage rate for depreciation will be greater than that for the improvements.

Assisted living facilities also have a component for personal property or furniture, fixtures, and equipment (FF&E). At the minimum, the project will be furnished with kitchen, dining, housekeeping, maintenance, office, and common area equipment and furnishings. In most projects the residents will bring in their own personal furniture and necessary household items. This is a variable factor, however, and it is not uncommon for resident rooms to be fully furnished. The cost of FF&E can be quite substantial but so can the amount of depreciation due to the relatively short life expectancy of this type of property.

An example of a cost approach analysis is shown in Figure 6.4.

Sales Comparison Approach

As stated earlier, it is often difficult to find recent sales of similar assisted living facilities. Successful projects are rarely sold as full going concerns unless a special motivation is involved (e.g., typically they are not being operated to their full potential). Similarly, there will be very few transactions involving leased facilities relative to physical assets. Therefore, it is necessary to extend the geographic area for investigation. The appraiser also should be extremely careful about dealing with time adjustments. It is acceptable to use sales of congregate housing projects as long as they do not represent the only source of comparison and they are properly adjusted. Valuation indications may be based upon price per bed, price per square foot of building area, or a gross revenue multiplier. In laying out a grid, the appraiser typically considers factors such as terms of sale, time, square feet of project area per bed, quality of construction, condition, location (as reflected in the rate structure), operating expense ratio, and financial capability.

In most respects the financial capability of the property, i.e., net operating income per bed, is a controlling factor. However, most reviewers expect a grid to deal with physical, functional, and economic factors, and therefore the test of the appraiser's ability is to put proper weight on the key factors. It is best to use more than one valuation indicator in the sales comparison approach. However, the expediencies of developing and explaining a single grid are such that this is not practical in many instances.

Unless comparables are unusually abundant or unless there is a comparable involving a virtually similar property, appraisers commonly recognize that a sales comparison approach is only capable of developing a valuation range. This type of valuation result should be preferred. An example of a sales summary appears in Table 6.10, which develops a variety of unit value indicators. The appraiser should have inspected each of the comparables, provided one or more photographs, interviewed the key parties involved in the operation and transaction, and properly analyzed the economics of the business.

The most recent *The Senior Care Acquisition Report*[6] includes statistics on over 700 transactions for a five-year period from 1991 through 1995. Statistics for 1995 include 89 nursing home transactions and 53 dealing with retirement housing/assisted living facilities. Assisted living projects have increased substantially in desirability in the last couple of years, and their unit prices now exceed those paid for unlicensed retirement/congregate facilities by 15%. The average unit price reported for ALFs was $43,500 in 1994 and $59,600 in 1995. *The Senior Care*

---

[6] *The Senior Care Acquisition Report* (New Canaan, CT: Irving Levin Associates, Inc., 1996).

Component/Item	Units (SF or #)	Cost (SF or Unit)	Replacement Cost—Total
Direct Costs[1]			
Indicated base cost (above ground)	44,171	$87.65	$3,871,588
Indicated base cost (basement area)	18,521	$22.28	$412,648
Paving and landscaping	18,435	$2.00	$36,870
Total Direct Costs	62,692	$68.93	$4,321,106
Indirect Costs			
Operational overhead/fees	4.00%	Direct Cost	$172,844
Legal/Other	62,692	$0.32	$20,000
Permanent Loan Fees	2.00%	$5,600,000	$112,000
Total indirect costs	62,692	$4.86	$304,844
Subtotal (Direct/Indirect)	62,692	$73.79	$4,625,950
Furniture/Fixtures/Equipment (FF&E)	135	$5,000	$675,000
Other/Miscellaneous	0	$0	$0
Total FF&E	135	$5,000	$675,000
Subtotal (Direct/Indirect)	62,692	$84.56	$5,300,950
Add: Entrepreneurial Profit	15.00%	$12.68	$795,143
Total Improvement Cost New	62,692	$97.24	$6,096,093
Less depreciation:			
Improvements (physical)	-20.00%	($16.97)	($1,063,969)
Improvements (functional)	0.00%	$0.00	$0
Improvements (economic)	0.00%	$0.00	$0
FF&E (physical+economic)	-50.00%	($6.19)	($388,125)
Total depreciation	62,692	($23.16)	($1,452,094)
Improvement depreciated value	62,692	$74.08	$4,643,999
Add: Land/site value	39,196	$35.00	$1,371,860
Total depreciated fee simple value	62,692	$95.96	$6,015,859
Rounded to:	62,692	$95.71	$6,000,000
Fee simple value per bed	135		$44,444
Fee simple value per room	114		$52,632

Figure 6.4 — Cost Approach Summary of 114-Unit, 135-Bed Assisted Living Facility

[1] *Marshall Valuation Service,* "Homes for Elderly" (Section 11, p. 17). All other figures from the author.

Table 6.10

Improved Sales Comparables Summary Chart

Name	Number of Rooms	Sales Date	Sales Price	Price per Room	Year Built	Size (GBA)	Price per SF	Gross Avg. Unit Size	Gross Oper. Inc.	Net Oper. Inc.	NOI/ Room	OAR	GIM	Occ. at Sale	% of Exp.	Unit Income/ Month
Comparable A	110	10/91	$5,250,000	$47,727	1975	50,000	$105.00	455	$1,573,296	$550,654	$5,006	10.49%	3.34	80%	65%	$14,303 $1,192
Comparable B	140	6/91	$7,300,000	$52,143	1988	108,116	$67.52	722	$1,855,578	$805,578	$5,754	11.04%	3.93	62%	57%	$13,254 $1,105
	140	7/94	$6,785,000	$48,464	1988	108,116	$62.76	772	$1,855,578	$805,578	$5,754	11.87%	3.66	62%	57%	
Comparable C	64	2/91	$2,325,000	$36,328	1972	32,291	$72.00	505	$637,200	$254,880	$3,983	10.96%	3.65	92%	60%	$9,956 $830
Comparable D	34	Pending Sale 6/94	$2,400,000	$70,588	1985	21,000	$114.29	618	$892,800	$312,480	$9,191	13.02%	2.69	91%	65%	$26,259 $2,188
Comparable E	138	3/90	$13,300,000	$96,377	1987	90,000	$147.78	652	$3,427,835	$1,683,067	$12,196	12.65%	3.88	75%	51%	$24,839 $2,070
Comparable F	119	3/90	$10,000,000	$84,034	1988	85,760	$116.60	721	$2,989,550	$1,349,000	$11,336	13.49%	3.45	70%	54%	$24,358 $2,030
Comparable G	132	3/90	$13,000,000	$98,485	1988	119,400	$108.88	905	$3,367,876	$1,627,609	$12,330	12.52%	3.86	67%	52%	$25,514 $2,126
Comparable H	114	12/92	$4,200,000	$36,842	1985	70,216	$59.82	616	$1,746,086	$615,130	$5,484	14.88%	2.35	92%	67%	$15,317 $1,276
Subject	82				1989	44,117	N/A	538	$2,327,392	$967,436	$11,798			97.56%	56.24%	$28,383 $2,365

Acquisition Report also includes separate ALF data for capitalization rates and effective gross income multipliers (*EGIM*). The average *EGIM* for ALFs in 1995 was 2.9.

Income Approach

Primary emphasis is given in virtually all assignments to the valuation results indicated by income capitalization. It is typical to use a direct comparison technique for a well-established assisted living facility and a discounted cash flow technique for one that has not reached a stabilized level of operation or is undergoing a highly irregular level of operating results. The two primary sources of revenue are monthly rentals and charges for ancillary services. Other income may be derived from rentals and services, etc.

The analysis of income producing potential begins with a survey of the competition and a comparative study of rental amounts on an aggregate and square foot basis (see Table 6.11).

Table 6.11			Comparable Rental Survey								
Rental	Units	Unit Size (SF)	Monthly Rent/ Private Room	Private Room Rent/SF	Semi-Private Rooms	Private Pay (% Res.)	SSI Residents (% Res.)	Reported Occupancy	Facility Age	Remarks	
1	76	225	$1,400	$6.22	Only 2	98%	2%	95%	1978		
		350	$1,800	$5.14							
2	90	240	$1,050	$4.38	Yes	65%	35%	90%	1977/	New wing added 1992	
		400	$1,800	$4.50					1992	Remodeled old wing	
3	125	468	$1,250	$2.67	Yes	90%	10%	100%	1977		
		648	$1,500	$2.31							
4	164	200	$1,250	$6.25	None	100%	0%	90%	1977		
		350	$1,650	$4.71							
5	102	275	$950	$3.45	Only 2	100%	0%	96%	1977		
		400	$2,500	$6.25							
6	88	360	$1,700+	$4.72+	None	100%	0%	95%	1990		
		520	$2,600+	$5.00+							
		720	$3,000+	$4.17+							
7	100	413	$2,595	$6.28	None	100%	0%	92%	1991		
		464	$2,995	$6.45							
		600	$3,995	$6.66							
Subj.*	82	285	$2,475	$8.68	None	100%				Double rooms with double occupancy.	
		296	$2,358	$7.97							
		303	$2,405	$7.94							
		314	$2,312	$7.36							
		354	$2,588	$7.31							
		423	$3,175	$7.51							
		445	$3,050	$6.85							
		606 (av)	$3,895 (av)	$6.43 (av)							

* The subject property's rental rates are actual and are increased annually by 3% on the anniversary of the tenant's move-in date.

Operating expenses fall into the categories of nursing care, dietary, housekeeping, laundry and linens, recreation, social services, general and administrative, repairs and maintenance, utilities, taxes, insurance, management, and reserves. When all operating expenses are included, typical ratios will be in the range of 55% to 70%. The primary component of operating expenses is salaries, which can represent as much as two-thirds of all operating expenses. In the income approach example here (Table 6.12) the revenue and expense categories have been set out by department. Since most of the expenses are fixed in nature, the break-even point is typically in the 70% occupancy range. The average ALF expense ratio was 68% in 1994 and 1995, as reported in *The Senior Care Acquisition Report*.[7]

Capitalization rates are difficult to derive because of the lack of usable transactions and the fact that few if any investor yield surveys are conducted on a continuing and reliable basis. Capitalization rates must reflect a component for the business, which means that apartment houses and independent housing transactions are really not appropriate. However, with proper investigation, capitalization rates derived from sales of congregate housing projects as well as skilled nursing facilities can be applicable if the projects have a similar degree of economic performance and future outlook. Based on a recent informal survey conducted by the author, capitalization rates for assisted living projects were in the range of 11.5% to 13% for good properties. The average ALF capitalization rate was 11.59% in 1994 and 11.1% in 1995, according to the Levin report.[8]

Conclusion

Assisted living projects have an important role to play in the provision for senior housing. An assisted living facility is not a hospital and it should provide a home-like atmosphere that emphasizes the individual requirements of each resident. Contribution of management is critical to the success of such enterprises. Facilities with an established reputation and solid history of profitable operating performance can have substantial business or goodwill value.

The market for assisted living facilities is larger than most people realize. The future outlook is excellent because a large portion of the elderly will require the level of care that is only available in assisted living projects. These facilities are also much less expensive to occupy than skilled nursing facilities, and they represent an environment that is conducive to good health and a longer life. There are unrecognized markets for assisted living facilities as well as niche arrangements where there is an overabundance of, say, congregate housing or where a large number of residents have been unnecessarily placed in skilled nursing facilities.

Successful assisted living facilities can be relatively modest in size and new projects can be successful with as few as 50 beds. The traditional rest home is much smaller than this, but the level of care involved in such operations is not comparable to the types of projects that have been developed in recent years.

It is important for the analyst and appraiser to understand the operations of such facilities. Through a study of available literature as well as visits to a variety of facilities and interviews with management representatives, one can recognize the elements of success and become a specialist in this growing field of elderly and disabled housing.

---

[7] Ibid.

[8] Ibid.

Table 6.12	Income Approach Summary - An Upscale Project		
	Total Amount	**As a % of EGI**	**$ Amount Per Bed**
Rental income	$2,302,392	104.13%	$28,078
Other income	$25,000	1.13%	$305
Total gross income	$2,327,392	105.26%	$28,383
Less vacancy (@5%)	$116,370	5.26%	$1,419
Effective gross income	$2,211,022	100.0%	$26,964
Less expenses (by department)			
General and administrative	$122,363	5.53%	$1,492
Management	$110,551	5.00%	$1,348
Advertising/marketing	$22,110	1.00%	$270
Accommodations/housekeeping	$275,831	12.48%	$3,364
Utilities	$91,463	4.14%	$1,115
Maintenance/repairs	$62,393	2.82%	$761
Activities/transportation	$8,488	0.38%	$104
Dietary	$315,934	14.29%	$3,853
Real estate taxes/licenses	$91,758	4.15%	$1,119
Insurance	$87,777	3.97%	$1,070
Reserves	$44,220	2.00%	$539
Miscellaneous	$10,698	0.48%	$130
Total expenses	$1,243,586	56.24%	$15,166
Net operating income	$967,436	43.76%	$11,798
Capitalization rate	12.00%		
Indicated value by income approach	$8,061,967		
Rounded	$8,100,000		

C H A P T E R
S E V E N

Subacute and Alzheimer's Care Facilities

Among the variety of special medical facilities that exist today, those offering subacute and Alzheimer's care are growing rapidly in aggregate number and attracting the increasing attention of medical entrepreneurs. With the new focus on integrated health care delivery systems (see Figure 1.2), large numbers of freestanding subacute and Alzheimer's projects and units within hospitals have been developed in recent years or are in the pipeline. Estimates are that at least 10% of all nursing homes have special units for the care of Alzheimer's patients, and subacute care generates revenues of $7.5 billion per year, close to 10% of the total nursing home market.

Appraisal and market feasibility assignments involving subacute and Alzheimer's care facilities (either freestanding or integrated within a facility) are becoming more common. While detailed operating and financial data are scarce, an attempt has been made to compile enough information in this chapter to provide readers with the capability to conduct well-reasoned analyses, studies, and appraisals of these unique health care property types.

Subacute Care Facilities

Definition

A widely recognized definition of subacute care was developed by the Joint Commission on the Accreditation of Healthcare Organizations:

> Subacute care is comprehensive inpatient care designed for someone who has had an acute illness, injury, or exacerbation of a disease process. It is goal-oriented treatment rendered immediately after, or instead of, acute hospitalization to treat one or more specific active complex medical conditions or to administer one or more technically complex treatments, in the context of a person's underlying long-term conditions and overall situation.
>
> Generally, the individual's condition is such that the care does not depend heavily on high-technology monitoring or complex diagnostic procedures. It requires the coordinated services of an interdisciplinary team including physicians, nurses, and other relevant professional disciplines, who are trained and knowledgeable to assess and manage these specific conditions and perform the necessary proce- dures. Subacute care is given as part of a specifically defined program, regardless of the site. Subacute care is generally more intensive than traditional nursing facility care and less than acute care. It requires frequent (daily to weekly) recur-

rent patient assessment and review of the clinical course and treatment plan for a limited (several days to several months) time period, until a condition is stabilized or a predetermined treatment course is completed.

Subacute care encompasses a broad range of services, including cardiac, neurological, and physical rehabilitation; infectious disease management; wound care; and orthopedic, pre- and post-transplant, and pulmonary care. Subacute patients are well enough not to require the services of an acute care hospital (ACH), but sick enough to require care that exceeds the services of an skilled nursing facility (SNF) or home care. According to *The Genesis Report,*

> Subacute patients typically need highly technical pre- or postoperative care, intravenous treatment, or extensive monitoring of physiological activities. Ancillary services such as cardiac rehabilitation, physical rehabilitation, infectious disease treatment, wound care, neurological rehabilitation, orthopedic programs, and pre- and post-transplant and pulmonary care are also provided for subacute patients whose conditions are more serious. In some cases, subacute units use sophisticated equipment such as telemetry monitoring needed for intensive treatment, but they are not equipped to the extent of intensive care units and cardiac care units, because subacute patients are medically stable.[1]

Rationale for Subacute Care

Subacute care is driven by economics. Changes in Medicare, the growth of managed care, and the rapidly growing elderly population are major factors influencing subacute care. Because DRGs limit the time patients can stay in hospitals, SNFs with special treatment programs and facilities become the logical next stage in the healing process. Also managed care payers are demanding lower cost solutions than those provided by ACHs. Subacute care is provided at a cost that is 30% to 60% less than at an acute care hospital, and yields three to four-and-a-half times more revenue per patient day than a skilled nursing facility. Further, pretax profit margins per bed are typically double or triple those of SNFs.

With these types of numbers, subacute care beds have had enormous growth in the past decade. Interest in the subject is so great that warnings are being issued to providers about potential abuses and overdevelopment. Nevertheless, the market is expected to increase by at least $500 million per year until it reaches $10 billion in 2000.

The International Subacute Healthcare Association (ISHA) has more than 500 members, representing over 12,500 subacute beds. However, the total market is much larger (probably by a factor of five) but cannot be accurately measured because subacute beds are not separately licensed and various long-term care organizations or entities define them somewhat differently. The ISHA estimates there are about 2,500 dedicated subacute units and facilities in the nation. Subacute provider types include long-term care PPS-exempt hospitals, nursing facility units, skilled nursing units in hospitals, rehabilitation hospitals, subacute nursing facilities, and swing bed programs in acute hospitals.

Diagnostic Categories

Subacute care referrals typically fall into seven diagnostic categories: cardiology, general surgery, neurology, oncology, orthopedics, pulmonology disease, and renal disease. They represent about 55% of first-listed diagnoses of persons discharged from acute care hospitals, which is another indication of the breadth of the market. Based on the experience of one of the nation's largest nursing home chains, the range of diseases and injuries of patients released to

---

[1] "Subacute Care: Halfway between Sick and Well," *The Genesis Report,* November 1994, 2.

subacute facilities is much narrower than the range for the majority of patients released from acute care hospitals. The analyst can use this type of data, which should be representative of the entire industry, to estimate the potential market (in terms of patient days) for a subacute facility in a defined service area. Orthopedic, complex medical, stroke, and cancer services account for slightly under 90% of patient days. The remainder, accounting for about one out of 8.5 patient days, includes brain injury, cardiac, and neuromuscular diagnoses (see Table 7.1).

Table 7.1	Characteristics of Subacute Care Delivery		
Diagnoses	Average Days Length of Stay	Average Age of Patient	Percent of Total Subacute Admissions
Orthopedic	24.3	72.8	31%
Complex medical	30.4	71.5	30%
Stroke	34.4	71.3	21%
Cancer	23.7	64.4	9%
Brain injury	45.7	45.7	3%
Cardiac	19.9	72.2	2%
Neuromuscular	50.3	58.0	2%
Other*	32.7	66.3	2%

* Includes amputee pain, spinal injury, and arthritis
Source: The Hillhaven Corp; POV Inc. "The Evolving Long-Term Care Market ... Business Opportunities and Threats 1994," *The Genesis Report,* November 1994.

Site Evaluation

In this context site evaluation refers to the entire environment of a subacute care facility. Location in a medical campus environment is most desired because it provides the facility close ties with an acute care hospital. New facilities should always be in close proximity to other medical facilities, including doctors' offices. For existing facilities an analysis should consider such factors as capability to remodel and expand, status of available technology, and layout of units in addition to appearance and age considerations.

To develop subacute care beds in an existing SNF requires an investment of about $15,000 per bed for equipment and technology (e.g., piped-in oxygen and air monitoring equipment, occupational therapy testing and treatment equipment, isolation rooms, individual bathrooms with showers, and handicapped facilities) as well as for functionality (e.g., architectural features that differentiate the unit in appearance from a typical nursing home). The characteristics of the target patient market relative to diagnostic categories to be treated and to age range should be determined before a particular design is adopted.

The ideal subacute unit of an acute care hospital or skilled nursing facility has been described by one writer[2] as having the following:

---

[2] K.T. Anders, "Is Subacute Right for You?," *Contemporary Long Term Care,* June 1994, 42.

- separate entrance

- separate reception-admitting area

- separate ambulance entrance

- separate nurses' station

- separate dining area

- dedicated rehabilitation space (at least 1,000 square feet)

- respiratory workroom and office near the nurses' station

- social services office for admissions and discharges

- office for unit coordinator

- family room

- motorized beds

- nurse call system

- piped-in oxygen and suction

- physician's office with dictation equipment

- at least seven private rooms and six or seven semi-private rooms

Due to requirements for higher-technology equipment and treatment/therapy space, subacute facilities will require more floor area than a skilled nursing facility of similar bed size. The likelihood is that the floor area ratio will be doubled.

Market Evaluation

Most subacute facilities have contractual or other arrangements with an acute care hospital, HMO, managed care company, or a physicians' group. Since the referring source of patients is an acute care hospital, the discharge characteristics of ACH patients by diagnosis must be studied to determine the potential number of available patient days at a subacute facility. The focus should be on those diagnoses that account for virtually all subacute admissions (orthopedic, complex medical, stroke, and cancer).

An environmental (or market) analysis recommended by one writer[3] includes these categories:

1. *Demographics*–breaking down the population service area by age, race, employment, education, medical status, and income

2. *Physician survey*–gathering such information as physicians' names, types of practices and medical specialties, lengths of practice in the area, referral procedures, numbers of referrals per week, and rates of satisfaction with existing facility care

3. *Hospital survey*–obtaining a general profile of the local facility, its specialty services and programs, most common diagnoses, payer mix, referral process, and rate of satisfaction with facility care

4. *Insurance industry survey*–identifying the companies by name and gathering a company profile and information on their referral processes, number of referrals per week, primary diagnosis referred, contractual agreements, and rate of satisfaction with facility care

5. *Case manager survey*–gathering names, profiles, medical specialties, referral processes, number of referrals, and overall satisfaction with existing facility care

---

[3] Robert J. Dahl, "Elements of a Site Evaluation," *Transitions*, November/December 1994, 24.

6. *Legislative and regulatory issues*–tracking changes influencing governing organizations

7. *Community attitude and value survey*–analyzing the community's cultural background and issues relating to the facility's medical specialties

8. *Competitive analysis*–determining competitors' names, profiles, census, payer mix, occupancy percentage, overall aesthetics, special features, medical specialties, and market share by specialty

A rule-of-thumb type of methodology, based on population, uses four steps to estimate bed demand.[4]

1. Apply 0.5 to 0.6 beds per 1,000 population of the service area.

2. Adjust ratio for service area demographic variations from the national distribution.

3. Identify existing subacute care providers/beds in the service area.

4. Subtract existing beds from estimated demand to determine net need.

A more accurate model using discharge data measures the patient day market by multiplying the average length of stay for the corresponding diagnosis by the number of potential patients and measuring the strength of the competition by patient day capability with the same DRGs.

Financial Analysis

Subacute care is highly attractive for financial as well as medical reasons. For one thing it is 30 to 60% less expensive than comparable treatment provided in an ACH (see Table 7.2). The cost efficiencies of subacute care are due not only to a lower level of health care but to savings advantages from lower plant and equipment costs and in lower operational and management overhead as compared to ACHs. The financial advantage of subacute beds over the traditional nursing home operation is equally dramatic. An SNF bed with $100 daily revenue, operating expenses of 90%, and an occupancy rate of 95% will produce a cash flow of $9.50 per day. A subacute care bed with $350 daily revenue, operating expenses of 80%, and an occupancy rate of 75% will produce a cash flow of $52.50 per day. This may be an extreme example, but it is representative of the huge differential between the two categories of health care.

Table 7.2	Daily Cost Comparisons: Subacute Care vs. Traditional Care		
Level of Care	Hospital Care	Subacute Care	Percent Savings
Medically complex	$1,250	$490	60.8%
Medically fragile, but stable	$780	$430	44.9%
Stable with rehabilitation	$750	$400	46.7%
Stable, near discharge	$750	$390	48.0%
Minimal care	$750	$320	57.3%
Source: The Genesis Report/MCx 1994			

---

[4] Laura Hyatt, *Subacute Care* (Chicago: Richard D. Irwin, 1995), 35.

Most comparative studies of the financial advantages of subacute units involve the partial conversion of nursing home beds. An example of the impact on profitability where 10 and 30 beds of a 125-bed SNF are converted to subacute care beds is shown in Figure 7.1. Another comparison of SNFs and subacute care facilities by operating parameters is shown in Table 7.3.

Table 7.3	Comparison of Subacute and Skilled Nursing Care	
Care Available	**Subacute Care**	**Skilled Nursing**
Admission criteria	Program-specific with clear outcome potential (orthopedic, neurology, cardiology, etc.)	Any diagnosis; Medicare skilled criteria
Average length of stay	7 to 21 days	90 to 180 days
Average charge/day	$300 to $700	$100 to $200
Physician visit	Average 1 to 3 times per week; consulting	1 time per month; limited consulting
Nursing care/day	4.5 to 8.0 hours direct care; high uses of aides, nonprofessional	2.5 to 4.0 hours
Rehabilitation therapies	Programmatic with specific goals; usually more than 1 hour per day	Limited in scope; usually less than 30 minutes per day

Source: Laura Hyatt, *Subacute Care* (Richard D. Irwin) 1995, 94.

Income and Expenses

Revenues are derived from daily charges for room, board, nursing care, and ancillary services, which include therapies (diagnostic radiology, laboratory, occupational, speech, intravenous, and respiratory) as well as supplies and medications. A conceptual estimate of revenue for a 20-bed subacute unit is given in Table 7.4. In this example total charges are about $400 per patient day and actual revenue is about $340 per patient day.

Cost and expense categories for subacute units should be the same as the standardized classifications for SNFs, except that daily charges for nursing services are about double and ancillaries much more (by as much as 12 times). Typical expense ratios for subacute care units are about 75% to 85%. The reader is encouraged to conduct individualized analyses for each project in the absence of an actual operating history.

Conclusions

Because they offer a cost-effective alternative to acute hospitalization, subacute care facilities are expected to be a major beneficiary of health care reform. They are not, however, something that can be created in the typical nursing home due to factors such as the nursing home's age, size, condition, location, competition, and service area demographics. Subacute units must be designed for function and image. Strong links with hospital discharge planners, physician groups, and other postacute businesses such as home health and outpatient therapies are necessary.

The attractive economics of subacute care will create a tendency to overdevelop a market or convert SNF beds without understanding where the facility fits in the local health care spectrum. Subacute care units can be specialized and even provide a broad spectrum of settings and services within a given hospital service area. Patients must be differentiated by diagnosis; sicker

Figure 7.1. Impact of Subacute Units on Nursing Facility

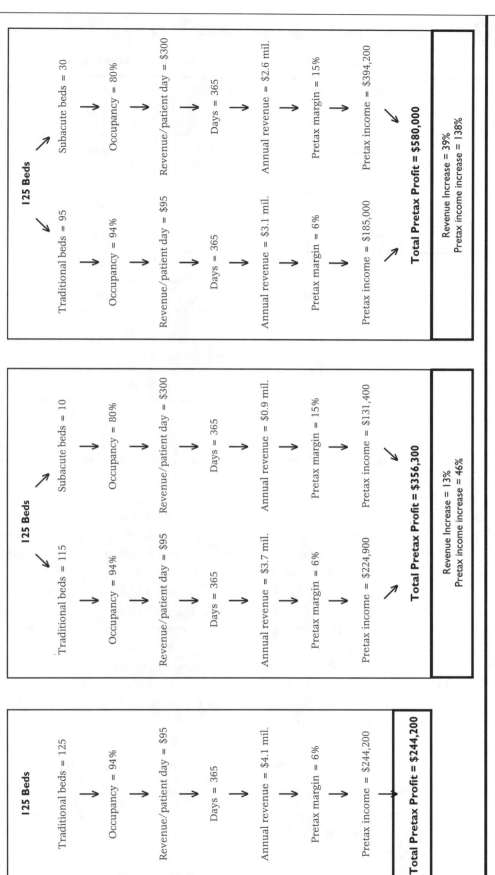

Traditional Facility

125 Beds

Traditional beds = 125 → Occupancy = 94% → Revenue/patient day = $95 → Days = 365 → Annual revenue = $4.1 mil. → Pretax margin = 6% → Pretax income = $244,200 →

Total Pretax Profit = $244,200

Facility with Small Subacute Unit

125 Beds

Subacute beds = 10 → Occupancy = 80% → Revenue/patient day = $300 → Days = 365 → Annual revenue = $0.9 mil. → Pretax margin = 15% → Pretax income = $131,400 ↘

Traditional beds = 115 → Occupancy = 94% → Revenue/patient day = $95 → Days = 365 → Annual revenue = $3.7 mil. → Pretax margin = 6% → Pretax income = $224,900 ↗

Total Pretax Profit = $356,300

Revenue Increase = 13%
Pretax income increase = 46%

Facility with Larger Subacute Unit

125 Beds

Subacute beds = 30 → Occupancy = 80% → Revenue/patient day = $300 → Days = 365 → Annual revenue = $2.6 mil. → Pretax margin = 15% → Pretax income = $394,200 ↘

Traditional beds = 95 → Occupancy = 94% → Revenue/patient day = $95 → Days = 365 → Annual revenue = $3.1 mil. → Pretax margin = 6% → Pretax income = $185,000 ↗

Total Pretax Profit = $580,000

Revenue Increase = 39%
Pretax income increase = 138%

Source: POV Inc., "The Evolving Long-Term Care Market...Business Opportunities and Threats," *The Genesis Report*, 1994.

Table 7.4 Subacute Care Unit Revenue Estimate

Category	Charge Per Day	Patient Days	Total Revenue
Room, board, and nursing ancillaries	$250	5,475	$1,368,750
Radiology	16	2,190	35,040
Laboratory	18	3,285	59,130
Respiratory	30	1,095	32,850
Therapy	100	4,380	438,000
Medical supplies	30	4,900	147,000
Pharmacy	20	5,475	109,500
Other	1	1,600	1,600
		Total	$2,191,870
	Less contractual adjustments and discounts		328,780
		Net unit revenue	$1,863,090

Source: Author

patients should be in a unit that is within an acute care or rehabilitation setting while others are better off in a freestanding or SNF setting.

The market is expected to be more competitive in the future, not only because of an expected increase in beds but the expected revenue squeeze from the efforts of managed care to seek the lowest cost provider and capitated contracts. Market feasibility studies should be conducted in all instances of a proposed project, not only to identify the competition but to analyze and forecast the numbers of potential patients by diagnosis and average length of stay.

Appraisers should be aware of these potential circumstances when appropriate because this modest adjustment in highest and best use can have a very significant impact on overall unit value. The high profit margin potential of ancillary services should not be overlooked. Again, they are a function of diagnostic categories, which requires an in-depth investigation of the market. Subacute facilities should be part of an integrated network (see Chapter 1) that provides a continuum of care. When providers are independent, they should develop relationships with acute care hospitals, HMOs, PPOs, managed care organizations, and physician groups.

In analyzing a subacute facility, the appraiser might apply the following questions, which were originally developed to answer the question, "Should you start a subacute unit?"[5]

1. Are there any license or reimbursement categories for subacute in this state?
2. Does Medicaid negotiate special rates?
3. Does the payer mix include managed care, insurance, health maintenance organizations, and preferred provider organizations?
4. Can the facility make the commitment to more aggressive marketing?

---

[5] Mary Marshall, Management and Planning Services, Inc., Atlanta, Georgia.

5. Can the physical facility accommodate, or be modified to accommodate, the needs of the subacute unit?

6. Is staffing available?

7. Is there ancillary staff available to support the unit?

8. Will therapy be staffed by employees or contractors?

9. Can the pharmacy company handle the extensive pharmacy services?

10. Are adequate consulting and pharmacy services available?

11. Is the facility located near an acute care hospital to generate patients and to facilitate interaction?

12. What other facilities have subacute units in the area?

13. What happens to the very sick Medicare patient currently?

14. Is the facility Medicare-certified?

15. Has the billing office had experience with billing and collecting from insurance companies?

16. Is medical staff available to support a nursing-facility-based unit?

17. Is there a commitment to understanding clearly the costs of delivering subacute services so that appropriate rates can be developed and negotiated?

18. Is cash flow available to develop the new business?

19. Does the facility have available reserves, investment sources, and funds to cover working capital for a period of approximately three years?

20. Does the current staff understand the proposed changes, and are they willing to take on the difficulties of new demands and a new authority structure?

Alzheimer's Facilities

The rapid growth in the number of patients suffering from Alzheimer's disease or other forms of dementia (estimated by some to be slightly more than one out of two nursing home residents) has spurred the development of freestanding projects and special or expanded units within or attached to existing SNFs. Alzheimer's patients used to be considered the black sheep of a nursing home, and because of their sometimes disruptive behavior, they were often isolated and overmedicated. These drastic control practices are not now allowed. Advocates of specialized facilities say by segregating the Alzheimer's population, the medical staff can better minister to them, keep them calm, and preserve some quality of life.

Further, it is now recognized that Alzheimer's patients have an illness that varies in intensity, and varied levels of care can be effectively applied depending on the stage of the disease. This can mean considerable savings if a patient can be lodged in an assisted living facility rather than an SNF. Estimates are that as much as $10 to $20 per day can be saved, which over a nursing home population of close to 2 million can mean enormous potential savings.

The idea of environment as therapy has many adherents. In the early and middle stages of the disease, patients can be effectively managed by altering their physical environment and by providing specially trained staff and programs. An "ideal" freestanding unit should have an alarm system for wanderers, a residential type of atmosphere with soft colors and no-shadow lighting, activities to stimulate physical, cognitive, and social skills, and ways to involve family members in patient care.

Various studies[6] have measured the prevalence of the disease by age group ranges:

Age Bracket	Number Suffering from Forms of Dementia
65-74 years	1% to 3%
75-84 years	7% to 18.7%
85+ years	25% to 47.2%

SNF vs. ALF Environment

Alzheimer's patients go through phases which require different levels of care. In the mid-term phase (between home care and skilled nursing), the patient can benefit from an assisted living or residential care environment (referred to in this chapter as a RAALF — Residential Assisted Alzheimer's Living Facility). A comparison of key differences between SNFs and RAALFs appears in Table 7.5.

Table 7.5	Comparison of Key Features of a RAALF and SNF	
	RAALF	**Skilled Nursing Facility**
Philosophy	Homelike, emphasizing privacy, resident choice, active participation in daily routine tasks, supplemented with scheduled activities.	Unit-based, emphasizing structured daily programming and activities; nonindividualized.
Physical Plant	Small-scale (42 units), largely private rooms; homelike, self-contained "houses" (14 beds per house).	Institutional setting, self-contained large unit (24-30 beds), shared common spaces, few private rooms.
Front Line Staff	Fully cross-trained, multifunction (resident care, programming, light housekeeping, laundry, meal service). RAs empowered for primary caregiving.	Specialist, single function; minimal cross-training (resident care and programming only). Supervisors direct caregiving tasks.
Management	Lean; no staff functions; high reliance on systems.	Staff functions (bookkeeper, HR, admissions)
Care Planning	Simplified, practical, tied to pricing.	OBRA driven.
Pricing	All-inclusive rates.	Base rate plus ancillaries.
Food Service	Simplified "homestyle" menus and service; limited special diets, small-scale kitchen (42 residents)	Extensive diet and preparation variety; larger-scale kitchen (120-200 residents).

Design Considerations

The philosophy that controls the design of RAALF projects is based on the following:

- small-scale, home-like setting
- secure, simple, and flexible living environment
- maximum freedom of choice for residents to extent possible (structured freedom)
- individualized care with an emphasis on the whole person

---

[6] The lower estimate appeared in *Losing a Million Minds: Confronting the Tragedy of Alzheimer's Disease and Other Dementias*. The higher estimate is based on a study by Denis A. Evans, et al., published in *The Journal of the American Medical Association*, November 1989.

- enhancement of resident capabilities and interests through resident participation in daily routine and schedule programming

- supportive and enabling staff

- involved families and caregiver support groups

Alzheimer's patients have typically been housed in separate sections or wings of skilled nursing facilities. Increasingly, the trend has been toward special freestanding care facilities or special wings of multiphased senior health care projects that have been designed or remodeled to reflect the unique care requirements of patients suffering from Alzheimer's or other forms of dementia.

Current RAALF projects are of a residential type of construction generally of one story and with a "pod" or unit design. Most accommodations are private rooms with toilet and vanity, and there are shared common areas for activities and dining. The emphasis is on providing a "homey" decor and comfortable/functional furnishings. The typical project has limited back-of-the-house support space; some have enclosed courtyards.

The primary components of the common area are a multipurpose room, lobby/reception area, nurses station, offices, central kitchen, and areas for various support services. Located off the common area are the patients/residents' rooms, which in some designs are divided into modular units. A typical room will be large enough for one bed, a large lounge chair, dresser, bedside table, and an open water closet/sink area. A common bath and shower room(s) serves all residents of the individual facility or wing.

Integral with the project program is the need for a secured area in which residents can wander, e.g., a landscaped walkway which uses most of the parcel's open space. For security and control purposes a common porch can be designed to overlook the pathway; the porch can be made accessible from the common lounge area and from the patient room unit. The secured portion of the site should be entirely enclosed with a six-foot high solid fence.

Determining Market Demand

Facilities for Alzheimer's patients tend to have a total target market area within 15 to 30 miles of the site. This radius indicates a reasonable driving distance for relatives and friends. However, where the population is spread over a larger geographic area such as a rural area, the radius can be extended. More important than a strict definition of market area based on distance is the overall character of the development's environment, whether it be urban, suburban, or small town/rural, where driving times might extend up to one to two hours.

Two separate methods of analysis can be used to derive an estimate of demand. The first is a market saturation analysis, which views the potential population by qualifying income levels augmented by an overlay of age brackets. This method gives only the number of available households from which a small portion will form the potential resident nucleus. A second method analyzes a general target population with a focus on the percentage of the senior population that falls into the statistical pool of those stricken with dementia. Both of these methods can then be reconciled to a conclusion.

Example of a Market Saturation Analysis

To measure the theoretical size of the subject's target market, demographic statistics from the 1990 U.S. Census Bureau were obtained for the relevant target area (25-mile radius). Population estimates and projections for 1993 and 1998 were also obtained. Saturation rates were then calculated as follows, the results of which are shown in Table 7.6. The steps included:

Table 7.6	**Market Saturation Analysis for Proposed 42-Unit Alzheimer's Facility (25-Mile Radius)**				
			Saturation Rates*		
	# Head of Household**	**W/O Subject (305 Units)**	**W/Subject (347 Units)**	**Subject Only (42 Units)**	
1993 Estimate:					
$50,000	2,054	14.8%	16.9%	2.0%	
$50,000-$75,000	1,219	25.0%	28.5%	3.4%	
$75,000+	835	36.5%	41.5%	5.0%	
1998 Projection:					
$50,000+	3,027	100%	11.4%	1.4%	
$50,000-$75,000	1,848	16.5%	18.7%	2.3%	
$75,000+	1,179	25.8%	29.4%	3.5%	

*Market saturation rates represent the percentage of total market demand which is necessary to absorb a) existing units not including the subject or b) existing units including the subject.
**Number of income- and age-qualifying senior households within 25 miles of site (per Claritas/NPDC).

Evaluation of saturation rates:

Penetration Level	Estimate of Overall Market Demand
0-10%	Conservative
10-20%	Moderate
20%+	Aggressive

1. Determining the number of households over a minimum age of 75, and minimum income requirements of $50,000 and $75,000 from the 1993 and 1998 projections. The minimum income bracket is based on residents' ability to pay 80% of their effective gross income. The parameters establish the different scenarios for calculating the market saturation rates.

2. Calculating the total market saturation rate required to fill the proposed subject's 42 units and all other existing competitive properties.

3. Analyzing the feasibility of the subject property given the calculated market saturation rates.

The parameters of the saturation analysis are specifically chosen to reflect the targeted population. According to our research seniors are willing to pay up to 80% of their effective gross income (*EGI*). The target *EGI* therefore is set at $50,000. Geographically, a 25-mile radius provides the maximum statistical rate of return for a resident's proximity to his or her original residence. Absorption rates are estimated for 1) the market area without the subject, 2) the market area with the subject, and 3) the subject only. Comparing the 1993 estimated population with the 1998 projected population allows one to observe any trends. In this case there is a favorable trend in the percentage of total market demand necessary to absorb existing units including the subject — from 16.9% in 1993 to 11.4% in 1998. The lower the absorption rate the better.

Based on experience from other comparable markets, saturation rates of 15% or less usually indicate an adequate feasibility for a proposed residential care facility. As shown, the calculated saturation rate of 16.9% for the subject property is not significantly above 15% when considering income-qualifying seniors 75 years of age and older who represent the subject's demand market. However, it is important to keep in mind that the saturation rate analysis is only an estimate of the total saturation of elderly units within a market area. Saturation rate analysis cannot take into account the advantages or disadvantages of any one facility. For example, a development with a superior marketing campaign and superior construction or amenities could be successful even in a highly saturated market. This analysis is made only as a general measure of the degree to which the subject market may be overbuilt. Given the calculated saturation rates for the subject's primary market area, it appears competitive but probably not overbuilt. Stabilized occupancy is a case in point regarding the variables associated with this analysis. To maximize itself, the subject must maintain a well-focused marketing campaign stressing its competitive advantages.

In summary, key characteristics for the feasibility in this example of a proposed 42-bed Alzheimer's project include:

1. Market saturation rates that indicate feasibility for the subject. This example suggests longer absorption periods, based on the competing facilities' low ratio of private-pay residents and higher vacancy of those facilities dedicated to private-pay residents.

2. The subject's new construction, specific architectural programming, extra staffing, and its philosophical uniqueness, which allow it to compete more effectively with older residential care and skilled nursing facilities for those persons with dementia.

3. Of the facilities listed in the census, most enjoy high occupancy rates suggesting adequate long-term demand and steady absorption of units over time. This would be true for the subject example due to its private-pay posture.

4. In this example, since only private-pay residents will be sought for this new, high-quality project, targeting residents will require some market education and focused, tactical marketing. Such marketing is imperative because RAALF projects overlap both traditional in-home care and that offered in skilled nursing facilities (see Figure 7.2)

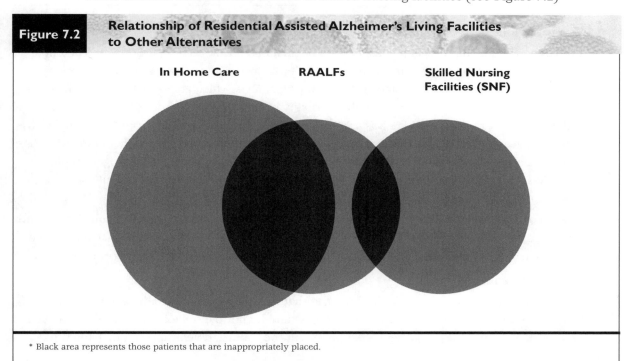

Figure 7.2 | **Relationship of Residential Assisted Alzheimer's Living Facilities to Other Alternatives**

In Home Care   RAALFs   Skilled Nursing Facilities (SNF)

* Black area represents those patients that are inappropriately placed.

Determining Size of Competitive Market

The first step is to determine the number of units competitive to the subject project by estimating the percentage of overlap of each of the competitive facilities and comparing their primary market area to the subject's primary market area based on distance and mobility patterns of the elderly within the region. Due to the overt institutional atmosphere of SNFs and level of individual care, the majority of SNF beds can be viewed as noncompetitive. Once dedicated facilities are in operation, they will likely drain the other existing institutions of their private-pay population. In this example, the subject's primary market area has approximately 305 existing beds, but only 71 competitive beds (see Table 7.8).

Table 7.8	Analysis of Competition - Existing Projects				
Comp. No.	Facility	No. of Residents	% of Market Overlap	No. of Total Beds	No. of Competitive Beds
1	A*	99	100%	99	33
2	B	20**	100%	26	26
3	C*	59	100%	59	0
4	D*	59	100%	59	0
5	E	50	100%	50	0
6	F	10	100%	12	12
Total existing estimated beds				305	71

* Indicates skilled nursing facility
** Full occupancy has been achieved in the past

Example of Target Population Analysis

A target population analysis estimates the total population and allocates a portion to the potential market relative to the supply of beds. In taking the entire estimated market area population, certain assumptions are made based on statistical relationships. These calculations include the percentage of the general population that have a high probability of suffering from various forms of dementia. In this example a multiple of 2.1% was applied (see Table 7.9). The derivative of 14,789 people was further reduced by a factor of 54% to indicate the portion of those in the mid stage of those diseases, which totaled 7,986. The number of potentially qualified residents, however, is only 10.4% of the total mid-stage population. Assuming that 25% of the qualified population will actually be placed in an RAALF, the total number of beds needed is estimated at 208.

A second method, based on national statistics, shows a demand for 207 beds. Reconciling the two methods of calculation yields a confident range of about 200 to 210 beds needed. Since the number of available competitive beds is 71, the example shows that a favorable market opportunity exists.

Appraisal Process

The appraisal process for RAALFs is similar to that for assisted living facilities. Some key differences are higher per resident income/rents and higher overall expense ratios. An annual income statement for a proposed 44-bed project in the stabilized year appears in Table 7.10.

Table 7.9 — Target Population Analysis for Proposed 42-Bed Alzheimer's Facility

A. Market Size

Market area population (1993 est.)	704,250
Percent with dementia, including Parkinson's and vascular*	× 2.1%
	14,789
In mid stage*	× 54%
Total mid-stage population	7,986
Percent income-qualified @ $50,000+	× 10.4%
	831
Percent likely to be placed in RAALFs	× 25%
Total RAALF bed demand	208

*extracted from estimates from local sources.

B. By Market Opportunity

Market Characteristic	National Estimate	Market Area Estimate
Age- and income-qualified (75+ years, $50,000+)	2,500,000*	11,818
Percent with mid-stage Alzheimer's	× 7%**	× 7%
Target market size	175,000	827
Percent likely to be placed in RAALFs	× 25%	× 25%
Total RAALF bed demand	43,750	207
Current competitive beds		71
Market share (based on 42 beds @ 92% occupancy)		20%

* National Planning Data Corp estimates
** U.S. Congress, Office of Technology Assessment

Table 7.10   44-Bed RAALF Project (New) Stabilized Year (Estimated)

Revenue		
Rents (44 x $3,250/mo. x 12 mos. x 95% occupancy)	$1,623,200	
Miscellaneous/ancillary (5%)	81,510	
Total		$1,711,710
Expenses		
Advertising	$ 9,600	
Bad debts	8,172	
Employee benefits	85,080	
Food service	63,360	
Housekeeping	65,700	
Insurance	21,997	
Laundry	5,832	
Maintenance	72,000	
Food supplies	64,240	
Recreation supplies	5,760	
Property taxes	40,000	
Wages–fixed	202,604	
Wages–variable	257,879	
Reserves	51,351	
Management	85,000	
Miscellaneous	34,000	
Total		$1,072,575
Net operating income		639,135
Capitalized at 14%		$4,565,250
Rounded		$4,565,000

Notes: Private room residents = 32; semi-private room residents = 12; private rate = $113.75/day; semi-private rate = $89.70/day

C H A P T E R
E I G H T

Medical Office Buildings

Powerful forces have recently emerged that will affect the future of the medical office building (MOB) market and that could change the physical characteristics and financial aspects of the MOB. This dynamic and changing environment presents unique opportunities for the development, investment, and management communities.

Prospective reform of national health care is not expected to have a detrimental impact on the existing stock of well-located MOBs. Those properties with strong hospital locations are expected to benefit from such trends as:

1. the anticipated broadening of responsibilities of general practitioners and pediatricians in the hospital setting;

2. the geographic centralization of hospital services;

3. the increased referral of "unprofitable" patients by general practitioners to specialists under prospective payment system reimbursement schemes;

4. reduced physician resources for relocating their practices;

5. the elimination of noncompetitive hospitals and the downgraded desirability of their attendant medical office buildings; and

6. the increased importance of patient referrals.

Changing Market Forces

Prospective Payment System (PPS)

In 1983 Medicare, followed by other third-party payers, changed from funding health care on a retrospective reimbursement basis to a prospective payment system (PPS). Prior to 1983 medical expenses were paid on a "cost-plus" basis, allowing care providers to be reimbursed for their actual cost plus a reasonable profit by third-party payers. Clearly, the higher the cost the higher the profits, and rapid growth ensued, especially within hospitals. Under PPS, however, health care providers are reimbursed a predetermined price, based upon an average regional price for a particular procedure. If a provider's cost is less than the specified price, the provider retains the difference as profit; conversely, if the cost exceeds the established price, the provider sustains the loss.

When PPS was initiated, it applied only to inpatient services; as a result outpatient services continued to enjoy the more favorable retrospective reimbursement system. Since outpatient services are frequently performed within the MOB, this expanded the demand for MOB space and had major impacts on the characteristics/design of such space.

Now PPS has been extended to outpatient procedures, and the need for efficient space and facilities has become more evident. Design features being emphasized are those that improve efficiency, provide flexibility, increase accessibility, and enhance physician productivity.

Many types of outpatient venues are gaining popularity, and the trend toward outpatient services has made the health care industry reconsider the financial viability and use of MOBs. Since these buildings offer lower construction and operating costs, outpatient services in such facilities are lower in cost compared to those in hospitals. Outpatients also respond more favorably to the MOB environment because it lacks the negative psychological associations of the hospital environment.

Physician Population

The dynamics of the physician population also affect the market for MOB space. The number of physicians practicing in the United States increased substantially from 1960 to 1990, when it stood at 533,000, resulting in an increase in overall demand for space. Also, physicians are forming larger group practices due to higher operational costs and increased competition, which has resulted in a shift in demand from smaller (500 to 1,500 square feet) to larger (2,000 to over 8,000 square feet) office areas. Increased competition, however, is making physicians increasingly cost conscious, resulting in lower space requirements per physician.

Hospitals, experiencing downward pressure on patient revenue, are seeking to increase patient volume. This has resulted in increased competition among hospitals. Since a physician typically decides what hospital a patient will use, the physician is the hospital's primary "customer." Providing competitively priced, high-quality MOB space is one technique employed by hospitals to attract physicians. Hospitals, therefore, often become a significant force in the supply and pricing of MOB space. Unfair MOB rental pricing by hospital owners, however, can result in legal and tax challenges.

Another trend is for hospitals to acquire physician practices and to integrate physicians into hospital management to some degree. In 1993, almost 14% of hospitals surveyed had a formal physician/hospital organization, 7% had a management services organization, and 4% had a foundation that negotiated managed care contracts on behalf of the hospital and physicians as a unit (see Table 8.1).

Medical Technology

Medical technology has contributed to the increased demand for MOB space by expanding the feasibility of outpatient diagnosis and treatment. It has also placed new demands on the physical characteristics of MOBs, furthering the need for new facilities and renovation of existing structures.

Patient Demographics

Finally, such national demographics as an expanding and aging population with a longer life expectancy and greater health consciousness have and will contribute to the continued expansion of demand for MOB space in future years.

Factors Affecting Success

The foremost factor affecting the success of any medical office building is clearly the supply and demand characteristics of the specific market segment. Beyond these, other key factors will also affect the successful development and operation of an MOB.

Proximity to Hospital

Reduced travel between office and hospital allows for more efficient use of a physician's time and results in higher earnings for the physician and lower overall health care costs. Increased

Table 8.1	Hospital-Physician Organizations, by Hospital Category, 1993					
		Organization (in percent)				
Hospital Category*	**Number of Hospitals**	**Any Joint Venture**	**PHO**	**MSO**	**Foundation**	**IHO**
Total	1,495	30.2%	13.6%	6.9%	4.1%	2.7%
Atlantic	400	33.3	18.3	6.5	5.3	2.3
East Central	391	34.8	13.8	7.2	4.6	2.8
West Central	404	24.3	10.3	5.1	2.4	2.0
Far West	300	32.7	11.3	9.3	4.3	4.3
Urban	736	47.0	21.5	10.7	6.4	4.6
Rural	759	14.0	5.9	3.2	2.0	0.9
Teaching	233	41.2	18.5	6.9	7.7	6.0
Non-teaching	1,262	28.2	12.6	6.8	3.5	2.1

Note: PHO = physician/hospital organization; MSO = management services organization; IHO = integrated health organization
* Atlantic includes the New England, Middle Atlantic, and South Atlantic census divisions. East Central includes the East North Central and East South Central census divisions. West Central includes the West North Central and West South Central census divisions. Far West includes the Mountain and Pacfic census divisions. Teaching hospitals are those with more than 5 percent professional time spent teaching.
Source: Survey of Hospital-Physician Relations conducted by MACRO International Inc., under contract to ProPAC.

earnings more than offset higher rental rates charged for prime office space. Physicians also prefer to be situated near the most prominent hospital in the area. This increases their status and indirectly affects their income.

Success of Local Hospital

The hospital and its surrounding MOBs are synergistically linked and typically referred to as a "campus." As a hospital expands, so does the demand for surrounding medical office space. This is an increasingly important factor today, as many hospitals consolidate operations to contain costs and meet the competition.

Tenant Mix

An effective selection of physicians and specialties will result in a strong core of doctors situated within one location. In turn they will attract other doctors because of the advantages of close medical associations and efficiencies of intraoffice and interoffice referrals. Physicians who are recognized as leaders within the local medical community generally are signed up early in a development program to enhance the success of an MOB.

Attracting Group Practices

Medical group practices are usually made up of five or more physicians who share a medical practice and primarily treat regularly scheduled patients. While some group practices may have 30 or more physicians, more than half of all group practices have fewer than 10 physicians. Group practices are likely to be in a strong bargaining position as health care reform proceeds, but will face challenges in financial management, staffing, and increased government regulation. Leading specialties among group practices are internal medicine, family practice, obstetrics/gynecology, pediatrics, and cardiology. Group practices are often associated with other health care facilities and services. It has been reported that 75% offer diagnostic imaging services, 59% have on-site clinical laboratory services, and 56% perform outpatient surgery.[1]

Physician Relations and Management

The success or failure of many MOBs has been largely attributed to relations between physicians and the developers and management of the MOB. The presence on the development team of individuals disliked by physicians, the insensitivities of management, or other negative considerations will spread quickly through a tight-knit medical community. MOBs typically are not managed by large property management firms but rather by employees of the medical ownership entity because they are unique properties and personal relationships and networks are considered important factors.

Design

Some buildings have architectural features that will result in long-term operating efficiencies. Examples include clear span space, which results in a greater degree of space availability and flexibility; tall clear heights to accommodate specialized equipment and permit changes to mechanical systems above the ceiling; a high ratio of net usable space to gross building area; ample elevators; and efficient traffic patterns.

Design and Typical Characteristics

Medical offices should be planned with "universal design" principles in mind so that they are accessible to all people, not just the able-bodied. More and more buildings are adopting these principles in the wake of the Americans with Disabilities Act of 1990 (ADA). However, ADA provides only minimum requirements for access; providing additional accommodations can make disabled patients more comfortable and build practice volume. Recently, much greater emphasis has been placed on waiting rooms, work stations, interior layouts, colors, and lighting. Generic structural dimensions for offices don't work for medical buildings.

In the layout for a small building shown in the upper part of Figure 8.1, bays are designed to be 27 to 29 feet or 45 to 48 feet in depth to optimize efficiency of patient care. The corridor layout shown allows both optimum office depths.

Spacious and color-coordinated waiting rooms with artwork make people feel more at ease, but individual specialties have unique requirements. For example, the office of a neurologist who sees patients who may be confused, dizzy, or unsteady should avoid highly contrasting surfaces, busy patterns, or bright colors. The office should be soothing and comfortable and offer no surprises. A radiology suite might be high tech. For a general practice, the design might be more homey and personal because the physicians see their patients more often and they are not dealing with specialties.

Making patients feel more comfortable is one of the benefits of a properly designed office. Attention should also be given to where the employees do their work. It is not uncommon to find "work stations" so small that they resemble pigeonholes. Several people may work elbow to elbow, all simultaneously on the phone, in a small space that also includes a copy machine and storage for supplies and medical charts. Two factors often tend to stall improvements in medical offices: 1) employees tend to say they are happy with their work space even when they are not; and 2) it is often difficult to measure the improvement to a practice, in dollars and cents, when the front office is upgraded.

Good working conditions pay dividends to physicians' practices. Excellent lighting is more important than wallpaper or anything else. If the office is viewed as a flexible tool, rather than a static setting, it becomes possible to imagine a number of environmental amenities that can and

---

[1] "Physician Center Market Encompasses Over 12,000 Sites," SMG Marketing Group, Inc., *Market Letter*, April 1994, p. 1.

Figure 8.1 **Medical Building Floor Plans**

A. Overall Floor Plan

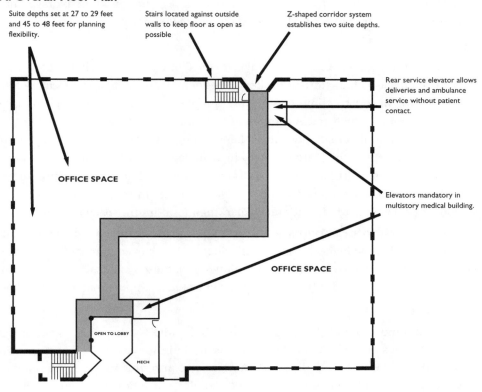

Suite depths set at 27 to 29 feet and 45 to 48 feet for planning flexibility.

Stairs located against outside walls to keep floor as open as possible

Z-shaped corridor system establishes two suite depths.

Rear service elevator allows deliveries and ambulance service without patient contact.

Elevators mandatory in multistory medical building.

OFFICE SPACE

OFFICE SPACE

OPEN TO LOBBY

MECH

B. Individual Suite Design

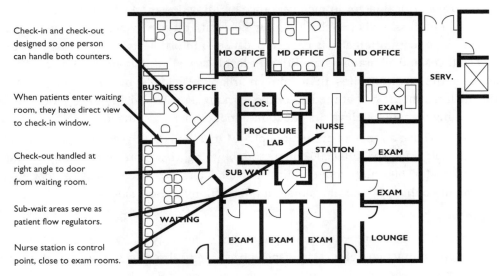

Check-in and check-out designed so one person can handle both counters.

When patients enter waiting room, they have direct view to check-in window.

Check-out handled at right angle to door from waiting room.

Sub-wait areas serve as patient flow regulators.

Nurse station is control point, close to exam rooms.

MD OFFICE   MD OFFICE   MD OFFICE

SERV.

BUSINESS OFFICE

CLOS.

EXAM

PROCEDURE LAB

NURSE STATION

EXAM

SUB WAIT

EXAM

WAITING

EXAM   EXAM   EXAM   LOUNGE

Source: "Building Doctor's Offices: A Lucrative—but Specialized—Opportunity," *Professional Builder and Remodeler,* January-March 1992.

do impact performance. Some consultants recommend a management audit of the practice, which is really a time and motion study, to design spaces for the way doctors and their staffs work. The impact on the income stream can be directly measured. For example, a poorly designed examining room can cost a doctor 30 seconds per patient. Over a day, that might translate to 24 minutes, or the opportunity to see two more patients. At an average charge of $50 per patient, the doctor is loosing $100 per day, or $24,000 per year.

Typical Size

Although substantial variations exist, most major medical office buildings being constructed today share many basic physical characteristics. They are generally 30,000 to 60,000 square feet, low- to medium-rise, ranging in construction type from fireproof steel for large buildings to masonry and wood for smaller low-rise structures. As land near hospitals becomes scarce, MOBs are frequently developed to the maximum density permitted. Land-to-building ratios are primarily controlled by MOB parking requirements, which are typically high since most patients arrive by automobile and there is a high rate of short-term turnover. Typical ratios are four to six parking spaces per 1,000 square feet of net usable or leasable area. Some buildings in very valuable and densely developed locations have resorted to attendant parking for optimum space utilization.

The ratio of net leasable area to gross building area is one measure of building construction and layout efficiency. Ideally, the highest possible ratio should be achieved to receive the greatest economy of operation from the relatively high construction cost of these facilities. The ratio for most new buildings ranges between 80% to 90%; a desirable level would be approximately 85% or more.

Special Features

As medical services move out of the hospital and into the MOB setting, MOBs adopt more of the physical characteristics of the hospital. Some MOBs are built to withstand disasters, with independent water and energy supplies and emergency communications equipment. Surgery suites, recovery rooms, and specially constructed radiology or medical imaging rooms are not uncommon. As some MOBs move toward 24-hour operation, electronic security becomes important as does a "smart" HVAC system, which is activated when a tenant enters a suite.

Elevators are a critical factor in medical office building design. An MOB requires more elevators than a professional office building. By necessity these elevators move at a slower speed. A higher concentration also is needed because of interfloor traffic, i.e., patients between the doctor's offices and laboratories on different levels as well as data from laboratories and X-ray facilities to the medical suites. In downtown urban areas MOBs may have a high degree of traffic during lunch hours and at the end of the working day. The higher degree of elevator use necessitates a higher ratio of elevators per square foot of total building area.

New buildings have a range of approximately .04 to a high of .06 elevators per 1,000 square feet of net leasable area. For a 100,000-square-foot building, this represents a range of four to six elevators, or for a 30,000-square-foot building, two elevators. For a 50,000-square-foot building, the range would be three to four elevators, rounded off on the high side.

Types of MOBs

Most medical offices are designed for multiple tenant occupancy. However, as the tendency toward larger group practices, clinics, and specialized medical services increases, this single-business design characteristic represents a specialized appraisal problem because of the inflexibility of the space for multiple tenancy. Here, the market analysis as well as the business evaluation become critical since the viability of the single tenant is an underwriting characteristic that can affect the valuation of the property and its potential marketability.

Entire buildings that have specialized medical activities are increasing. They may be termed ambulatory care centers, urgent care centers, imaging centers, surgery centers, etc. Most of these activities have higher tenant improvement cost requirements than typical MOBs, which is another appraisal consideration. For example, a surgery center tenant in an MOB may have a rental value requirement that is 25% to 35% higher than the typical medical suite in the same building.

A description on a component basis of a typical two-story medical office building is shown in Table 8.2.

Table 8.2	Description of Medical Office Building	
System component	**Specifications**	**Unit**
Foundations		
Footings & foundations	Poured concrete; strip and spread footings and 4 ft. foundation wall	S.F. Ground
Excavation & backfill	Site preparation for slab and trench for foundation wall and footing	S.F. Ground
Substructure		
Slab on grade	4" reinforced concrete with vapor barrier and granular base	S.F. Slab
Superstructure		
Columns & beams	Included in elevated floors	-
Elevated floors	Open web steel joists, slab form, concrete, columns	S.F. Floor
Roof	Metal deck, open web steel joists, beams, columns	S.F. Roof
Stairs	Concrete filled metal pan	Flight
Exterior Closure		
Walls	Concrete block, insulated (70% of wall)	S.F. Floor
Exterior wall finishes	Stucco on concrete block (70% of wall)	S.F. Wall
Doors	Aluminum and glass doors with transoms	Each
Windows & glazed walls	Outward projecting metal (30% of wall)	Each
Roofing		
Roof coverings	Built-up tar and gravel with flashing	S.F. Roof
Insulation	Perlite/urethane composite	S.F. Roof
Openings & specialties	Gravel stop and hatches	S.F. Roof
Interior Construction		
Partitions	Gypsum board and sound deadening board on wood studs with insulation (6 S.F. Floor/L.F. Partition)	S.F. Partition
Interior doors	Single leaf wood (60 S.F. Floor/Door)	Each
Wall finishes	50% paint, 50% vinyl wall coating	S.F. Surface
Floor finishes	50% carpet, 50% vinyl asbestos tile	S.F. Floor
Ceiling finishes	Mineral fiber tile on concealed zee bars	S.F. Ceiling
Interior surface/exterior wall	Painted gypsum board on furring (70% of wall)	S.F. Wall
Mechanical		
Plumbing	Toilet and service fixtures, supply & drainage (1 fixture/160 S.F. Fl.)	Each
Fire protection	N/A	-
Heating	Included in cooling	-
Cooling	Multizone unit, gas heating, electric cooling	S.F. Floor
Electrical		
Service & distribution	100 ampere service, panel board and feeders	S.F. Floor
Lighting and power	Fluorescent fixtures, receptacles, switches and misc. power	S.F. Floor
Special electrical	Alarm systems and emergency lighting	S.F. Floor

Source: *Means Square Foot Costs, 1991*, R.S. Means Company, Inc., Kingston, MA., p. 153.

Location Factors

There are no specific rules of thumb for rating location, but for valuation purposes a medical campus location is considered the best. On-campus locations are preferred because of the need for physicians to use their time to the highest degree of efficiency. Studies have shown that three out of four doctors choose a medical office facility that is either in a hospital or within an easy walk of one.

The demographics of an area have become more important to doctors when choosing where to locate their medical offices. While rental price is an obvious factor, choosing an area based on population growth rate and composition may be more important to attract patients. General care physicians should consider areas with high growth rates, while gerontologists and orthopedic surgeons should choose neighborhoods with older populations. Furthermore, some medical practices should be located near hospitals while others may profit more from locations in residential districts.

Various factors must be considered to ensure the success of an MOB such as the development of quality medical office facilities, provision of space for outpatient procedures, location of offices of leading physicians, potential expansion and movement of more practicing medical groups into the system, and the ownership structure between hospitals, physicians, and developers.

Market Analysis

The market analysis starts with defining the medical neighborhood or patient service area. In many areas the state government will have established health facilities planning areas (HFPAs), for which statistics and demographic data are available.

The analysis and study of supply should include existing and proposed MOBs that are competitive with the subject property. The analyst needs to determine the size of each building, its occupancy rate, and many other factors (see Table 8.3)

The study of demand should consider the space requirements per physician. This can be accomplished through a survey of medical office buildings considered similar to the subject in size and location. A recent study of a highly concentrated urban location found a range of 700 square feet to slightly over 1,000 square feet per physician and an average of about 800 square feet.

The amount of medical office space within a hospital campus or surrounding area that has not been constrained or limited in size due to outside factors may be analyzed to determine the relationship between occupied beds, physicians on staff, and the supply of MOB space. One such study found 1,021 square feet of MOB space being used for every occupied bed. Where MOB space has been limited or undersupplied, the lack of physicians (who are truly the clients of the hospital) can limit the admissions potential of the hospital. Additional MOB space could improve the hospital performance. Given the trend toward outpatient health services, the ratio of MOB space to hospital beds will likely continue to increase.

Another measure of MOB demand is the number of physicians per 1,000 civilian population. Statistics can be derived from state medical associations to compute ratios for cities, counties, and states. In urban areas, well-served populations have ratios ranging from 2.5 to 6 or more physicians per 1,000 persons where there are major medical centers and teaching hospitals.

Ratio analysis is a macro technique for analyzing proposed projects and unsatisfied demand for physicians, which can be converted to absorption rates for additional MOB space. This absorption, however, is predicated on proper and professional marketing. The medical community does not behave in a fashion typical to many other commercial markets. It possesses special professional, psychological, political, and financial needs, which must be addressed in the marketing program employed. For example, physicians typically prefer equity participation in their building of tenancy when a new project is being proposed. Developers need to be sensitive to the idiosyncrasies of the MOB market and its participants.

Data Required for Appraisal

A questionnaire may be prepared to gather data on the subject property or comparables. It will enable the analyst to obtain detailed information on rental prices, characteristics of occupants, quality of improvements, locational rating, improvement description, supply and demand factors, past and future absorption rates, etc. A specially designed questionnaire, as in Table 8.3, covers subject categories such as physical elements, absorption performance, rent schedule, tenant profile, competition, construction costs, and operating expenses.

The Appraisal Process

Medical office buildings are typically appraised using the three approaches to value. Primary weight should be given to the results indicated by the income approach since an MOB is an investment property. New projects or ones that are underutilized may require a discounted cash flow analysis to the point in time when the project is stabilized.

The cost approach may have more weight in the valuation of MOBs because of their scarcity in many circumstances, combined with the difficulty of developing a new project. This is especially true in a growing market where a project has a unique locational advantage such as an on-campus or close-to-hospital location. For a new project an adjustment for the status of occupancy should be made in the cost approach to provide for the income stream until stabilized occupancy is reached.

The sales comparison approach can be quite important because unit prices (presented on the basis of per square foot of net rentable area) can be used to appraise a subject property as well as to compare the prices paid for MOBs with those for typical professional buildings of a nonmedical nature. Where MOB comparables are limited, the difference between unit prices typically paid for MOBs and high quality professional buildings can be used as an adjustment factor. Differences between MOB comparables and the subject can be analyzed in terms of rental rates, net income per square foot of rentable area, gross revenue multiplier, and even price per physician/tenant under certain unique circumstances. It is proper to extend the geographic area for medical building comparables to a much larger area than would be typically used for professional buildings because of the way they are concentrated around certain, primary hospitals. Furthermore, arm's-length sales of MOBs are generally lacking because the well-managed ones are excellent investments for which owners are unwilling to relinquish control.

Cost Approach

The first step in the cost approach is the land valuation. In addition to a traditional land analysis on the basis of comparable sales converted to a price per square foot of land area, it is recommended that equivalent weight be given to a study of land prices for competitive projects converted to a price per square foot of gross or rentable floor area. The latter calculation will show land as a project cost input on a unit basis in the same manner as building improvements, and will reveal whether the land cost or value is at a proper level. It also provides an automatic adjustment for differences in project densities. Other factors such as time and location must be calculated by the appraiser.

On-campus locations will have a higher land value than off-campus locations. Corner sites are preferred, and locations that can attract related retail tenants such as a pharmacy on the ground floor should be given careful consideration.

On medical campuses, land for MOBs is usually leased by the primary hospital to the developing partnership on a fully subordinated basis for at least 75 years. Covenants typically

Table 8.3   **Medical Office Building Survey**

Physical Elements

1. Land area
2. Architectural style
3. Condition of building
4. Air conditioning
5. Number of floors
6. Number of elevators
7. Special features that enhance the building's serviceability, including unique design features
8. Special features/conditions that interfere with building operations
9. Number of parking spaces
10. Building's completion date
11. Gross building area
12. Square feet of net rentable space:
    a. Occupied by commercial tenants
    b. Occupied by other nonmedical tenants
13. Number and type of nonmedical tenants

Absorption Performance

1. Number of square feet/percentage of rental space committed upon opening
2. Number of square feet/percentage of rental space occupied:
    a. Within six months of opening
    b. Within one year of opening
    c. At present
3. Length of time after opening building was:
    a. 50% occupied
    b. 90% occupied
4. Key elements causing building to fill up as quickly as it did or kept it from filling up more quickly
5. Type of inducements used to attract physicians to the building:
    a. Tenant improvements allowance per square foot
    b. Free rent for _____ months
    c. Buy-out of existing leases
    d. Other
6. In addition to allowance for tenant improvements, average (estimated) amount spent by each physician to complete office, excluding equipment

Rent Schedule

1. The rental rate schedule for the building has been:
    a. Average rents on opening
    b. Average rents at present

2. When rent increases occurred
3. Periodic rental adjustments
4. Is rent for building higher than for other medical office buildings in same market area?
5. If so, is this higher rent attributable to:
    a. Hospital-oriented location?
    b. Newer facility?
6. Utilities and janitorial services, if any, included in rental
7. Is parking included in rent?
8. If not, monthly parking costs for tenants
9. Do tenants provide free parking to patients, using validation stamps, etc.?
10. Length of most leases
11. Is there is an escalation clause to provide for:
    a. Property taxes?
    b. Building operating costs?
12. Amount of last increase per square foot due to escalating costs

Competition

1. Competitive medical office buildings in the same market area:
    a. Name and location
    b. Rental rates
    c. Services

Total Cost of Building

1. Cost per square foot
    a. MOB
    b. Parking structure/other

Operating Expenses

1. Operating expense ratio (actual expenses exclusive of depreciation and interest as a percentage of stabilized gross)
2. Is there is a trend in operating ratios (up, down, or stabilized)?

General

1. Any knowledge of square-foot rental paid by doctors in space occupied before moving to this building
2. If doctors have indicated any change in admittance or referrals since moving into this building

Source: Author

included in the ground lease restrict the use of the building to tenancy by the hospital's medical staff and give the hospital the right of first refusal if the building is sold. Hospital-sponsored projects may also feature long-term leases from the primary hospital for a substantial portion of the building rentable area as well as cash equity in the project.

MOB construction costs typically exceed those of equivalent quality professional buildings by about 20%. Specialized interior areas, e.g., surgery centers (see Chapter 4), can add another $75 to $100 per square foot for the area occupied by the function. Other specialized areas such as imaging centers should be analyzed on a component basis or by a separate contractor's estimate.

Table 8.4 provides a detailed cost study of a proposed good quality medical office building. It illustrates current cost levels and relationships between hard costs and indirect costs. The proposed property is a four-story medical office building containing approximately 42,000 square feet of gross floor area with surface and structured parking for 277 cars (a ratio of 6.5 spaces per 1,000 square feet) situated on an existing hospital site. The appraised value of the land is $1,750,000, or approximately $42 per square foot of total gross medical office space area.

The total cost of the medical office building is based on the sum of the costs of the building shell and tenant improvements. In this example, the building shell and core cost $2,281,000 and tenant improvements cost $1,231,000. The balance of the total cost is represented by interim interest, loan fees, architectural and engineering, project management and leasing, legal and accounting, physician marketing expenses, miscellaneous costs and fees, and, finally, the developer's fee.

Tenant improvements are a considerable item, and allowance for them at various building rate levels varies from one project to another. Typically, this allowance runs from $35 to $60 per square foot of rentable area. In many projects the developer will provide a basic tenant improvement allowance, and then individual tenants will spend larger amounts to provide for a completed suite. This allows each physician to pay special attention to modifications that might be required because of the physician's professional specialty (e.g., interior partitioning, ceilings, carpeting, lighting, plumbing, cabinet work, decorative wall finishes).

In the example, additional cost items for developing the entire project include indirect or soft costs of $1,501,000, or slightly over 24% of the total cost of $6,219,000. The hard costs of the building shell, site development, and tenant improvements amount to $4,247,000, or about 68% of project costs. Not much can be done about loan fees (except a dose of hard bargaining), but interim interest charges can be reduced through faster construction timetables. The total project cost (exclusive of land) amounts to about $150 per square foot of gross floor area.

Recently compiled data indicate that good to high quality medical office space has been constructed in the range of $165 to $175 per square foot, not including land. Careful analysis should be made of cost comparables because they may include specialized facilities such as surgical suites or an imaging center with a much higher unit cost.

Medical Building Leases

Rental rates for good to excellent medical office buildings generally range from $1.25 to $2.50 per square foot per month on a full-service basis; however, many medical buildings are rented on a triple net basis where the tenants pay all of the operating expenses for the building over and above a base rate for the underlying real property. For comparative purposes the appraiser must be able to adjust leases from gross to net or net to gross, depending on the existing or planned lease basis for the subject property. In setting up medical office building leases special factors to consider include inflation, escalation clauses, parking requirements, type of ownership, tenant improvement allowance, and location. Table 8.5 is a grid of rent comparables on a triple net basis.

When buildings have been open for a period of time, management must have some means to increase rental income such as tying the basic rental rate to the Consumer Price Index or to

Table 8.4	Physicians Center Cost Breakdown		
Project Costs	**Cost**	**Per Square Foot**
Shell and core	$2,281,000	$54.31
Tenant improvements	1,231,000	29.31
Site development	735,000	17.50
Architecture & engineering	209,000	4.98
Loan fees	211,000	5.02
Construction period interest	387,000	9.21
Physician marketing expenses	246,000	5.86
Construction management	127,000	3.02
Permits, fees, bonds	60,000	1.43
Leasing commissions	211,000	5.02
Syndication costs	50,000	1.19
Development fee	311,000	7.40
Miscellaneous and contingency	187,000	4.45
Total project costs	$6,219,000	$148.07

other tax and escalation clauses. To facilitate initial lease-up, rents should be set at a moderate but competitive level.

A parking space for each doctor is often included in the basic rent at no additional cost. The controlling factor is usually the cost of providing parking facilities. Where land values are high, the doctors may be charged an additional monthly amount for parking in a costly garage. Very few doctors provide free patient parking (using a validation system or tokens). In some cases patients pay for parking at an hourly rate.

Rental rates for MOBs vary according to type of ownership. Generally, privately developed and investment-oriented buildings receive more in monthly rental rates compared to hospital-owned buildings. Hospitals often subsidize developments by various means so that their rates will be lower. This is done by charging a rate that is substantially lower than the fair market rental for the land on which the building is located. This practice may be illegal, but appraisers should allow for proper adjustment. Buildings situated adjacent to these hospitals will lease more rapidly at higher rental rates than similar buildings without this characteristic.

Income Approach

In the example in Table 8.6, project income was comprised of income from the rental of office space. Office space income production is calculated by standardized space times rate applications. The rental survey in Table 8.5 supported a rental conclusion of $2.05 per square foot per month, triple net.

Although the leases are on a triple net basis, it is necessary to analyze these costs to determine total occupancy costs for the physician tenants. Operating expenses include such catego-

Table 8.5			Physicians Center Rental Rate Adjustment Grid						
Comp. No.	Effective Rate	Rate/Usable Sq. Ft.	$35 Tenant Improvement Adjustment	NNN Adjustment	Parking Adjustment	Physical/ Age	Location		Adjusted NNN Rate
1.	$2.25	$2.50	+$0.05	-$0.55	+$0.09	+5%	-5%		$2.09
2.	$2.00	$2.00	+$0.10	$0	$0	0	-5%		$2.00
3.	$1.62	$1.78	+$0.13	$0	$0	0	+5%		$2.01
4.	$2.09	$2.34	+$0.10	-$0.55	$0	+10%	0		$2.08
5.	$2.15	$2.15	+$0.10	-$0.55	+$0.03	+10%	0		$1.90
6.	$2.15	$2.48	-$0.03	-$0.55	$0	0	+5%		$2.00
7.	$2.70	$2.70	+$0.05	-$0.55	+$0.08	0	-10%		$2.05
8.	$1.90	$1.90	+$0.15	-$0.45	$0	+10%	+15%		$2.00
9.	$1.70	$1.87	+$0.15	-$0.45	$0	+15%	+10%		$1.96

ries as cleaning, electricity, heating and air conditioning, water, management, maintenance and repairs, insurance, gardener, scavenger service, real estate taxes, reserves for replacement, elevator maintenance, and miscellaneous items. The expenses may be analyzed in terms of:

1. Cost per square foot of rentable area for categories that are a function of the size of the building. *The Office Building Experience Exchange Report,* published annually by BOMA International, provides operating expense statistics for medical office buildings by downtown and suburban location (see Table 8.7). Operating expenses for MOBs exceed those of similarly designed professional buildings usually by 15% to 30%.

2. Percentage of effective gross income for those items that vary with the volume of business.

3. Direct contract costs for categories that are based on contract services, e.g., elevator maintenance.

4. Comparison with other facilities.

In the last category, real estate taxes may be computed on the basis of tax per square foot of net rentable area as they are applied to comparable MOBs in the area, or the taxes can be put into the capitalization rate if state law requires that properties be assessed at market value or sale price.

Capitalization of Income

In the final step in this analysis the total net income is converted into a value estimate. The capitalization rate could be based on a function of the mortgage financing cost and equity return requirements, comparable sales of other MOBs, or investment surveys of experts in the field. In the example shown here, a capitalization rate of 9.5% was used, which resulted in a total property valuation of $6,200,000, as of completion, and $7,500,000 as of stabilization (see Table 8.6).

Sales Comparison Approach

The sales comparison approach compares a subject property to recent sales and/or listings of other MOBs in the area of the subject property or in competing areas. Each of the sales must be analyzed

Table 8.6	Discounted Cash Flow				
Item	Mos. 0-6	Mos. 7-12	Mos. 13-18	Mos. 19-24	Year 3
Rental rate per sq. ft. per month	$2.05	$2.05	$2.05	$2.05	$2.15
Leased area	26,373	28,571	30,769	32,967	35,164
Potential gross income	$162,194	$175,712	$189,229	$202,747	$907,231
Less: Vacancy & collection loss (5%)	Scheduled	Scheduled	Scheduled	Scheduled	$45,362
Effective gross income	$162,194	$175,712	$189,229	$202,747	$861,869
Expenses					
Nonreimbursed fixed ($0.15/S.F./Mo., +5%/year)*	$23,735	$25,714	$27,692	$29,670	$66,502
Management (5% effective)	$8,110	$8,786	$9,461	$10,137	$43,093
Lease commissions (25% initial leases)**	$51,361	$51,361	$51,361	$51,361	0
Reserves for replacements (2% potential)	$3,244	$3,514	$3,785	$4,055	$17,237
Total expense	$86,450	$89,375	$92,299	$95,223	$126,832
Net operating income (loss)	$75,744	$86,337	$96,930	$107,524	$735,037

Value at Completion		Stabilized & Reversion Values	
Present value NOI (Months 0-24) @ 12%	$313,692	Year 3 NOI	$735,037
Plus: Present value reversion @ 12%	$5,910,744	Capitalized @ 9.5% (Stabilized Value)	$7,737,232
Value at completion	$6,224,466	Less: 3% Commission (Reversion Value)	$7,505,115
Rounded	$6,200,000	Rounded	$7,500,000

* Computed on basis of occupied space at end of period.
** Based on total lease commissions to reach 95% occupancy, divided evenly during the first four six-month periods

to establish the elements of comparability. The reliability of this technique depends on 1) the degree of comparability between the subject and the sale property; 2) the length of time since the sales were consummated; 3) the accuracy of the sales data; and 4) the absence of unusual conditions affecting each sale. In comparing sales to the subject property, adjustments are typically made for location, quality, date of sale, tenancies, parking, status of the primary hospital (if the MOB is on a medical campus) as well as the financial status of the tenants. Obviously, this type of analysis goes far beyond what is typically made for a conventional office building.

Properties are typically analyzed on a price per square foot of net rentable area and then adjusted for the factors listed above. It should be recognized that MOBs are unique investments and do not follow the trends of the conventional office market. Under proper conditions they are considered to be outstanding real estate investments because of such factors as a limited supply or a growing physician market. Other considerations include physician tenant mix,

Table 8.7   Medical Building Income and Expense Averages

Medical Buildings
ALL SUBURBAN

	# BLDS	TOTAL BUILDING RENTABLE AREA				TOTAL OFFICE RENTABLE AREA			
69 BLDS		4,124,781 SQ. FT.				4,068,206 SQ. FT.			
		DOLLARS/SQ. FT.		MID RANGE		DOLLARS/SQ. FT.		MID RANGE	
INCOME	BLDS	AVG	MEDIAN	LOW	HIGH	AVG	MEDIAN	LOW	HIGH
OFFICE AREA	66					16.56	15.24	12.24	19.79
RETAIL AREA	9	15.95	17.48	11.13	21.86				
OTHER AREA	2	6.63	6.61						
TOTAL RENT	67	16.41	15.11	12.38	19.83				
NET PARKING INC	20	2.06	.88	.10	2.64				
MISCELLANEOUS	37	.09	.05	.02	.11				
TOTAL INCOME	67	17.44	15.54	12.61	19.94				
EXPENSE									
CLEANING	65	1.06	1.03	.82	1.27	1.07	1.04	.84	1.27
REPAIR/MAINT	69	.91	.85	.64	1.11	.91	.85	.64	1.12
UTILITIES	64	1.86	1.80	1.54	2.17	1.87	1.81	1.54	2.17
RDS/GDS/SEC	69	.41	.36	.23	.56	.42	.36	.23	.56
ADMINISTRATIVE	69	.99	.78	.61	1.10	1.01	.78	.61	1.10
TOTAL OPER EXP	62	5.24	5.24	4.33	6.12	5.31	5.32	4.41	6.21
FIXED EXPENSES	66	1.76	1.59	1.20	2.01	1.79	1.68	1.20	2.01
TOTAL OPER+FIX	60	7.01	6.88	6.02	8.14	7.12	7.05	6.04	8.14
LEASING EXP	58	1.53	.79	.22	2.36				
TOTAL PAYROLL	58	.71	.45	.29	.83				
TOTAL CONTRACT	35	2.09	2.17	1.71	2.62				

OCCUPANCY INFO.	AVERAGE	BLDS
SQFT/OFFICE TENANT	2634	61
SQFT/RETAIL TENANT	1507	13
SQFT/OFFICE WORKER	318	40
SQFT/MAINT STAFF	56,249	41
OFFICE OCCUPANCY (%)	87.5	69
RETAIL OCCUPANCY (%)	99.3	13
YR-END RENT ($)	18.97	55
NET PARKING INC/STALL ($)	492	19
PARKING RATIO (SF)	248	44
RENTABLE/GROSS SQFT	.90	46

DETAIL*	AVERAGE	BLDS	DETAIL*	AVERAGE	BLDS	DETAIL*	AVERAGE	BLDS	DETAIL*	AVERAGE	BLDS	DETAIL*	AVERAGE	BLDS
OFFICE RENT			**REPAIR/MAINT**			PURCH CH WTR	.77	2	**ADMINISTRATIVE**			**LEASING EXPENSES**		
BASE RENT	15.49	66	PAYROLL	.36	60	COAL			PAYROLL	.63	24	ADV/PROMOTION	.03	29
PASS-THROUGHS	2.77	23	ELEVATOR	.11	57	WATER/SEWER	.15	63	MGMT FEES	.61	62	COMMISSIONS	.43	40
OPER COST ESCAL	.89	25	HVAC	.17	64				PROF FEES	.10	25	PROF FEES	.10	23
BASE RENT ESCAL			ELECTRICAL	.05	60	**RDS/GDS/SEC**			GEN OFC EXP	.09	46	TENANT ALTS	1.51	41
LEASE CANCEL			STRUCT/ROOF	.05	37	RDS/GDS TOTAL	.21	63	OTHER ADM EXP	.06	43	BUY-OUTS		
RENT ABATEMENT	.17	4	PLUMBING	.02	58	RDS/GDS PAYROLL	.19	9				OTHER LEASING	.10	13
TENANT SVCS INC	.05	17	FIRE/LIFE SAFETY	.05	44	RDS/GDS CONTRACT	.17	55	**FIXED EXPENSES**					
			OTHER MAINT/SUP	.18	61	RDS/GDS OTHER	.07	43	REAL ESTATE TAX	1.59	66	**OTHER CONTRACTS**		
CLEANING									BLDG INSURANCE	.17	66	REPAIR/MAINT	.29	35
PAYROLL	.39	6	**UTILITIES**			SECURITY TOTAL	.28	50	PERS PROP TAX	.57	13	ADMINISTRATIVE	.64	64
CONTRACT	.88	62	ELECTRICITY	1.61	64	SEC PAYROLL	.17	6	OTHER TAX	.04	16			
SUP/MAT/MISC	.08	58	GAS	.12	40	SEC CONTRACT	.27	45						
TRASH REMOVAL	.07	58	FUEL OIL			SEC OTHER	.03	13						
			PURCH STEAM	.36	2									

*Income calculation based on office rentable s.f.; Expense calculation based on total bldg. rentable s.f.

©1996 BOMA Experience Exchange Report

SUBURBAN LESS THAN 50,000 SQ. FT.

	# BLDS	TOTAL BUILDING RENTABLE AREA				TOTAL OFFICE RENTABLE AREA			
21 BLDS		667,831 SQ. FT.				661,784 SQ. FT.			
		DOLLARS/SQ. FT.		MID RANGE		DOLLARS/SQ. FT.		MID RANGE	
INCOME	BLDS	AVG	MEDIAN	LOW	HIGH	AVG	MEDIAN	LOW	HIGH
OFFICE AREA	20					14.30	15.10	12.69	16.57
RETAIL AREA									
OTHER AREA	2	6.63	6.61						
TOTAL RENT	20	14.24	14.92	12.69	16.19				
NET PARKING INC	2	.18	.27						
MISCELLANEOUS	5	.05	.02	.01	.18				
TOTAL INCOME	20	14.28	14.92	12.69	16.21				
EXPENSE									
CLEANING	20	1.21	1.10	.81	1.39	1.21	1.10	.83	1.39
REPAIR/MAINT	21	1.04	1.01	.77	1.34	1.05	1.01	.77	1.34
UTILITIES	21	1.80	1.71	1.45	2.27	1.80	1.71	1.45	2.33
RDS/GDS/SEC	21	.33	.32	.23	.46	.34	.32	.23	.46
ADMINISTRATIVE	21	.74	.74	.54	.82	.75	.74	.54	.82
TOTAL OPER EXP	20	5.18	5.15	4.26	6.47	5.23	5.15	4.26	6.48
FIXED EXPENSES	21	1.97	1.59	1.24	2.20	1.99	1.64	1.24	2.26
TOTAL OPER+FIX	20	7.21	6.82	5.53	8.25	7.28	7.10	5.53	8.29
LEASING EXP	15	1.26	.59	.25	.85				
TOTAL PAYROLL	17	.52	.42	.28	.60				
TOTAL CONTRACT	13	2.06	1.84	1.52	2.77				

OCCUPANCY INFO.	AVERAGE	BLDS
SQFT/OFFICE TENANT	2589	17
SQFT/RETAIL TENANT	937	3
SQFT/OFFICE WORKER	259	12
SQFT/MAINT STAFF	42,360	8
OFFICE OCCUPANCY (%)	86.7	21
RETAIL OCCUPANCY (%)	100.0	3
YR-END RENT ($)	16.39	16
NET PARKING INC/STALL ($)	27	2
PARKING RATIO (SF)	216	13
RENTABLE/GROSS SQFT	.86	12

DETAIL*	AVERAGE	BLDS	DETAIL*	AVERAGE	BLDS	DETAIL*	AVERAGE	BLDS	DETAIL*	AVERAGE	BLDS	DETAIL*	AVERAGE	BLDS
OFFICE RENT			**REPAIR/MAINT**			PURCH CH WTR			**ADMINISTRATIVE**			**LEASING EXPENSES**		
BASE RENT	12.12	20	PAYROLL	.37	17	COAL			PAYROLL	.44	8	ADV/PROMOTION	.06	6
PASS-THROUGHS	4.80	9	ELEVATOR	.09	17	WATER/SEWER	.16	21	MGMT FEES	.53	19	COMMISSIONS	.32	9
OPER COST ESCAL	.61	5	HVAC	.28	21				PROF FEES	.01	3	PROF FEES	.09	7
BASE RENT ESCAL			ELECTRICAL	.10	21	**RDS/GDS/SEC**			GEN OFC EXP	.07	12	TENANT ALTS	1.71	8
LEASE CANCEL			STRUCT/ROOF	.09	15	RDS/GDS TOTAL	.29	21	OTHER ADM EXP	.05	12	BUY-OUTS		
RENT ABATEMENT			PLUMBING	.03	19	RDS/GDS PAYROLL	.20	2				OTHER LEASING	.16	2
TENANT SVCS INC	.07	5	FIRE/LIFE SAFETY	.05	16	RDS/GDS CONTRACT	.20	21	**FIXED EXPENSES**					
			OTHER MAINT/SUP	.15	20	RDS/GDS OTHER	.14	12	REAL ESTATE TAX	1.76	21	**OTHER CONTRACTS**		
CLEANING									BLDG INSURANCE	.20	21	REPAIR/MAINT	.41	13
PAYROLL			**UTILITIES**			SECURITY TOTAL	.07	13	PERS PROP TAX			ADMINISTRATIVE	.50	20
CONTRACT	1.01	18	ELECTRICITY	1.37	21	SEC PAYROLL			OTHER TAX	.06	4			
SUP/MAT/MISC	.17	18	GAS	.27	16	SEC CONTRACT	.07	12						
TRASH REMOVAL	.10	17	FUEL OIL			SEC OTHER	.02	4						
			PURCH STEAM											

*Income calculation based on office rentable s.f.; Expense calculation based on total bldg. rentable s.f.

©1996 BOMA Experience Exchange Report

Source: *1996 Experience Exchange Report*, Building Owners and Managers International, Washington, DC. Reprinted with permission.

availability (or lack thereof) of outpatient services and competing projects, reputation or name of the building, and demographics of the trade or service area. An example of a sales summary and adjustment grid is shown in Table 8.8.

Conclusion

A medical office building requires a high degree of expertise to develop and to analyze. Many MOB projects have highly unique or monopoly-type locations close to primary hospitals, which has resulted in extremely high rentals and appraised values. In general, however, building prices and rentals have tended to stabilize in recent years due to the state of the economy and the inability of physicians to increase their revenues beyond the rate of inflation. A recent wave of MOB development has incorporated new design features and construction techniques that have resulted in increased efficiency and income producing potential.

Studies have indicated that the cost of space is relatively insignificant when compared to the total income and operating costs of a doctor's practice. Physicians are motivated to make efficient use of their time. A small savings of 30 minutes per day in travel time can result in an annual income potential of as much as $50,000. This compares to a typical annual rent of $20,000 at current prices for a good quality, 1,000-square-foot office space. Thus, the trend to locate medical office buildings as close as possible to primary hospitals is based on economics which are likely to prevail in the future.

Other trends taking place in the MOB market include the development of condominium medical office buildings and sale-leasebacks of MOBs by hospital owners. The latter allows hospitals to release capital tied up in real estate for other purposes, including balance sheet considerations, and to relieve perceived conflicts. MOB development will also be affected by the continued introduction of new design standards to maximize physician productivity.

Development of MOBs is beyond the scope of the typical real estate entrepreneur who has capabilities in the commercial investment market. Evidence indicates that larger firms with research expertise, medical and health care knowledge, the ability to work with specialized tenants, and with contractual or close relationships with HMOs, PPOs, and hospital systems will have a very substantial advantage.

Table 8.8

Improved Sales Summary Grid

	Comparable 1	Comparable 2	Comparable 3	Comparable 4	Comparable 5	Subject
Price	$4,650,000	$8,594,635	$12,750,000	$5,200,000	$12,316,980	
Size (rentable SF)	32,086	47,604	71,206	25,684	55,300	57,812
Price per SF	$145	$181	$179	$202	$223	
Date of sale	3/28/95	7/21/94	1/14/94	12/16/93	4/1/93	
Year built	1968	1992	1984	1987	1988	1962
Type of construction	steel frame	concrete tilt-up	concrete & steel/concrete tilt-up (2 bldgs.)	steel frame	concrete & steel	concrete & steel
Site area (acres)	1.38	3.15	2.56	0.34	2.79	1.90
Parking ratio (per 1,000 S.F.)	2.7	4.9	4.9	3.7	5.6	2.4 (3.7 with adjacent spaces)
Occupancy at sale	70%	100%	93%	96%	100%	100%
Gross income	$596,796	$1,096,800	$2,078,029	$647,237	$1,000,800	$1,502,224 (projected)
GRM	7.8	7.8	6.1	8.0	12.3	
NOI, adjusted	N/A	$937,764 (est. at 90% occ.)	$1,228,937 (est. at 94% occ.)	$382,882 (est. at 96% occ.)	$855,684	$899,813 (projected)
NOI per SF	N/A	$19.70	$17.26	$14.91	$15.47	$15.56 (projected)
Overall rate, adjusted	N/A	10.9%	9.6%	7.4%	6.9%	

(continued)

Table 8.8   Improved Sales Summary Grid (continued)

	Comparable 1	Comparable 2	Comparable 3	Comparable 4	Comparable 5
Adjustment Grid					
Price	$4,650,000	$8,594,635	$12,750,000	$5,200,000	$12,316,980
Financing terms	0.0%	-5.0%	0.0%	0.0%	-10.0%
Conditions of sale	0.0%	0.0%	0.0%	0.0%	0.0%
Cash-equivalent price	$4,650,000	$8,164,903	$12,750,000	$5,200,000	$11,085,282
Date of sale	0.0%	0.0%	0.0%	0.0%	0.0%
Time-adjusted price	$4,650,000	$8,164,903	$12,750,000	$5,200,000	$11,085,282
Location	0.0%	-15.0%	-10.0%	0.0%	0.0%
Access/exposure	0.0%	0.0%	0.0%	0.0%	0.0%
Building age/condition	10.8%	5.0%	0.0%	0.0%	0.0%
Amenities	0.0%	0.0%	0.0%	-12.9%	0.0%
Total adjustments	10.8%	-15.0%	-10.0%	-12.9%	-10.0%
Adjusted price	$5,150,000	$7,348,413	$11,475,000	$4,528,000	$11,085,282
Adjusted price per SF	$161	$154	$161	$176	$200

C H A P T E R

N I N E

Adaptive Reuse of Medical Facilities

The adaptive reuse of medical facilities necessarily addresses highest and best use questions related to a given facility. Attention to this type of analysis is significant since the useful economic life of certain types of facilities, especially acute care hospitals, commonly ends due to financial reasons even though the physical facilities are sound and usually can be used for other economically productive purposes. Although these are special-purpose properties, appraisal errors can occur if the analyst is overwhelmed by the original purpose and nature of the building and fails to question if that purpose is still economically viable. The necessary analysis requires two primary areas of concern: 1) can the facility continue to be profitable in its present or past role given current market conditions and trends? and 2) if not, what are the adaptive reuse possibilities short of demolition? This chapter offers special suggestions for analyzing and understanding market conditions, particularly the difficulties facing hospitals, and provides a simplified "ladder" of probable reuse possibilities as a reference point for a given property.

Nature of the Problem

The rate of hospital closures could increase in the future if proposed cuts in health care spending now being debated in Congress become a reality. According to the National Association of Urban Critical Access Hospitals, "The Medicare changes called for by the Congressional budgets would have a devastating impact on America's urban hospitals, leading to sharp cutbacks in service, and would even close the doors on many established facilities." Although the hospital industry has tended to overstate the threat of closures due to government cutbacks, this factor will have to be closely watched.

Each of the medical facilities discussed in this book tends to exist within its own market context unless specifically linked by some special circumstance. For example, medical office buildings can be considered in the larger context of a town or an extended neighborhood unless they are located on a hospital campus. In such cases they are "linked" to a variety of policies and practices of the primary hospital as well as to the general trends, fortunes, and specialties of the hospital. Medical practices are similarly affected and analyzed. Skilled nursing facilities, rehabilitation hospitals, and a variety of clinics also may have an interrelationship with hospitals or other patient-channeling entities. These linkages, if they have relative permanence, usually affect value in a positive way and must be probed and analyzed.

Unfortunately, many of the relationships between given facilities and how they obtain patronage are subtle and often purposely kept secret. General hospitals tend to be the most complex and expensive facilities and also the most highly regulated. As such, they are also the most reviewed, reported, and difficult to understand, but they are related in significant ways to the other medical uses and facilities discussed in this book. Thus, to some extent, they can be viewed as a convenient exemplar to explain characteristics applicable to some other medical facilities for which complete and regular information is unavailable.

A continuing review of medical industry literature indicates an interplay for more than half a century between government policy and the economics of the health care industry in the United States. While the rhetoric changes as do the policies and methods of subsidization, a relatively steady investment of new capital in medical facilities of various kinds has occurred in recent years despite numerous hospital closures and a popular media perception that the health care industry is in danger. Clearly on a national basis there is a vast oversupply of available hospital beds, but bed supply and occupancy are only one of many relevant factors.

An American Hospital Association study of hospital closures from 1980 through 1993 showed that the number of closures varied widely from 1980 to 1988 but thereafter leveled out at approximately 60 per year (see Figure 9.1, Table 9.1. and Table 9.2) . In 1993, 34 acute care hospitals and 28 specialty hospitals—mainly rehab and psychiatric facilities—closed. These closing rates would suggest a shrinkage in the total number of hospitals, especially in an overbedded world. However, the other side of the equation—new hospitals opened—shows that in 1993, 23 new specialty hospitals and 17 new acute care hospitals opened. Of the 34 acute care hospitals that closed, 16 continued to offer some form of ancillary health care.

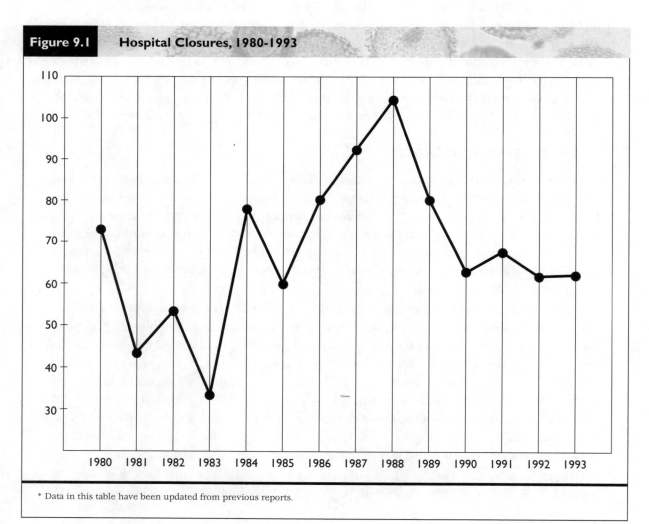

Figure 9.1   Hospital Closures, 1980-1993

* Data in this table have been updated from previous reports.

Table 9.1	Hospital Closures, 1980-1993		
Year	Total	Community	Non-Community
1980	73	45	28
1981	43	27	16
1982*	53	24	29
1983*	34	24	10
1984	76	45	31
1985*	59	47	12
1986*	80	68	12
1987*	93	77	16
1988*	106	85	21
1989	80	65	15
1990	63	50	13
1991	67	45	22
1992	60	39	21
1993	62	34	28
Total	949	675	274

* Data in this table have been updated from previous reports.

Source: American Hospital Association, *Directory of Multihospital Systems, 1980-1987, AHA Guide,* 1988-1993, *Financial Growth and Diversification of Hospitals and Multihospital Systems,* 1988, *Data Book on Multihospital Systems,* 1980-1985, *Hospital Statistics,* 1992-93, and *Annual Survey of Hospitals,* 1992.

Table 9.2	Urban/Rural Hospital Closures, 1980-1993					
	Urban			Rural		
Year	Total	Community	Non-Community	Total	Community	Non-Community
1980	51	30	21	22	15	7
1981	30	16	14	13	11	2
1982*	29	9	20	24	15	9
1983*	24	17	7	10	7	3
1984	49	27	22	27	18	9
1985*	36	27	9	23	20	3
1986*	42	32	10	38	36	2
1987*	50	37	13	43	40	3
1988*	57	39	18	49	46	3
1989	30	21	9	50	44	6
1990	32	22	10	31	28	3
1991	34	16	18	33	29	4
1992	34	18	16	26	21	5
1993	42	15	27	20	19	1
Total	540	326	214	409	349	60

* Data in this table have been updated from previous reports, based on additional information received during the routine canvass for information on closed hopsitals.

Source: American Hospital Association, *Directory of Multihospital Systems, 1980-1987, AHA Guide,* 1988-1993, *Financial Growth and Diversification of Hospitals and Multihospital Systems,* 1988, *Data Book on Multihospital Systems,* 1980-1985, *Hospital Statistics,* 1992-93, and *Annual Survey of Hospitals,* 1992.

| Table 9.3 | Multihospital Systems, 1979-1992 |

Year	Number of Systems	Number of Hospitals in System	Percent of All Hospitals
1979	267	1,797	27.1%
1980	256	1,877	28.4
1981	256	1,924	29.2
1982	243	1,958	29.8
1983	249	2,050	31.3
1984	250	2,208	33.8
1985	268	2,477	37.9
1986	278	2,514	38.7
1987	303	2,567	39.6
1988	303	2,572	40.0
1989	307	2,901	43.2
1990	311	2,906	43.7
1991	309	2,873	43.3
1992	300	2,826	43.2
Percent change, 1979-1982	12.4%	57.3%	

Note: Increases between 1988 and 1989 reflect, in part, inclusion of federal hospitals in 1989 and thereafter.

Source: American Hospital Association, *Directory of Multihospital Systems, 1980-1987, AHA Guide,* 1988-1993, *Financial Growth and Diversification of Hospitals and Multihospital Systems,* 1988, *Data Book on Multihospital Systems,* 1980-1985, *Hospital Statistics,* 1992-93, and *Annual Survey of Hospitals,* 1992.

Perhaps most important, at those times since 1980 when it appeared that closure rates were rising, the dollar value of new hospital construction was also rising. Thus, most of the closures represent normal recycling of facilities due to changes in style, technology, and other forms of obsolescence as well as the effects of normal business mergers and consolidations and the growth of hospital systems (see Table 9.3).

It should be noted that standard building cost and age-life references (e.g., *Marshall Valuation Service*) estimate the typical life of hospital buildings at 35 to 50 years depending on design. Nevertheless, it is common in the real market to see 30-year-old buildings at the end of their useful lives as hospitals. This latter reality is well supported by the American Hospital Association,[1] which estimates building lives between 20 to 40 years depending on design type (see Table 9.4). The time when a specific building actually reaches a point of sufficient obsolescence to require replacement and/or reuse is quite variable depending on facility finances and local market and competitive conditions. Clearly, noncompetitive situations can result in vastly

[1] *Estimated Useful Lives of Depreciable Hospital Assets,* 1988 edition (Chicago: American Hospital Association).

Table 9.4

Item	Years	Item	Years
Building Components		**Buildings**	
Automatic doors	10	Boiler house	30
Canopies	15	Garage	
Ceiling finishes	12	Masonry	25
Computer flooring	10	Wood frame	15
Cubicle tracks	20	Guardhouse	15
Designation signs	5	Masonry building, reinforced concrete frame	40
Drapery tracks	10	Masonry building, steel frame	
Floor finishes	10	Fireproofed	40
Folding partitions	10	Not fireproofed	30
Handrails	15	Masonry building, wood frame	25
Interior finishes	15	Metal-clad buildng	20
Loading docks	15	Multilevel parking structure, masonry	25
Overhead doors	10	Reinforced concrete building, common design	40
Partitions, interior	15	Residence	
Partitions, toilet	20	Masonry	25
Railings	15	Wood frame	25
Roof covering	10	Storage building	
Storefront construction	20	Masonry	25
Wall paint	5	Metal garden-type	10
Wallpaper	5	Wood frame	18

Table 9.4   Estimated Useful Lives of Building Components and Buildings

Source: American Hospital Association, *Estimated Useful Lives of Depreciable Hospital Assets*, 1988 edition. Copyright by the American Hospital Association.

extended building lives whereas competitive urban situations can result in even relatively new buildings being recycled when, for example, efforts to break into a new market have not succeeded. While such facilities can often be sold to a competitor and recycled without a change in use, such situations often cause an older nearby facility to be retired.

Similar factors and circumstances affect other medical facilities. To the extent that properties are unspecialized, more customary notions of building life prevail as are typically reported in the general commercial market. Following are some broad statements concerning potential reuse of specific types of medical facilities:

1. *Medical Office Buildings.* Rarely recycled. Due to limited supply and growing physician population, usually a medical-related occupancy is available for vacated spaces, even in older buildings. In rare situations, buildings can be used for general office types of activities.

2. *Psychiatric Hospitals.* Recently sold facilities that are relatively new are being acquired by local government agencies for outpatient purposes or by former competitors for continued use as designed. The market is recognizing a substantial decline in value in these circumstances.

3. *Nursing Homes.* Rarely recycled. Due to continued and growing demand for long-term care beds even the oldest SNF can be profitable with a very high ratio of beds occupied by Medicaid-reimbursed patients. Older SNFs may be periodically upgraded to meet current standards or codes, and even if they are shut down or empty, usually an operator is ready and willing to do a start-up operation except in extraordinary circumstances. SNFs are sometimes converted to a higher use such as a rehabilitation hospital (which typically requires only a skilled nursing license).

4. *Assisted Living Facilities.* Most are too new to have experienced a possible change in use. Former unlicensed congregate housing facilities for the elderly are being upgraded in design requirements to ALFs. In oversupplied markets, facilities that have undergone foreclosure are typically acquired by efficient operators and down-priced in terms of monthly fees to broaden the market reach.

5. *Surgery Centers.* Rarely recycled. Only a few examples of failures of freestanding operations exist. SCs situated in MOBs can be reconverted to normal medical office use.

6. *Rehabilitation Hospitals.* Many of these were formerly used as community hospitals or SNFs. If they fail in their rebirth, they are likely to be reused for some type of outpatient activity related to substance abuse or child care or as a public clinic, or they may be converted to low-cost institutional space for general office use.

7. *Other Specialty Hospitals.* Hospitals catering to specific health problems (e.g., eye and ear hospital) have been "blindsided" by recent changes in health care delivery. Factors such as managed care, capitation of fees, cutbacks in Medicare payments, and changes in technology are likely to put an end to these types of facilities.

Identifying Problem Properties

Closed facilities clearly represent problem properties but do not always indicate the necessity for adaptive reuse. However, in most cases the author has observed, the mere closing of a facility, in the absence of some clear reason to refute the assumption, almost certainly indicates that demolition or adaptive reuse is in order. A common appraisal mistake in such cases involves failure to adequately analyze and understand the reasons for the closure. The error is compounded if it is falsely assumed that readiness of the facility for the older use is deemed sufficient reason to apply average industry profit ratios after adjustments for reopening costs and absorption. Where a hospital has closed and the license has terminated or the fixtures and equipment have been sold, it is almost certain that it is not feasible to restore the old use. (As an aside regarding the value in-place of equipment, a common rule of thumb for value is 10% of original cost. Typically, professional hospital equipment buyers will inventory the equipment and bid a fixed price with the right to price and resell or auction to the public over a period of, say, 30 days. Should an analyst conclude that a rule-of-thumb approach is insufficient, companies that specialize in the disposal of such property should be consulted.)

Recognizing problem properties that are still in operation is basically a typical business analysis that considers the characteristics of the market in which the subject property is operating, trends and directions of the market, and the specific performance of the subject property.

Each of the medical facility types discussed in this book tends to have its own market characteristics. In most cases medical facilities are relatively local businesses, but this is not always the case. Certain diagnostic hospitals are nationally and world famous. Similarly, a few drug rehab centers have widespread fame (usually attributed to celebrity guests). The extent of the market is usually obvious from the method of referral and/or marketing. Certain niche medical operations can be found in the hospital field where, for example, weight-control programs have been marketed regionally or nationally. Similarly, some psychiatric hospitals have functioned on a fairly wide regional basis with referrals from a variety of clinics and other hospitals. Congregate care facilities for the elderly are typically local businesses but exceptions occur where marketing is done on a religious or other basis without local limitations. Within the limitations of the typical marketing mechanism, it is important to know the extent and nature of competing facilities and the general supply of available facilities compared to demand. In some states, a needs determination is necessary for licensing a facility. Where this is the case, the relevant state agency typically maintains the necessary information and conclusions. When it is necessary to do this analysis independently, the guiding factor is evidence of a significant level of unsatisfied demand. Other chapters have discussed specific methods and rules of thumb for analyzing market demand.

In some cases trends and directions in the local market can make a difference in predicting a change in the present performance of a property. For example, facilities of various types clustered around and dependent on a hospital operation will clearly suffer if the hospital closes or changes its business operations in a substantial way. Commonly, population growth and direction are significant to businesses in developing areas. Such growth characteristics may very well offset current poor performance if simple shortage of demand is a critical factor. Conversely, the aging and economic decline of neighborhoods are likely to affect adversely what may be a currently viable operation.

Analysis of the subject property must at least address the so-called "bottom line." Clearly an enterprise that is operating at a loss is a problem property unless it is in a planned absorption phase or some other factor can be identified that will bring an end to the losses. Another characteristic that must be studied is utilization. In hospitals this factor is typically reported as a bed-occupancy rate although in some cases a variety of outpatient and other activities may offset the simple implication of an occupancy rate. Occupancy or other tests of utilization should be noted over at least a three-year period to ascertain trends in the performance of the subject property. To the extent possible, management performance should also be studied.

Monitoring and reporting services are available for some types of facilities.[2] Approximately 1,100 facilities nationally (about 20% of the total) have recently been designated as financially distressed. During the last four years (to mid-1994), the percentage of financially distressed hospitals has not changed significantly. Average characteristics of distressed hospitals appear in Table 9.5. Once these types of characteristics have been analyzed and a problem property identified, the issue of adaptive reuse is automatically raised. It can also arise from other circumstances not specifically obvious in the foregoing analysis. Some of these factors include

---

[2] Since 1990 Health Care Investment Analysts, Inc., has compiled a list of distressed hospitals on a quarterly basis. HCIA specifically monitors occupancy rate, average days in accounts receivable, long-term debt to total assets, operating profit margin, and total profit margin. It then identifies hospitals as distressed "if they showed substantial adverse changes in utilization, payer mix, profitability, capital structure or liquidity."

Table 9.5	Common Characteristics of Distressed Hospitals	
	1993	**1994**
Occupancy rate	30.43%	30.21%
Medicare and Medicaid discharges	71.57%	83.29%
Days in accounts receivable	83.22	83.29
Long-term debt to total assets	0.49	0.46
Debt per bed	$168,969	$176,408
Days cash on hand	11.02	13.41
Return on assets (%)	0.88	1.37
Operating profit margin (%)	0.78	0.18
Total profit margin (%)	0.88	1.22

Source: Health Care Investment Analysts, Inc. All figures represent median values derived from Medicare cost reports. The figures are those for the lowest 25th percentile.

probable new competition in the market area, consolidation or merger of facilities resulting in an excess or a specifically surplus facility, and possible FTC divestiture orders.

Highest and Best Use Analysis

Highest and best use as currently defined as:

the reasonably probable and legal use of vacant land or an improved property, which is physically possible, appropriately supported, financially feasible, and that results in the highest value.[3]

To the extent that the principles and methods of determining highest and best use are readily available in other professional publications, no effort will be made to duplicate such material. The intent of this chapter is to supplement such resources regarding special problems or applications relevant to medical facilities that might intervene or affect the normal analytic process. Some medical facilities (typically the most expensive or most specialized) will require the most comment.

Legally Permissible Uses

While the analysis of this element is largely straightforward and traditional as applied to medical facilities, local planning and political policies should be specially investigated. Traditionally, medical office buildings and some clinic facilities have been zoned commercial whereas most hospitals, convalescent homes, and skilled nursing facilities are often placed in residentially, medically, or publicly zoned areas. Special and often unique political considerations can override all other elements in predicting the reasonableness of a given use.

---

[3] *The Dictionary of Real Estate Appraisal,* third edition (Chicago: Appraisal Institute, 1993).

Example 1

An obsolete and failed hospital in a declining neighborhood had an economically viable reuse as a drug and alcohol rehabilitation facility. County health care planners favored this goal and had uses for the facility and funding to support it for the indefinite future. However, the neighborhood chamber of commerce associated the proposal with a methadone clinic and not only strongly opposed it but obtained commitments from leading city council members to oppose the plan. Careful investigation and questioning of health officials, planners, politicians, and the head of the chamber of commerce led to the conclusion that a medical reuse of the facility was not possible. As a result, the value conclusion was equal to land value less the cost of demolition.

Example 2

In another case of an obsolete hospital, the value of the property as improved was exceeded by the value of the land for housing development, and demolition was mandated according to market principles. While the city government was not adverse to demolishing most of the hospital, it wished to preserve a small portion which had been the original hospital and contained quaint architectural features. As a condition of reuse of the entire property, the city designated that this portion be preserved as a historic building, including its deep and beautifully landscaped front setback. This condition substantially lowered the available square footage of land and the potential number of new housing units. It also generated extra costs to renovate the historic building and bring it into modern code compliance. Although the value effects were complicated, they were readily definable and calculable, but the appropriate value conclusion was again dependent on a thorough investigation of the political possibilities.

Example 3

A federal hospital in a large city closed and was declared surplus and available. Due to its desirable location and extensive facilities, a number of federal, state, and local agencies as well as some nonprofit charitable programs sought to obtain control of the facility for a variety of purposes. The political complexities at every level of government eventually frustrated use of the property for any purpose, and it has stood empty for more than 10 years. In attempting to estimate the value of the property at any given time an appraiser would find it necessary to analyze and predict political events, which are nearly unpredictable and cannot be reasoned. This example is mentioned to emphasize the appraiser's need for clear and thorough statements of conditions about any conclusions, alternative possibilities, and at least the possible value effects if other results occur.

Aside from the investigations suggested by the above examples, since most medical facilities are required to be licensed, the appraiser should know not only the status of existing licenses pertinent to the property but the policies of any licensing authority regarding a potential highest and best use. If the facility is currently closed, the appraiser should know the terms (if any) to reinstate its license. Most states allow a reasonable period of time (e.g., one to three years) to reinstate a license after activities have been terminated. Direct costs of reinstatement can be determined based on the requirements and conditions of the licensing authority. Indirect costs of reinstatement can be estimated and must also be analyzed. In many cases, if reinstatement cannot be accomplished and a new license application is required, changes in building codes and other requirements (including a needs test in some states) may eliminate the former use legally, economically, and physically. Time considerations may also be a factor in reinstatement where, for example, essential equipment has been stripped and sold, and time would be insufficient to re-equip and staff the facility or meet other reinstatement requirements.

Physically Possible Uses

This issue is always potentially present whenever one contemplates a change from an existing use to a new use. Nearly all changes in use involve some physical modifications, which can and must be costed and considered against the functional and economic appeal of the final product. Many obsolete hospitals have been successfully converted to elderly housing facilities, and this idea for reuse typically arises. Whether or not the facility can be modified to be competitive in the new use can be a very subtle question. The answer depends either on having a high degree of familiarity with the market for and characteristics of facilities in the new use or on holding appropriate interviews with people experienced in developing and marketing facilities of the proposed use. Most hospitals are configured in such a way that it is difficult to use the full amount of the improved space effectively to create residential rooms with light and air. Development of light wells or other means of providing light and air do not provide an acceptable or competitive level of appeal. In buildings where most rooms are usable in respect to light and air, the cost of relocating plumbing and toilet facilities may make the project prohibitive if the quality of the result is not optimal. Thus, while many of these matters can be reasoned through, it is desirable to confirm such an analysis with experts in the utilization or marketing of the proposed use.

Financially Feasible Uses

Financial feasibility relates the capital investment required to achieve a specified use with the income that will be realized from that use. Financial feasibility analysis is discussed in various valuation texts (e.g., *The Appraisal of Real Estate*) where the concept of internal rate of return (*IRR*) has been introduced as the measure of the relationship between investment and income. A proposed use is considered feasible if the *IRR* meets or exceeds the benchmark yield requirements of the market (see Figure 9.2).

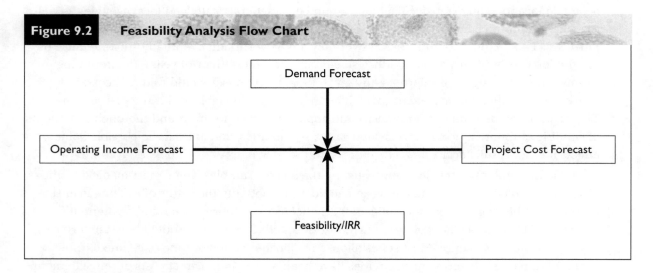

Figure 9.2   Feasibility Analysis Flow Chart

Demand Forecast

Operating Income Forecast

Project Cost Forecast

Feasibility/*IRR*

Maximally Productive Uses

Several different uses may be feasible, i.e., may produce an *IRR* equal to or greater than a typical investor's requirements, but the use that offers the highest *IRR* is maximally productive. If this use meets the other three criteria, it represents the property's highest and best use. It is important to remember that the use with the highest *IRR* is the maximally productive use only if its level of uncertainty and risk is equivalent to that of the alternative uses considered. Uncertainty relates to the likelihood of an outcome, while risk relates to the level of loss or reward associated with an outcome.

Consider two alternative uses, each with an *IRR* of 15%. One investment has a 95% probability of meeting or exceeding this *IRR,* the other has an 85% probability. The first use, which has greater certainty, would most likely represent the highest and best use. If, however, the first project requires an investment of $3.9 million and the second requires only $1.1 million, the situation becomes more complicated. The uncertainty remains equivalent, but the risk is different, so the choice for highest and best use is less clear. Problematic forecasting and risk analysis, which address such a situation, are beyond the scope of most appraisal assignments and of this text. Uncertainty and risk are relevant to the appraisal process, however, so the appraiser should be familiar with the concepts.

At a minimum, when comparing alternative uses, the income and expenses of all alternatives must be forecast with the same level of certainty. If the most likely income level is projected for one alternative, while the income of another is projected conservatively, the basis for effective comparison is eroded.

Based on the characteristics of the subject property and its environment, an appraiser determines the highest and best use to which the subject may be put. The property is then valued at that use using comparables which also reflect that use. The highest and best use determination serves as the bridge between factual data on the subject and its environment and the valuation process.

Various chapters in this text address the application of the three approaches used to estimate value. In the cost approach, value is estimated by determining the cost to develop an equivalent facility, including land, and deducting the depreciation evident in the subject property. Because it is founded on the principle of substitution, the availability of entitlements is critical to the usefulness of this approach. The income approach assumes that value is based on the price the market would pay to receive the financial returns that the subject property will produce. In the sales comparison approach, value is estimated by analyzing unit prices paid for similar, comparable properties.

Typically, all three approaches are employed and each yields a value indication. These three value indications are then reconciled into a final opinion of value. The appropriateness and accuracy of each approach depends on the characteristics of the subject property, the purpose of the assignment, the quantity and quality of data available, and the valuation methodologies used by investors in the subject's market. Based on these criteria, the appraiser may conclude that one or two approaches are less appropriate, and exclude them from the analysis. More commonly, all three approaches are employed and when their value indications are analyzed, they are weighted based on the above criteria and reconciled into a final value estimate.

Special Considerations

Highest and best use and related value concepts solely address economic concepts, i.e., computations of dollars. However, the delivery of medical services in many cases is fraught with eleemosynary considerations in terms of benefits to the public. Accordingly, payment for medical services typically comes from many sources and is subsidized in a variety of ways both directly and indirectly. Similarly, ownership is structured in a variety of ways including both profit and nonprofit corporations as well as government entities. Nevertheless, to equate one alternative with another, the foregoing considerations must be ignored, neutralized, or provided with a specific dollar adjustment. A comparison of alternatives requires that each be analyzed as a profit enterprise with adjustments made in dollars to the extent possible for any public benefit subsidies. To attract medical facilities many municipalities will donate land, street improvements, and other benefits including bond underwriting at favorable municipal rates.

Each of these benefits typically can be valued by traditional methods and must be identified and considered in the comparative equation of alternative uses.

Depending on the age of the facility, physical factors such as those dealing with contamination (e.g., asbestos, underground tanks, contaminated plumbing or parts of a site) could be highly significant. In certain geographic areas, seismic upgrading considerations may be needed at enormous cost. Building codes for health care facilities are among the most stringent, and a closed hospital is a prime target for building code updates and compliance with the latest disability and access regulations. Elevators, electrical, and HVAC systems should not be overlooked.

In some states the certificate of need process may have to be considered for certain types of alternative uses. Just because a hospital once had a license does not mean that it will automatically qualify for a different type of license for a related activity. Loss of a license may trigger an entirely new regulatory requirement that heavily impacts financial feasibility.

Valuation and Elements of Comparison

The valuation of particular medical facilities is described in detail in their respective chapters in this text, and the general principles of valuation are presumed to be known to the reader. However, from the valuation of each use, including the present use if relevant, a small number of basic elements should be quantifiable as follows:

1. Net operating income (*NOI*) for each alternative
2. Appropriate capitalization rate for each alternative
3. The value of public benefit subsidies (if any) for each alternative
4. The capital needed to accomplish all changes required for each alternative
5. The internal rate of return (*IRR*) required by any specific investors

This information, derived from the valuation process, can be presented in a comparison table (see Table 9.6). In Comparison 1 market alternatives with comparative values related to market capitalization rates for specific uses are emphasized. This manner of presentation lends itself well to the inclusion of the demolition alternative where the market value of the cleared land can be presented. In some situations, the market value of the land will exceed the value of the improved property in its present form. This is common when the existing improvements are relatively old and subject to various forms of depreciation and obsolescence.

An alternative method of presentation, Comparison 2, emphasizes the *IRR* desired by a particular group of investors rather than the capitalization rates appropriate to different alternative uses. Presenting the information in this form emphasizes the specific net operating income amounts for each use and applies an appropriate part of the income to cover conversion costs at the common *IRR* figure. The table results in a comparative value for each use at the acceptable level of return desired by the particular investors.

Final Comment and "Ladder of Uses"

When valuing and studying a medical property for adaptive reuse, the most favorable reuse possibility is often within the medical industry. At the very minimum, this is suggested by the past or existing use, which has already established the specific location as a place for the delivery of medical services of some kind. This is helpful not only in marketing new medical services, especially if they are related to the old use, but in obtaining or extending use permits and other political approvals. With few exceptions adaptive reuse for nonmedical purposes has

	Present Use (if relevant)	**Alternative Use A**	**Alternative Use B**	**Demolition Alternative**
Table 9.6 — **Use and Feasibility Analysis**				
Comparison Table 1				
Capitalized *NOI*				
Plus public benefit subsidy (if any)				Land value
Less conversion cost				Cost of demolition
Residual comparative value				
Comparison Table 2* (alternative approach)				
Net cost of conversion				
NOI				Not applicable
Income to conversion cost at X%**				Not applicable
Residual income capitalized at X%				Not applicable

* All comparisons must be equated to the same date and absorption costs properly recognized.
** At *IRR* desired by investors.

an infinite variety of possibilities. These are largely beyond the scope of this book and are approached by conventional appraisal techniques.

As a simplified aid to thinking about adaptive reuse, a ladder of uses is presented here (see Figure 9.3), which shows a variety of medical uses and a few categories of nonmedical uses. It is organized with the most specialized (and usually the most expensive per square foot) at the top. The steps are not uniformly in order from most specialized to least specialized but are divided between uses requiring overnight stays and those that do not. In general, an existing or former use on the ladder is not likely to be adaptable to a use higher on the scale. Thus, wherever the beginning use is found, one should generally look below that on the ladder for possible alternative uses. The ladder is offered to assist readers in considering the possibilities. It is not intended to be precise or predictive since many other factors as discussed earlier are relevant.

Figure 9.3   **Ladder of Alternative Uses**

1. General Acute Care

    a. Medical/Surgical

    b. Pediatric

    c. Intensive/Coronary/etc.

    d. Prenatal

    e. Rehabilitation

    f. Psychiatric

2. Specialty Care

    a. Burn Center

    b. Trauma Rehabilitation

3. Long-Term Care

    a. Skilled Nursing

    b. Subacute Care

    c. Intermediate Care

    d. Mentally Disordered

    e. Developmentally Disabled

4. Alcohol/Chemical Dependency

5. Assisted Living (minimal health care)

6. Congregate Care Living (nonmedical)   **Places where lodging is provided**

7. Ambulatory Care (outpatient)   **Places where lodging is *not* provided**

    a. Surgery Centers

    b. Psychiatric Counseling

    c. Dialysis Centers

    d. Urgent Care Centers

8. Medical Office Buildings/Clinics

9. Nonmedical Office Buildings

10. Other Retail and Commercial Uses

C H A P T E R
T E N

Medical Practices and Related Entities

As noted earlier in this text, important shifts have taken place in the amounts of expenditures going to different segments of the health care services industry. These shifts have been the result of both public and private sector efforts to contain the growth of health care costs in the United States.

A major factor changing health care delivery is the increased emphasis on outpatient services. Other factors are the continuous growth of prepaid health care, an increased number of physicians (since 1960, 40 new medical schools have been established), and the number of foreign medical school graduates entering U.S. practices, which figure grew more rapidly than the U.S. graduate output of physicians. Between 1970 and 1993 the number of physicians in practice increased by 102% to 703,700, and the ratio of foreign-trained physicians (MDs and DDSs) as a percentage of all active MDs went from 5.8% in 1950 to 23.0% in 1993 (Table 10.1).

Increasing competition among health care providers has resulted in the application of business and financial management techniques and strategies to most areas of the health care industry. Consequently, the valuation of medical practices, physical therapist practices, and other medical entities can now appropriately parallel the value analyses of general business entities. In turn, closer attention is being paid to both current and future earning power. This approach represents a departure from the traditional view that the nontransferable value attributed to the personal goodwill of medical practitioners essentially accounted for the value of many provider entities.

Health management organizations (HMOs) and preferred provider organizations (PPOs) continue to grow in importance. HMOs provide all prescribed health services for a fixed premium or fee on a group or an individual basis. PPOs negotiate fee schedules with providers and provide incentives to member patients to use these preferred providers. The U.S. Department of Commerce has estimated that as many as 25% of the U.S. population now look to managed care organizations (HMOs and PPOs) for their health care needs.[1] Evidence of a consolidation in and integration of medical practices and other specialized entities (e.g., solo physician practices, home health care agencies, physical therapy practices, etc.) has created investor awareness of business and financial opportunities in these fields.

These trends suggest that patients increasingly are less concerned about who provides for their health care needs and more concerned about the cost and availability of services. Who the individual medical practitioner is, is less likely to be the overriding directional motivation in patients' propensity to seek medical services.

---

[1] U.S. Department of Commerce, *1990 U.S. Industrial Outlook.*

Table 10.1   Physicians, by Selected Activity, 1970 to 1993

[In thousands. Through 1985, as of Dec. 31; thereafter, as of Jan. 1, except as noted. Includes Puerto Rico and outlying areas. See also Historical Statistics, Colonial Times to 1970, series B 275-280]

Activity	1970	1980	1985	1989	1990	1992	1993
Doctors of medicine, total	334.0	467.7	552.7	600.8	615.4	653.1	670.3
Professionally active	311.2	435.5	511.1	549.2	560.0	594.7	605.7
Place of medical education:							
U.S. medical graduates	256.8	343.6	398.4	428.3	437.2	460.4	466.6
Foreign medical graduates[1]	54.4	91.8	112.7	120.8	122.8	134.3	139.1
Sex:							
Male	289.8	386.7	436.3	458.4	463.9	484.6	488.5
Female	21.4	48.7	74.8	90.7	96.1	110.1	117.2
Active Non-Federal	281.7	417.7	489.5	528.8	539.5	575.5	584.0
Patient care	255.0	361.9	431.5	477.2	487.8	520.2	531.7
Office-based practice	188.9	271.3	329.0	350.1	359.9	387.9	398.8
General and family practice	50.8	47.8	53.9	56.3	57.6	58.6	58.1
Cardiovascular diseases	3.9	6.7	9.1	10.2	10.7	11.4	12.1
Dermatology	2.9	4.4	5.3	5.7	6.0	6.3	6.5
Gastroenterology	1.1	2.7	4.1	4.9	5.2	5.7	6.3
Internal medicine	23.0	40.5	52.7	56.9	57.8	65.1	67.3
Pediatrics	10.3	17.4	22.4	24.7	26.5	29.0	30.8
Pulmonary diseases	0.8	2.0	3.0	3.6	3.7	4.0	4.4
General surgery	18.1	22.4	24.7	24.7	24.5	24.9	24.3
Obsterics and gynecology	13.8	19.5	23.5	25.2	25.5	27.1	27.6
Ophthalmology	7.6	10.6	12.2	12.8	13.1	13.7	13.9
Orthopedic surgery	6.5	10.7	13.0	14.1	14.2	15.8	16.3
Otolaryngology	3.9	5.3	5.8	6.2	6.4	6.6	6.7
Plastic surgery	1.2	2.4	3.3	3.6	3.8	4.0	4.1
Urological surgery	4.3	6.2	7.1	7.3	7.4	7.7	7.8
Anesthesiology	7.4	11.3	15.3	16.7	17.8	20.0	20.6
Diagnostic radiology	0.9	4.2	7.7	9.0	9.8	10.9	11.9

Table 10.1   Physicians, by Selected Activity, 1970 to 1993 (continued)

Activity	1970	1980	1985	1989	1990	1992	1993
Emergency medicine	(NA)	(NA)	(NA)	8.0	8.4	9.4	9.8
Neurology	1.2	3.2	4.7	5.4	5.6	6.3	6.8
Pathology, anatomical/clinical		3.0	6.0	6.9	7.0	7.3	7.98.5
Psychiatry	10.1	15.9	18.5	19.6	20.0	21.8	22.3
Other specialty	18.2	31.9	35.8	27.8	28.8	31.7	32.4
Hospital-based practice	66.1	90.6	102.5	127.2	127.9	132.3	132.9
Clinical fellows	(NA)	(NA)	(NA)	8.3	8.2	6.8	5.9
Residents and interns	45.8	59.6	72.2	80.0	81.7	85.4	83.1
Full-time hospital staff	20.3	31.0	30.3	38.8	38.0	40.1	43.9
Other professional activity[2]	26.3	35.2	44.0	39.2	39.0	38.7	37.7
Not classified[3]	0.4	20.6	14.0	12.4	12.7	16.6	14.7
Federal	29.5	17.8	21.6	20.4	20.5	19.2	21.7
Patient care	23.5	14.6	17.3	15.9	16.1	15.0	18.8
Office-based practice	3.5	0.7	1.2	1.1	1.1	1.5	0.1
Hospital-based practice	20.0	13.9	16.1	14.8	15.0	13.5	18.7
Other professional activity[2]	6.0	3.2	4.3	4.4	4.4	4.2	2.9
Inactive/unknown address	22.8	32.1	41.6	51.6	55.4	58.4	64.7
Doctors of osteopathy[4]	14.3	18.8	24.0	29.6	30.9	33.5	33.4
Medical and osteopathic schools[5]	110	141	142	142	141	141	142
Students[5]	42.6	70.1	73.2	71.6	72.0	73.5	74.5
Graduates[5]	8.8	16.2	17.8	17.2	16.9	17.1	17.1

NA Not available. [1] Foreign medical graduates received their medical education in schools outside the United States and Canada. [2] Includes medical teaching, administration, research, and other. [3] Not classified established in 1970; however, complete data not available until 1972. [4] As of July. Total DO's. Source: American Osteopathic Association, Chicago, IL. [5] Number of schools and students as of fall; graduates for academic year ending in year shown. Based on data from annual surveys conducted by the Association of American Medical Colleges and the American Association of Colleges of Osteopathic Medicine.

Source: Except as noted, American Medical Association, Chicago, IL, *Physician Characteristics and Distribution in the U.S.,* copyright 1994. Reprinted with permission.

Non-Real Estate-Based Valuation Analyses

In the preceding chapters of this book specific types of health care entities requiring a considerable asset base were described and valued by appropriate appraisal approaches and methodologies. The central focus for the value determination in most of those cases was a specifically designed and/or developed facility required to advance the objectives of a well-defined health care enterprise.

Within the health care industry are entities that do not require uniquely designed facilities or a large asset base to provide services. Some of these entities may not require an optimum size or restricted facility design to function efficiently and effectively since only the personal service of one or a few individuals is involved. Physical property, therefore, is of lesser importance and the facilities used by such entities will be more general purpose in nature. Among the entities where ownership values tend to be less dependent upon real property are certain solo medical doctor professional practices and subspecialties, group medical practices, home nursing and personal care service agencies, physical therapy practices, some types of outpatient clinics, and other allied health services including dentists, optometrists, osteopaths, and chiropractors.

The differentiation of approaches for value determination among nonasset-based entities is primarily a function of their services and how they are performed rather than the facilities used. As a consequence, these entities are more appropriately valued from the perspective of a business valuation. This differs from the perspective of the highest and best use of a set of unique real property features present in the facility accommodating a given health care service. Business valuation incorporates more directly into its methodologies the business ownership rights (along with the relative strength of claims) of a commercial, industrial, or service organization pursuing economic activities for profit. Real estate appraisal, on the other hand, is primarily focused on physical assets and the attendant rights and benefits directly associated with the utility of real and personal property rights.

To appraise entities whose value is largely based on the use of physical facilities requires not only an intimate knowledge of property appraisal theory and practice but also an understanding of many aspects of engineering, architecture, real estate brokerage and financing, urban land economics, legal regulations relating to real property such as zoning, and specific statutes relating to real property ownership and its taxation. Where facilities are of a more generalized nature or of small ownership significance, an appraisal should emphasize the perspectives found in most operating business organizations. In these instances the preponderance of value may be found to be general business asset value (both tangible and intangible) rather than primarily real property value. In these cases, particular attention should be given to the projection of future earnings power, which is basically a function of products and services provided and not of the physical facilities in a fixed location used by such entities. The performance of a business valuation involves the theory and knowledge of corporate finance, business management, applied economics, security analysis, business organization behavior, accounting, marketing, and personnel. The intangible assets may represent the most important element of value.

Greater variations in the indicated overall ownership interest value can occur among similar nonasset-intensive health care entities than among those health care enterprises essentially recognized as asset intensive. With real property the elements of value tend to be more highly standardized and documented. With the nonasset-intensive entity the variance in value results from factors such as management techniques, service market economics, demographics, competition, specialties, referral bases, potential patient/customer/client flow, and individual practitioner characteristics and training.

A further noteworthy difference between business valuations and physical asset valuations is that business values are more likely to be affected by the business elements of a practice (e.g., the solo medical practitioner who discontinues practice, changes specialty, takes in a partner, emphasizes certain types of referral relationships, or initiates new management techniques). Value factors will be less standardized from one entity to another due to the potentially greater spectrum of business operating and performance characteristics. In valuing real property the focus is on demonstrating how the facility affects value.

The economic impact on facilities-based entities is often more muted in response to both general and specific business and economic developments than it is on nonasset-based entities. General business markets tend to be more volatile than real estate markets. This is demonstrated in the difference in the volatility of yields on general financial claims on business entities compared to the yields on financial claims on specific real property. Business appraisers, therefore, justifiably give more consideration to a variety of business elements than would be the case with real property appraisers at a given point in time.

The condition of the general financial markets (as opposed to that sector devoted primarily to property-based financial claims) should be taken into consideration when establishing business ownership interest value. This follows from the fact that the purpose of real property appraisals is to arrive at an indicated value for a subject property. In a business valuation the purpose is to establish the value of the overall ownership interest or a partial interest thereof, which would include real and personal property ownership rights.

In health care facility appraisals the difference between a property's depreciated cost and its value based on income may be identified by some real property appraisers as a bundle of business value or goodwill. When goodwill does not represent a relatively large amount, this is not of vital concern. It becomes of material concern, however, in those instances where income-based value materially exceeds replacement cost new. It can result in misleading interpretations or substantial overvaluation of real property if nonidentified business factors are essentially responsible for an entity's large or excess income rather than the real property being appraised.

To the extent that health care entities continue to adopt operating strategies or introduce business factors commonly found in nonhealth-related business enterprises, a business valuation approach is required in addition to or in conjunction with real property/facilities appraisals of such entities. A business valuation approach to determining total value for health care enterprises is expected to be a logical direction for the general appraisal services provided to this industry in the years to come.

Impact of Structural Changes in Health Services Expenditures

Changes in the relative share of health care expenditures accruing to various provider segments are illustrated in Table 10.2. Hospital care, physicians' services, and prescription drugs totaled $546.4 billion in 1993, an increase of more than 240% since 1980. Physicians' services grew the most, by 279%, to over $171 billion. Physicians' services are less asset-intensive entities (compared to hospitals) and are most likely to have substantial and greater relative intangible values generated by business and service factors.

As suggested in the preceding section, the value of an increasing number of health care entities will likely be influenced more frequently from the perspective of a business investor. And, as noted, this can result in ownership interest values considerably in excess of the tangible assets in place. In estimating the market value of ownership interests from the viewpoint of third-party investors, emphasis will be attached to the future earning power of health care entities. This is expected to bring more recognition to a larger amount of transferable owner interest value, when health service entities or group practices are sold or ownership is restructured, than has been the case traditionally. Historically, selling health practitioner(s) have

Table 10.2 Personal Health Care Expenditures, by State, 1993

[In millions of dollars. Data represent spending for services produced by each State's health care providers, as opposed to those consumed by State residents or supplied by State employees.]

State	Total	Hospital care	Physican services	Dental services	Other professional services	Home health care	Drugs[1]	Vision products[2]	Nursing home care	Other personal health care	Medicare PHC expenditures	Medicaid PHC expenditures
US	778,510	323,919	171,226	37,383	51,220	22,982	74,956	12,636	66,201	17,988	150,374	112,776
AL	12,060	5,301	2,631	456	641	602	1,247	155	703	323	2,625	1,276
AK	1,573	701	301	124	127	5	165	26	56	68	101	273
AZ	10,635	3,999	2,799	551	821	317	1,124	227	567	230	2,276	1,270
AR	6,111	2,723	1,244	242	332	145	684	56	558	127	1,422	1,007
CA	94,178	34,827	28,827	5,664	6,859	1,640	9,017	1,522	4,103	1,565	17,347	11,330
CO	10,066	3,932	2,452	605	751	195	919	226	661	327	1,556	957
CT	12,216	4,380	2,587	685	769	391	996	192	1,749	467	2,134	1,998
DE	2,260	937	466	104	156	51	214	35	217	79	377	249
DC	4,285	2,612	672	119	267	45	175	34	231	130	603	678
FL	44,811	17,131	10,498	2,029	3,505	2,323	4,450	872	3,089	912	12,484	4,697
GA	20,104	8,704	4,543	898	1,226	729	2,117	331	1,038	516	3,549	2,753
HI	3,485	1,450	771	235	222	32	416	64	181	104	496	354
ID	2,277	900	486	163	126	49	265	35	197	55	384	290
IL	34,747	15,621	6,980	1,588	2,063	853	3,263	604	3,148	636	6,404	4,609
IN	16,401	6,996	3,263	692	993	308	1,594	270	2,018	264	3,126	2,777
IA	7,341	3,111	1,376	341	431	137	743	148	927	127	1,447	960
KS	6,903	2,868	1,425	325	470	152	695	107	721	140	1,326	769
KY	10,384	4,515	2,038	369	691	357	1,196	141	850	228	2,143	1,683
LA	13,014	5,956	2,537	432	736	410	1,269	160	1,186	328	2,730	2,664
ME	3,433	1,376	601	157	210	104	333	46	453	153	605	722
MD	15,154	5,926	3,704	749	942	314	1,749	272	1,185	312	2,692	1,924
MA	23,421	10,034	4,442	1,022	1,524	835	1,961	269	2,737	597	4,712	3,689
MI	27,136	11,711	5,562	1,531	1,844	714	2,937	457	1,849	532	5,405	3,865
MN	14,194	4,796	3,617	741	933	414	1,146	277	1,884	386	2,164	2,229
MS	6,187	2,897	1,107	214	288	300	720	60	460	141	1,367	1,043
MO	15,949	7,652	2,958	602	1,013	347	14,20	244	1,368	346	3,439	1,648
MT	2,103	894	392	103	166	50	209	36	178	74	391	322

(continued)

Table 10.2   Personal Health Care Expenditures, by State, 1993 (continued)

[In millions of dollars. Data represent spending for services produced by each State's health care providers, as opposed to those consumed by State residents or supplied by State employees.]

State	Total	Hospital care	Physican services	Dental services	Other professional services	Home health care	Drugs[1]	Vision products[2]	Nursing home care	Other personal health care	Medicare PHC expenditures	Medicaid PHC expenditures
NE	4,400	2,003	825	191	225	74	421	80	482	99	746	561
NV	3,747	1,362	1,029	215	307	120	408	76	164	67	732	344
NH	3,452	1,388	780	177	269	71	319	43	268	136	473	446
NJ	25,741	10,312	5,776	1,460	1,870	718	2,452	457	2,128	570	4,838	3,857
NM	3,878	1,848	716	175	254	62	409	69	215	131	565	577
NY	67,033	28,001	12,003	2,837	3,717	3,562	5,081	1,090	9,106	1,635	11,872	18,041
NC	18,241	7,801	3,717	810	1,102	541	2,027	268	1,562	413	3,553	2,564
ND	2,021	903	445	78	93	16	160	28	246	52	374	269
OH	33,456	14,305	7,118	1,398	1,969	649	3,218	531	3,758	511	6,177	4,665
OK	8,041	3,329	1,640	356	504	273	874	121	748	196	1,665	1,013
OR	7,999	2,966	1,904	578	530	122	762	91	656	391	1,521	955
PA	41,521	19,540	7,460	1,634	3,005	796	3,519	617	4,153	798	10,056	5,116
RI	3,428	1,314	575	150	239	103	310	33	485	219	664	793
SC	9,029	4,221	1,685	387	472	216	978	115	638	317	1,541	1,324
SD	1,953	920	342	87	117	16	163	30	216	63	364	264
TN	16,203	7,208	3,137	609	1,166	899	1,635	228	1,085	235	3,549	2,183
TX	49,816	21,592	10,526	2,081	3,591	1,583	5,131	883	3,104	1,325	8,765	5,914
UT	4,118	1,743	864	276	220	100	439	117	260	99	624	477
VT	1,499	562	265	84	122	52	161	24	148	82	241	232
VA	16,682	7,031	3,769	863	970	368	2,015	295	976	395	2,736	1,621
WA	15,129	5,305	3,720	1,189	1,102	380	1,474	242	1,291	425	2,360	2,161
WV	5,197	2,346	988	182	326	150	574	74	365	192	1,106	1,075
WI	14,502	5,537	3,362	765	875	265	1,290	240	1,752	415	2,397	2,138
WY	998	417	160	57	68	29	113	17	83	55	150	137

[1] Includes other medical nondurables. [2] Includes other medical durables.

Source: U.S. Health Care Financing Administration, Office of the Actuary. Estimates prepared by the Office of National Health Statistics.

tended to find the value of their practices largely based on tangible assets with only minimal recognition given to goodwill and/or business value.

Home Health Agencies

One for-profit category that is growing as a result of the "cost containment effort" is home health care. Over 5 million disabled people in the United States require health services in their respective homes. The basic service of home health care, where feasible, is significantly less costly to both patient and insurer than would be the case in a traditional hospital. Home health care agencies (HHAs) offer significant profit opportunities to investors. In 1993 there were an estimated 13,951 HHAs in the United States, and about half of them were Medicare certified. These organizations are valued appropriately by business valuation methodology.

Physical Therapy Practices

Another important and growing health care segment is that of physical therapy practitioners, who provide service as private contractors to hospitals as well as to outpatients from their own respective locations. Rehabilitation is an emerging growth segment in health care, and much of the demand emanates from the growing proportion of elderly people who have impairments that can benefit from physical therapy. Population projections, documented elsewhere, indicate that the general population will increase 40% by 2030 while the number of persons 65 and older is expected to more than double.

The majority of outpatient therapy services (estimated to be over 80% of revenue) are provided by solo certified therapists or small groups of therapists organized similarly to medical group practices. In some instances, physical therapy outpatient clinics were owned by physicians who referred their patients to them for treatment. Since 1992, however, federal legislation prohibits physicians from sending their Medicare and Medicaid patients to any service entity in which they have an ownership interest. This is an example of a unique situation that could trigger a need for an entity valuation if the physician ownership interests in such an entity were sold or transferred as a result of this prohibition. Some major physical therapy provider organizations, particularly in larger metropolitan areas, are operated as investor-owned service enterprises and organized as closely held corporations. Hospitals have also been active in the acquisition of physical therapy practices as part of a policy to vertically integrate health care systems (see Chapter 1).

As a more active market develops from divestiture and consolidation of the ownership interests in adjunct health care entities, national firms can be expected to accelerate their acquisition of many of the small closely held health care entities. As with medical practices, because of costs, competition, and up-front financial requirements, etc., more of these entities will be bought and sold on the basis of professional third-party appraisals developed through business valuation methodologies. The larger practices and entities, where net revenue exceeds $150,000 annually, are particularly marketable.

Physician Practitioners

The most commonly identified and prevalent health care entities are office-based physician medical practices. Practices are found in a variety of residential as well as commercial locations that can have important differentiated demographic characteristics and varying levels of competition from other adjunct health-related providers and services.

In recent years the increase in medical school graduates has been a major contributing factor to the growth in the physician share of health care expenditures. This increase resulted from government programs that stimulated physician supply and a greater number of college graduates who entered medical schools. As these new physicians enter private medical practice, they are increasingly apt to purchase an existing practice rather than start a new one from scratch. Even though the pool of new entrants to medical colleges has decreased recently, a significant demand and supply relationship continues to exist that perpetuates a competitive environment for medical services not believed possible a decade ago.

Because of the increasingly competitive characteristics of medical practices, more attention is being given to the business management of practices and to their significance as valuable business entities. Competitive pressures have caused a relaxation of traditional ethical constraints on promotional activities by physicians. Physicians increasingly identify and appeal to patient needs and requirements with promotional and public relations strategies, which have stimulated patient flow. One study found, for example, that as many as 40% of the physicians surveyed had employed some marketing strategy.[2]

In today's cost containment environment, physicians are also employing a larger number of nonphysician personnel to bring about operating efficiencies that control costs as well as free themselves for more intensive patient care (flow), which is the primary source of practice revenues.

A physician's acquisition of an established practice or entrance into an association with an established practice offers attractive and feasible alternatives to that of creating a solo practice with its heavy up-front start-up financial outlays and patient flow development costs. It would be difficult in many locales today to establish a large patient base in a reasonable period of time. New physicians in some desirable and highly competitive service areas have been found to come and go with some regularity. The general risks associated with a start-up practice can largely be avoided by entering an established practice that enjoys good current and potential patient flow.

The creation of practitioner partnerships and other arrangements for group practices from existing solo practices is almost the norm today. It has been found that 1) the number of group medical practices increased 70% between 1969 and 1980 and by another 40% between 1980 and 1984; and 2) the number of physicians in group practice increased 60% between 1980 and 1984.[3] By 1995 there were about 5,240 group practices of five or more physicians, accounting for a total of about 104,300 physicians.

With today's cost containment realities, the economies of scale accruing to group practices frequently enable physicians to spread their fixed costs (such as those connected to stringent reimbursement systems) over a larger patient flow with resultant incremental earnings. Further, the number of visits per physician per week has been found to increase from 183 visits in a solo practice to an average of 213 visits in group practices. It is not surprising to find that as long ago as 1984 that over 44% of physicians were in group practices.[4] It was also determined that the average size of physician groups ranged from 26.6 members in multispecialty practices to 5.7 members in family or general group practices. Single-specialty group practices averaged 5.8 members.

The more intensive use of nonphysician support personnel in medical practices reduces administrative demands on physicians for the business management of a medical practice. The practice begins to take on many of the characteristics common to "business" entities. Studies of physician productivity relative to nonphysician employees indicate that the average solo physician (who employs 1.81 aides) could profitably employ twice as many auxiliaries as he or she currently does. Another study found that doubling allied health personnel in physicians' offices would result in a 20% to 25% increase in total patient visits per physician.[5] In such instances a practice's incremental income would exceed the incremental costs associated with the additional personnel.

---

[2] Ibid.

[3] American Medical Association, "Number of Group Practices Rising in U.S.," *American Medical News* (December 7, 1984), 17.

[4] Penny L. Havlicek, *Medical Groups in the United States, 1984* (Chicago: American Medical Association, 1985), 4-16.

[5] Uwe Reinhardt, "A Production Function for Physician Services," *The Review of Economics and Statistics* (February 1972), 60.

In addition to practitioner consolidation, many physicians are becoming salaried employees of for-profit outpatient organizations. For physicians with less than five years in practice, 25% are salaried.[6] Many of these physicians are likely to be employed by investor-owned entities rather than entities owned by other medical practitioners. The growth of investor-owned outpatient clinics and practices is another important explanation for shifts in health care services expenditures. Many hospitals have moved aggressively into such enterprises to combat the trend toward outpatient clinics. One of the strategies hospitals use is simply to purchase physicians' medical practices. A 1988 survey of 600 hospitals found that 18% of the hospitals were buying private medical practices while another 8% had such action under active consideration.[7]

These trends are leading away from the traditional solo physician-dominated health care system to health care entities that recognize consumer needs and preferences but are controlled by "bottom-line" expectancies. These entities are increasingly providing health services within the context of investor earning power objectives. Medical practices as well as other health care entities are, and increasingly will be, valued in the light of the business and economic elements found in most business enterprises in a free marketplace. Indeed, it is not unusual to hear practitioners themselves refer to their practice as their "business."

Most of the nonasset-intensive provider entities enumerated above can be appraised effectively from the perspectives of a business valuation. The approaches and data sources required in such valuations are quite similar. The following discussion, however, will be presented in terms of a physician-centered enterprise.

Business Valuation of a Medical Practice

The general factors considered in a business valuation are consistent with those determinants of business ownership value in connection with estate, gift, and income taxation issues as outlined in IRS Revenue Ruling 59-60. This ruling has been a common frame of reference for many court decisions regarding business ownership value in a variety of circumstances. It also provides a basic standard of value known as "fair market value." This concept of fair market value is used in the majority of business valuations as well as many other appraisal disciplines.

While the definition of fair market value is generally understood, considerable differences in value might be derived in different situations depending on the purpose of an appraisal. A substantial difference may be found in values estimated for the purpose of dissolving a marriage in different state jurisdictions. For instance, some state statutes, case law, and court decisions have concluded that goodwill in professional practices has no value or cannot be transferred to other parties. This position is based on the view that no direct investment was required to create the goodwill, and that the goodwill that exists is essentially "personal" rather than "commercial," which can have significant value in connection with the transfer or division of general business ownership interests. In other jurisdictions as well as in some situations where tax and estate issues are in contention, an opposite view may prevail. In such cases the medical practice activity is viewed as an economic activity and its value is defined in terms of "anticipated" earnings that are partially supported by the existence of business value or goodwill.

The general perspective common to most business valuations is included in Section 4 of the IRS Revenue Ruling 59-60:

---

[6] Roger A. Reynolds and Daniel J. Duann, eds., *1985 Socioeconomic Characteristics of Medical Practice* (Chicago: American Medical Association, 1985).

[7] "Patients for Sale—Warm Bodies," *Wall Street Journal* (February 2, 1989).

It is advisable to emphasize that in the valuation of the stock of closely-held corporations or the stock of corporations where market quotations are either lacking or too scarce to be recognized, all available financial data, as well as all relevant factors affecting the fair market value, should be considered. . .[and that valuation] in essence, [is] a prophecy as to the future and must be based on facts available at the required date of appraisal.

Further, the ruling provides that

The following factors, although not all-inclusive, are fundamental and require careful analysis in each case:

1. The nature of the business and the history of the enterprise from its inception.
2. The economic outlook in general and the condition and outlook of the specific industry in particular.
3. The book value of the stock and the financial condition of the business.
4. The earning capacity of the company.
5. The dividend-paying capacity.
6. Whether or not the enterprise has goodwill or other intangible value.
7. Sales of the stock and the size of the block of stock to be valued.
8. The market price of stocks of corporations engaged in the same or a similar line of business having their stocks actively traded in a free and open market, either on an exchange or over-the-counter.

Background for the Appraisal

The economic variable having an impact on a subject medical practice can only be determined within that practice's characteristics after development of a complete understanding of the economic environment in which the practice functions. A background review should include not only demographics but also the locale's trends in and levels of personal income, employment and its composition (e.g., payroll, salaried, professional, service, unskilled, manufacturing, etc.), labor force stability, education levels attained, business income, and general buying power.[8] A second basic set of background data should focus on those aspects of the health/medical care industry that relate most closely to that of the practice being appraised. Both county and state medical societies can provide a good deal of information regarding medically related areas that impact the practice of medicine in a given community. These data will provide insight on the number of hospitals/beds and their capacity utilization, the number of practitioners in each specialty or general practice, the number of HMOs and PPOs providing coverage, and the extent of that coverage along with fee schedules.

Competing practices and clinics should be identified. Medical societies should also be able to identify the types of specialties, education, years in practice, etc., of physicians in the area. The location of competing practitioners can be identified along with the length of time they have been at their present location.

After external data are gathered, specific internal information about the individual practitioner(s) and the day-to-day operation of the subject practice should be developed. This information should include practitioner(s) age, health, education, patient flow per unit of time, hours typically worked per week, practice history, characteristics of patient base, magnitude of

---

[8] *The CACI Sourcebook of Demographic and Buying Power for Every Zip Code* is an excellent source for these data. It is developed from U.S. Census summary data files and provides economic and demographic profiles for every county, census tract, and minor civil division in the United States.

referral patients, and average service duration of practice patients/clients. Additional fundamental information on nonphysician employees include their educational background, length of employment, compensation, work rules, responsibilities, etc. Specific duties and roles of nonphysician employees in practice functions must be understood.

Of particular importance in analyzing the nature of a practice is the intensity of the practitioner(s) work week, which should be correlated with practice revenue. Table 10.3 provides information on various medical practice characteristics such as mean patient visits per week, hours in patient care per week, net income, professional expenses and liability premium. For instance, in 1992 the average family practitioner obtained a net income of $111,800. However, there are vast differences in physician compensation. In Florida two family doctors reported joint practice gross earnings of "nearly $1 million a year." Both doctors worked between 60 to 80 hours a week. If their expenses approximated 50% of gross income, each would obtain an annual income of about $250,000 annually. Clearly, higher incomes will accrue to practitioners who work more hours than the average physician in their respective specialty and/or have higher patient flow. The risk of using broad averages to analyze specific practitioner incomes can be appreciated by noting that Denton Cooley, the famous heart surgeon, reportedly had an income of $10 million in 1988.[9]

Recent data on physician compensation are presented in Table 10.4. In 1993 the average net income of employed physicians increased 10.7% or four times the general rate of inflation. This is reportedly due to competition among health care employers such as hospitals, group practices, managed care plans, and others to merge the economic interests of physicians with their own. Mean compensation figures from various surveys vary substantially due to the type of group that is emphasized. For example, surveys that emphasize group practices will report higher incomes because group practices pay more than do hospitals or managed care plans. The AMA's figures generally are higher because it reports the net income of all physicians, including employed physicians.

The documentation from the practice may include financial statements and tax returns of the practice (if incorporated) and the practitioner(s) for the previous five years, copies of any loan agreements involving the practice, the practice fee schedule, appointment books, schedule of accounts receivable, equipment depreciation schedule, and insurance schedules. It should be determined if any practice assets are used totally or partially for personal activities.

Since most practices use cash basis accounting, balance sheets will have to be adjusted to reflect any accrued and unpaid expenses including any pension liabilities and payroll taxes, accounts receivable, or other assets (e.g., art work, luxury automobiles) that are not required in the performance of regular medical services. The income statement, likewise, should be adjusted to reflect any nonpractice income (e.g., interest income) included in practice income or expense that could be considered discretionary or inconsistent with the requirements of normal practice.

A thorough financial analysis and interpretation of the financial history of the practice is then performed. In addition to internal interpretations, a comparison to the financial characteristics of other provider entities should be made. Today, published sources of business financial statistics include most categories of medical/health care provider organizations. Comparisons will need to be made between the practice income and salary of the practitioner(s) relative to specialty peers.[10]

---

[9] *Washington Post* (October 24, 1989).

[10] The results of regularly updated surveys of medical practitioners by the American Medical Association and the Center for Health Policy Research appear in the publication entitled *Socioeconomic Characteristics of Medical Practice*. A second helpful source for this type of information is the periodical, *Medical Economics*.

Table 10.3   Medical Practice Characteristics, by Selected Specialty, 1985 to 1992

[Dollar figures in thousands. Based on a sample telephone survey of 4,000 non-Federal office and hospital based patient care physicians, excluding residents, with a response rate of 69.1% in 1990, 66.7% in 1991, and 64.4% in 1992.

Specialty	1985	1987	1988	1989	1990	1991	1992
Mean Patient Visits per Week							
All physicians[1]	117.1	119.3	121.1	121.6	120.9	118.4	114.8
General/family practice	138.1	138.3	145.6	143.0	146.0	144.4	138.4
Internal medicine	105.2	114.5	113.0	117.9	112.0	110.7	109.4
Surgery	108.2	107.8	105.0	107.7	107.6	106.9	101.6
Pediatrics	130.8	127.4	135.1	138.1	134.0	133.4	126.9
Obstetrics/Gynecology	112.0	112.7	118.9	115.6	120.0	112.2	110.5
Mean Hours in Patient Care per Week							
All physicians[1]	51.3	52.9	53.1	53.3	53.3	53.3	52.9
General/family practice	53.6	53.7	54.4	54.4	55.0	54.7	53.1
Internal medicine	52.4	56.0	56.2	56.8	55.7	56.3	55.5
Surgery	51.2	53.0	53.8	53.3	53.1	53.4	53.0
Pediatrics	50.6	53.6	52.5	53.4	52.4	52.4	52.6
Obstetrics/Gynecology	56.9	57.0	59.4	59.0	60.4	59.5	58.8
Mean Net Income							
All physicians[1]	$112.2	$132.3	$144.7	$155.8	$164.3	$170.6	$177.4
General/Family practice	77.9	91.5	94.6	95.9	102.7	111.5	111.8
Internal medicine	102.0	121.8	130.9	146.5	152.5	149.6	159.3
Surgery	155.0	187.9	207.5	220.5	236.4	233.8	244.6
Pediatrics	76.2	85.3	94.9	104.7	106.5	119.3	121.7
Obstetrics/Gynecology	124.3	163.2	180.7	194.3	207.3	221.8	215.1
Mean Professional Expenses							
All physicians[1]	$102.7	$123.7	$140.8	$148.4	$150.0	$168.4	$179.0
General/Family practice	96.5	121.2	122.3	128.5	134.5	146.4	156.3
Internal medicine	90.0	117.8	136.3	139.1	139.2	159.0	172.9
Surgery	135.7	164.7	188.2	203.2	201.0	215.6	238.6
Pediatrics	87.3	100.2	115.3	132.5	138.0	145.4	168.8
Obstetrics/Gynecology	131.9	173.2	189.6	197.4	212.6	236.2	234.8
Mean Liability Premium							
All physicians[1]	$10.5	$15.0	$15.9	$15.5	$14.5	$14.9	$13.5
General/Family practice	6.8	8.9	9.4	9.0	7.8	8.1	8.1
Internal medicine	5.8	8.4	9.0	8.2	9.2	8.0	8.5
Surgery	16.6	24.5	26.5	25.8	22.8	22.5	20.6
Pediatrics	4.7	7.1	9.3	7.8	7.8	8.4	7.8
Obstetrics/Gynecology	23.5	35.3	35.3	37.0	34.3	34.9	33.5

[1] Includes other specialties not shown separately.

Source: American Medical Association, Chicago, IL, *Socioeconomic Characteristics of Medical Practice,* copyright 1994. Reprinted with permission.

Table 10.4   **Physician Salary Surveys (1994)**

Specialty	No. of Surveys	Mean	Range of Means	Percent Increase in Mean over Previous Year
Anesthesiology	8	$203,326	$162,500-$262,327	0.3
Cardiology (noninvasive)	9	$207,690	$150,000-$262,057	5.4
Emergency medicine	9	$157,286	$128,300-$174,775	3.7
Family practitioners	10	$122,625	$100,000-$132,578	7.8
General surgery	10	$190,273	$150,000-$232,700	3.2
Internal medicine	10	$127,366	$100,000-$147,300	2.4
Neurology	8	$149,309	$125,000-$188,765	2.5
Obstetrics/gynecology	10	$204,752	$180,000-$231,565	7.8
Oncology	8	$173,655	$120,000-$229,184	N/A
Pathology	9	$175,048	$130,000-$210,070	N/A
Pediatrics	10	$121,776	$100,000-$135,855	6.0
Psychiatry	10	$130,267	$120,000-$139,000	0.9
Radiology	9	$209,150	$165,200-$291,251	(2.6)
Urology	9	$198,300	$140,000-$229,000	5.1

Source: *Modern Healthcare*, July 10, 1995.

Valuation Approaches

There is a wide variety of so-called approaches or methods to the appraisal of businesses. The Institute of Business Appraisers lists as many as 14 (see Figure 10.1). The following discussion will focus on two asset-based methods, four income-based methods, and two market- or sale-based methods.

Asset-Based Approaches

One method of valuation involves a determination of the value of adjusted net assets or adjusted book (market) value. A practice's equipment, instruments, accounts receivable, leasehold improvements, or owned facilities can be valued in a direct manner. Because of the technical nature and high costs of some equipment, it may be necessary to consult equipment appraisers and/or manufacturers or suppliers about current market values. Normally the hard assets would have an indicated value based on their depreciated replacement cost. The aggregate value of tangible assets would be decreased by any outstanding liabilities to arrive at a "fair market value" of an ownership interest on an adjusted net asset basis. This basic method is perhaps most appropriate for a newly established practice or one that has not established an earnings history or its growth potential. The value thus derived might also be looked upon as an approximate liquidating value. Unfortunately, the value obtained by this method gives no recognition to the prospects for the future earning power of the practice.

Figure 10.1   **Business Appraisal Methodology**

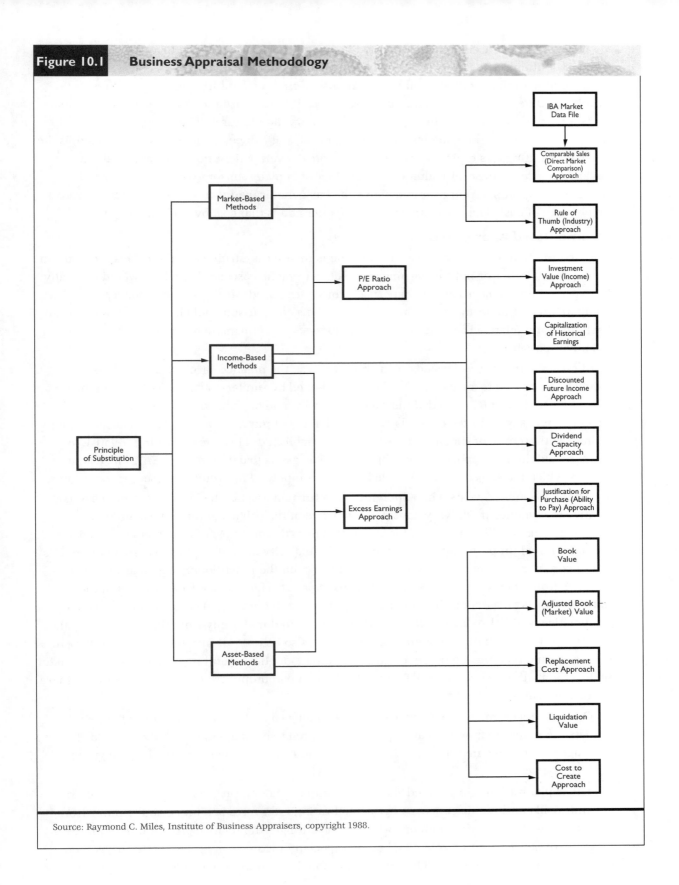

A second asset-based approach method has sometimes been referred to as the cost to create method. It attempts to determine the costs involved in starting up a new practice. The cost items used with this method include the expense of finding and hiring employees, the cost of locating and negotiating a lease or purchase of a facility to house the practice, and the normal costs incurred for new equipment, supplies inventory, and fixtures. The salary of the practitioner(s) also would be included. Another cost, if it can be adequately substantiated, is the normal operating loss typically accrued until a break-even patient flow is established that covers practice expenses. In addition, if the amount is material, some or all of the cost of practitioner(s) preparation over and above the basic medical education might be recognized as an element of cost. The disadvantage of such a method is that cost by itself is not value.

Income-Based Approaches

The first method of valuation based on income is the excess earnings method. This method can determine whether or not the earnings of a subject practice exceed that which would normally be expected in a subject's area of expertise. Here normalized earnings of the practice would be compared with the norms of similar practices.[11] This comparison could be made on an absolute basis and/or a relative basis and should use practices of comparable revenue and asset levels wherever possible.

If excess earnings were tested on an absolute level, the practice earnings before taxes (EBT) would be compared to an average level of EBT attained by similar practices. The amount by which the subject's EBT exceeded the expected level would be defined as "excess earnings." If excess earnings were tested on a relative level, the rate of return on assets (EBT/total assets) for a representative group of similar entities would be established. This rate of earnings relative to assets would then be applied to the subject's tangible assets to derive normal EBT. The extent, if any, by which the subject's EBT exceeded the just computed EBT would represent excess profits.

There are some caveats when applying the return on assets. The level of reported assets relative to revenues might vary considerably between the subject and the norm group of practices. This would be the case, for instance, where the principal of the practice owned substantial real property not usually found in the majority of similar practices. In addition, it is not uncommon for a practice, as a separate entity from the practitioner(s), to lease practice facilities from another entity owned by the principal(s). The practice facilities would, therefore, not show up as an asset on the financial statements of the practice. Lease payments made by the practice could also distort EBT if market rent differed materially from the actual rent paid. Important investment or nonoperating assets may also be present in some practices. These, of course, should be removed before calculations are made. If a careful investigation is undertaken in developing the practice's fundamental database and appropriate adjustments are made, these distortions can be avoided.

Once excess earnings are estimated, they would be capitalized at an appropriate rate that reflects the reality that excess earnings are considered to be at a higher risk than regular earnings on a passive investment. The resulting value is the value of goodwill or the group of intangible assets.

The capitalization rate selected should take into consideration the likelihood that the excess earnings will continue. Excess earnings capitalization rates have been reported to range from 20% to 100% with a median rate of 33-1/3%. The stronger the relative growth rate in practice revenue, the lower the rate selected. Relative specialty incomes and growth rates have been described previously (e.g., see Table 10.4). Additional insight into selecting an appropriate

---

[11] Financial data of this type are reported by such companies as Robert Morris Associates, Financial Research Associates, Standard & Poor's References, Media General Financial Services, and Dunn & Bradstreet.

capitalization rate might be related to the internal rate of return on the medical education investment experienced by practitioners over the life of their professional careers. Several studies have addressed this question; findings from them are shown in Table 10.5.

To arrive at an overall value for the ownership interest in the practice following this methodology, the fair market value of tangible assets is added to the capitalized value of the excess earnings and then practice liabilities are deducted. The result is the value of the overall ownership interest of the practice. Some appraisers do not consider this methodology completely satisfactory depending on the purpose of a given appraisal. Their concern is that the value thus derived is largely based upon historical costs and performance. They argue that the value of any economic good at a given point in time must be fundamentally weighted in favor of anticipated future benefits or the earning power available to an owner. Since this excess earnings methodology is essentially based on assets and past performance, it may not be prudent to rely heavily on it in some situations. The appropriateness of this methodology may depend on whether or not the goodwill is deemed to be "personal" or "commercial." The purpose of the appraisal and the jurisdiction involved should provide guidance in the application and relevance of this methodology.

The value of an economic good or ownership interest is, in theory and commonly in practice, a function of the discounted future benefits accruing to the ownership interest. Two discounted future income methodologies are based on *residual income* or *residual asset* value. To apply these methods it is necessary to project both the level of earnings and the level of assets over some future time period and their terminal value at a defined future point in time. Analysts disagree about the length of time that should be employed for these projections. Some appraisers believe that to project for more than three to five years represents questionable speculation, given the propensity for recurring changes or cycles in most economic environments. Others, however, insist that some types of economic activity such as medical practices are predictable for more extended periods of time, perhaps 10 to 15 years. For medical practices 10 years is not unreasonable if the external and internal circumstances and characteristics of a practice and its principal(s) support such a time frame.

To make projections with some confidence it is usually necessary to have at least five years of complete operating and financial data. These data should be adjusted on an annual basis to stabilize and isolate the true and relevant revenue, expenses, and assets of the practice. After the adjustments have been completed, the most statistically correct projection would be to calculate a separate least squares progression (trend line) for both revenue and major expense categories. The resulting *EBT* should be checked by applying normalized expense and profit ratios with internal and external norms, which may suggest some adjustments. The projected results should also be fine-tuned to reflect any known changes that will likely occur in the practice during the projected time period. The projected level of assets is usually expressed as one ratio of the gross revenue of the practice.

After projected values are established, a decision is required about the rate of discount to be applied to the future amounts. The rate can be arrived at by a subjective buildup of elements of the rate. This should take into consideration the risk-free rate of interest, inflation, required investment yields in the financial markets, degree of comfort with the projections, relative performance of the practice to professional norms, whether it is a solo or a group practice, degree of competition, etc. As noted earlier, the internal rate of return experienced in the medical profession (Table 10.5) could be considered a base, with an addition or deduction to the rate depending on the revenue growth rate of the subject practice compared to current experience in the profession. In some situations it may be appropriate to have some step-up in the discount rate for those years more distant in the future. The step differential would be of a subjective nature but should reflect the known characteristics of the practice and its operating environment.

Table 10.5	Internal Rates of Return of Physicians* 1955-1980	
Year	All Physicians	General Practitioners
1955	3.5%	9.1%
1959	4.7%	3.7%
1962	6.6%	N/A
1965	7.5%	4.1%
1970	2.0%	6.8%
1976	7.5%	16.4%
1980	4.0%	6.7%
Average	5.1%	7.8%

* The annual compound rate of discount required to equate practice net income with the cost of a medical education over the estimated career life of physicians.
Source: Taken from five studies reported in Paul J. Feldstein, *Health Care Economics*, 3rd ed., (New York: John Wiley & Sons, 1988), 361.

With the residual income method, present value factors of the selected discount rate(s) would be applied to the *EBT* of each of the projected years and summed. It is then assumed that the *EBT* will stabilize to perpetuity at the level of the last year of the projected time frame. This *EBT* value is then capitalized by a rate appropriate to a constant return investment keyed to a yield on intermediate or long-term investment grade bonds. The result of this capitalization is multiplied by the present value factor for the last year in the projected time period and added to the sum of the present values previously found for the annual EBT flows. The combined value would then be reduced to an after-tax equivalent by applying the appropriate individual or corporate income tax rates. The resulting amount would be an indicated fair market value of the practice.

The residual asset method is similar to the residual income method with respect to the annual *EBT* flows, but the terminal value would be the expected level of adjusted net assets in place at that time. This inherently assumes that the practice would be liquidated at the terminal point in time. The present value of the future level of assets would be added to the sum of the present values of the *EBT* flows and the income amount adjusted for taxes (this assumes no capital gains inherent in the assets) for an indicated fair market value of the practice.

A third basic method employs *price/earnings multiples*. The value of an investment is often described as a multiple of earnings or capitalization of earnings. The P/E relationship, in theory, provides a value that will return the cost of an investment plus a fair compensation to an owner for taking the risks of ownership. This is the most frequently used relative measure of value of earnings in the public equity markets. Factors derived from publicly traded equity interests (common and preferred stock) in an active and liquid public market are widely accepted as the most realistic fair market value indicators of equity ownership claims. Unfortunately, closely held professional practices do not enjoy such a direct market valuation of their worth to owners. Nevertheless, in business valuations of professional practices, an attempt should be made to correlate the value of the practices to investor demand yields (multiples) found in active financial markets involving similar types of enterprises.

Today, there are publicly traded firms that operate in the health care industry, and a careful search for companies providing direct patient medical services included in the U.S. Department of Commerce 8000 Standard Industrial Classification should be undertaken. Computer accessible and published databases will likely provide at least a minimal number of such firms. Those firms believed to be most like small, closely held entities that have some public trading and make public their financial data will usually be found in stock listings from the over-the-counter market published by financial reference services.

Once a list of publicly traded firms has been identified, each listing should be analyzed for the nature and size of the business, number of employees, years in operation, level of profitability, location, etc. When a qualified list of businesses (seldom more than 10) has been selected, their respective earnings and prices are noted. Depending upon the source of data, average five-year price/earnings ratios may be reported. This will make it possible to get a feel for current pricing compared to historical pricing. For the most part, however, the P/Es that exist close to the date of valuation are the ones that should be identified. Some business appraisers weigh each of the respective listed P/Es depending on how close their characteristics match those of the subject practice to derive a weighted P/E ratio rather than taking a simple average.

For purposes of valuing a practice, the earnings of the subject practice should be normalized if much variation exists in either revenues or earnings over the five-year base period. This would usually be the case in fairly new and growing practices or those located in environments undergoing significant demographic or competitive change. The next step in this method is to multiply the P/Es of similar companies by the subject's after-tax net income (adjusted for significant nonoperating items).

A final adjustment in this method is recognition of the lack of marketability of the ownership interest of the practice. The value obtained requires one final adjustment and this is for a marketability discount. This liquidity preference is served when an investment is traded in an ongoing and active market with frequent price quotations. This liquidity preference value is not present in most professional practice situations. A range of acceptable discounts for lack of marketability has been found in several research reports and case studies. These studies entail the pricing of "letter stock." Letter stock is similar in almost all characteristics to the traded stock of the same publicly owned company, but is restricted from being traded on the open market for a specified period of time. The spreads found between privately exchanged letter stock and standard traded stock values provide an excellent measure for the lack of marketability. These discounts for lack of marketability have been found to have a wide range (as high as 90%) but appear to fall frequently in the 30% to 50% range. The indicated fair market value of the ownership interest in a medical practice, therefore, with this method is:

$$\text{after-tax income} \times \text{P/E} \times (1 - \text{marketability discount}).$$

The disadvantage of this method is that P/E ratios vary substantially, the reasons for buying a stock are not the same as for buying a firm, and P/E ratios are generally based on the previous year's results.

Sales-Based Approaches

The comparable business sales method attempts to find recent sales transactions involving medical practices and identify appropriate value multiples such as the comparison of the entity's sale price to gross revenue, assets, net earnings, and/or excess earnings if this can be determined. Business brokers who may normally handle practice sales may be one of the best sources for this type of information. Several business broker trade associations maintain market databases for the benefit of their members. The Institute of Business Appraisers (IBA), for example, provides market data information for its members.[12] Some databases are maintained by large valuation firms and other professional valuation associations.

For example, a report from the Institute of Business Appraisers' database identified six medical practices that were sold in 1989. Included in the report were family, internal medicine, and obstetrics practices. The only usable multiple was selling price of the practice to gross revenue. Revenue ranged from $115,000 to $400,000 and transaction prices ranged from $45,000 to $125,000, producing transaction price/gross revenue multiples from .18 to .39. Both the highest and lowest multiple occurred with internal medicine practices. This is another indicator of the significant differences in value found between practices of even the same specialty.

As with many types of businesses, generalized indicators of value, usually related to the sales price of a practice, can be found. These so-called rules of thumb, however, seldom if ever take into consideration the significant differences among medical practices. At best these indicators serve only as a very rough point of reference for value derived by other methods based on a subject practice's unique external and internal characteristics and performance. For instance, one consultant with experience in the valuation of medical practices purports to have found that "many" practices sell for tangible assets plus three to six months' collections. Some CPAs have been known to suggest that a medical practice is worth one year's gross revenue (perhaps this is because accounting practices are sometimes sold on this basis). Another medical valuation consultant maintains he has never found a medical practice that sold for this high an amount. Again, even rules of thumb suggest a likely wide spectrum of value may be associated with medical practices.

Conclusion

The values produced by the various approaches discussed here prove that a *reasonable* indication of value should be included in the appraisal report of a medical practice. All such estimates, of course, must be clearly spelled out and the specific assumptions on which the methodologies are based should be apparent. It is questionable whether averaging of values can be defended adequately even though such practice is in common use. The largest difference in the derived values of the ownership interest of a highly successful and growing medical practice will be found between asset-based values and income-based values.

The development of background data and unique practice characteristics and trends should suggest which method is most appropriate. The income-based methods, theoretically, should set the parameters for the final estimate of value that is consistent with the purpose of an appraisal. The final value will be selected within that range, reflecting the appraiser's professional judgment and experience. Certainly the value selected for the subject will be as realistic as possible when such value reflects due consideration of the total set of external and internal factors affecting practice operations within those perspectives and perceptions common in business valuations.

An outline of the approaches, methods, and elements for an appraisal of a medical practice that can usually be adopted to any nonasset-based medical/health care entity is provided in Figure 10.2.

An example of a business valuation of a family medical practice appears in the following chapter.

---

[12] See Bibliography in Appendix E for sources of market data on actual sales of closely held businesses and published rules of thumb.

Figure 10.2	Outline of Business Valuation of a Medical Practice

I. **External Macro Information**

    A. National Economic Developments

    B. Industry Background Data

        1. Factors and States of Competition

        2. Significant Developments in Professional Sector

        3. Federal and State Legislative Developments

    C. Conditions in the Financial Markets

        1. Government Sector Securities

        2. Private Sector Securities and Claims

    D. Demographic Trends

        1. National

        2. Local

        3. Specific Aggregate Employment and Income Data

    E. Industry, Financial, and Performance Norms

II. **Practice Characteristics**

    A. Location and Competing Practices/Services

    B. Practice Historical Development

    C. Practice Principal(s) Characteristics

    D. Practice Employees

    E. Patient Profile

    F. Financial History and Adjusted Financials

    G. Existing Partnership or Buy/Sell Agreements

    H. Financial Projections

III. **Financial Analysis and Interpretations**

IV. **Asset-Based Approaches**

    A. Adjusted Net Assets

    B. Cost to Create

V. **Income-Based Approaches**

    A. Excess Earnings Method

    B. Residual Income Method

    C. Residual Asset Method

    D. Price/Earnings Multiples

VI. **Sales-Based Approaches**

VII. **Summary and Valuation Conclusion**

C H A P T E R

E L E V E N

Business Valuation Case Study:
Family Medical Practice

The purpose of this valuation is to obtain an indication of the fair market value of a solo family medical practice in contemplation of a sale of part of the practice.

The subject professional practice is located in a high-income, stable community. The subject's county has grown rapidly over the past 20 years. The service area of the practice, however, was well established prior to this high-growth period and the area has not grown as fast as some of the other municipalities in the county. Economic data indicate that 65% to 70% of the working population in the service area is white collar, 24% to 29% of its residents are college graduates, and 24% to 34% of household incomes exceed $50,000. Also, the likelihood that residents in the service area have investments is 22% to 32% greater than the national average.

The impact of national trends in the health care industry is expected to be only minimal on the subject practice in the short run (1-3 years). Federal health care policy changes are not a major concern. Since both the practice and its immediate service area have more stability and continuity than adjacent areas, competition from new entrants into family medical practice in the immediate locale is judged to be of minimal significance. Because of the entrenched nature of the subject practice and the characteristics of its service area, the value of the practice can be maintained indefinitely. If new physician entrants or medical service companies want to locate in the service area, it is believed the value of the subject practice should enjoy some premium above any large set or norm group of medical practice prices.

A major, private nonprofit general hospital is located less than one mile from the practice location. The subject physician is on the medical staff of that hospital. There are 14 other practices with family practice designations in the service area. Approximately half of these are group practices. Several well-established group practices with specialties other than family medicine are also located in the vicinity of the hospital. In recent years, some practices have extended office hours into the early evening five or six days a week. Some of the family practice physicians have more than one office in locations outside the primary practice service area. Because the subject practice is well established, competition is considered only moderate.

In addition to private practices two health maintenance organizations operate in the larger central area of the state. Several preferred provider plans are also available to employees of larger businesses and governmental agencies. Further, two "walk-in" clinics for general medical services have been in operation about five years. One is operated by the hospital previously identified and is approximately five miles from the hospital and beyond city limits. The other clinic is operated by a for-profit organization with an all-employee medical staff.

The appraisal subject is a solo general medical practice started by the physician owner in 1979. The physician is board-certified in family medicine and is 47 years old. The practice is located on one of the main thoroughfares in the middle of the primary community and is within walking distance of several affluent residential areas. The practice has continued to lease the same one-story, masonry, 4,000-square-foot facility since it first opened. In 1980 the practice was incorporated by the practice physician. Two years later the facility was personally purchased by the physician and remodeled. The incorporated practice (P.A.) has continued to lease the facility from the physician.

The practice maintains between 5,000 and 5,500 patient files, which is somewhat higher than found in the average solo practice. About 25% of the practice's patients are retired. Except for 5% of practice revenue that is derived from fees of hospitalized patients, all other practice revenue is office generated. The practice employs four office personnel and two nurses. In addition, the practice employs an X-ray technician and a lab technician who each typically average somewhat less than 40 hours per week. The physician works approximately 70 hours per week. He is considering the recruitment of a physician partner within the next three years, which would enable him to reduce his working hours while expanding the patient flow of the practice. The practice fee schedule is comparable to most other practices in the area but higher than some by 10% to 12%.

Financial Adjustments

Because the income statements in most closely held companies and professional practices are designed to reduce taxes rather than report a true economic picture of the company's performance, adjustments to the financial statements are generally necessary. In the case of the subject practice the following adjustments were needed.

1. Nondirect practice income (interest and dividends) was deducted from reported income in order to recognize only the operating activity of the practice.

2. Contributions and donations are considered a discretionary expense of the business and were therefore added back to net income.

3. Because of accelerated depreciation methods, excessive depreciation (accounting depreciation greater than economic depreciation) has been taken. To calculate and adjust for the excessive expense, the fair market value of the fixed depreciable assets was divided into the book value to determine the percentage of excess depreciation. This percentage was then multiplied by the annual depreciation expense to provide an estimate of the excessive depreciation expense taken.

4. Operating expense was adjusted to reflect the below-market rent paid by the practice.

In addition to the adjustments required because taxes are determined on a cash basis, adjustments are also needed to determine the fair market value of unrealized and tangible practice assets and to identify any assets owned by the practice that are not required in providing its services. In the subject case the balance sheet was adjusted for the value of accounts receivable, supplies and materials, and accrued liabilities not reported on tax returns.

Comparative Performance

The adjusted income statement and balance sheet as of December 31, 1990, was compared with the norms for a set of 219 medical practices having revenues of less than $1,000,000 annually. The following comparisons were obtained:

	Practice 12/31/90	Industry 12/31/90
1. Income Statement Percentages Summary		
Total revenue	100.00%	100.00%
Gross profit	100.00%	100.00%
Operating expenses	53.09%	56.60%
Physician's salary	37.09%	33.10%
Depreciation expense	3.85%	3.20%
Pretax operating profit	5.97%	7.10%
2. Balance sheet percentages summary		
Cash and equivalent	0.05%	16.20%
Accounts receivable	52.25%	20.70%
Inventory	3.54%	0.40%
Fixed assets (net)	43.04%	42.40%
Other current assets	1.12%	3.80%
Other noncurrent assets	0.00%	14.70%
Intangibles (net)	0.00%	1.80%
Total assets	100.00%	100.00%
Total liabilities	28.73%	65.90%
Total equity	71.27%	34.10%
Total liabilities and equity	100.00%	100.00%
Debt/tangible net worth	0.40	2.00
Earnings before tax/tangible net worth	19%	20%
Earnings before taxes/total assets	13%	6%
Sales/net fixed assets	14.54	12.10

The above comparison indicates that the subject practice is maintaining high liquidity (cash is an exception), less debt, and higher equity than the norm group of practices. Although the subject's percentage of assets in receivables is higher relative to its total assets, its collection period is only 45.9 days compared to the norm group's 61.9 days.

It is not uncommon to find that the higher the liquidity position is in the asset base of a professional practice, the less the earnings ratio on total assets will be. In this instance the before-tax earnings ratio on net worth is about the same as for the norm group (in spite of the fact that the subject practice employs considerably less leverage). However, the return on the assets employed in the subject practice, based on a before-tax earnings margin, exceeds that of the norm group by 7%. This resulted primarily because of the subject's lower operating expense ratio even though the physician's salary is above that of the norm group. The X-ray and lab capabilities also contribute to the higher profit of the practice.

Except for physician salaries drawn in medical practices, the largest remaining part of operating expenses tends to be fixed personnel costs. As a practice provides more hours of service or achieves a higher level of patient flow per unit of time, revenue per patient unit tends to be higher than that of the larger group of medical practices. If the norm group on the average is less efficient in handling patient flow, or generally does not offer in-office X-ray and lab support, the group's revenue per physician is likely to be less than that of practices similar to the valuation subject.

Valuation Methodology

The value of the subject practice is determined with a view toward the value of its assets, the value of its income flow, and its market value as a going concern. Book value and *adjusted net assets* consider the value of the business's assets. Income-based methods, which consider past, projected future, and excess earnings, concentrate on income flows as the principal determinant of value. The appropriateness of each of these methods was considered in developing an indication of value for the subject practice.

Asset-Based Approaches

Reported book value represents the "accounting value" of the business assets minus liabilities at the date of valuation. As of the date of valuation, reported book value of entity equity was *$374,592.* Because balance sheets are prepared in accordance with generally accepted accounting principles, the book value of a business does not usually reflect the fair market value of the underlying assets, future earning power, or "unbooked" market value appreciation.

The *adjusted net assets* are represented by the total equity as presented on an "economic" balance sheet as of the date of valuation. Adjustments are made to the assets and liabilities to reflect their fair market value. As an indicator of the total fair market value of the equity, the adjusted value has the disadvantage of considering the status of the business at only one point in time. Additionally, the adjusted value does not properly take into account the earning capacity of the business. In many respects, adjusted net assets represent the minimum benchmark value of the total assets of an operating business entity. On December 31, 1990, the adjusted book value of entity equity was *$794,969.*

The *cost-to-create method* of valuation is based on determining the cost that would be incurred to reproduce and initiate medical practice operations in terms of both tangible and intangible net adjusted values at a comparable location.

One of the first costs of creating a medical practice is organizational cost. This consists of accounting and legal fees, set-up costs, licenses and permits, and initial printing and supplies. Organization cost is estimated to be $5,000. Recruiting and training of personnel is estimated to be the equivalent of one month's office payroll. Acquisition of a leased facility is estimated on the basis of the commission a brokerage service would charge. This is estimated to equal one month's rental charge. In the case of the subject, the existing lease has five years to run and the below-market lease payments provide a residual lease value.

The cost of assembling the fixed assets is estimated at 5% of net fixed assets. The value of intangible assets accrues from the stream of income they produce or their cost to develop. In a number of transactions it has been found that an established solo medical practice often will have goodwill purchased at a value of from three to five months' collections. Four months was used for the subject case. The net tangible assets represent the adjusted book value of the tangible operating assets.

The result of the cost to create approach leads to a conclusion of business value of *$414,849* and a total entity value of *$942,599* at December 31, 1990.

Organizational costs	$ 5,000
Acquisition of personnel	10,311
Acquisition of lease	4,500
Acquisition of fixed assets	2,500
Residual leasehold value	8,453
Intangible asset value	200,000
Adjusted net tangible operating assets	184,085
Indicated business value	414,849
Plus nonoperating assets	527,750
Total entity combined value	$942,599

Income-Based Approaches

Using a capitalization of historic earnings methodology, historic earnings are weighted or normalized to determine a base, which is then divided by an appropriate capitalization rate to derive a total business value. Before-tax operating income was selected for capitalization to avoid tax differences among members of a comparison group of practices. These earnings are capitalized into perpetuity using a rate that reflects returns for the tangible and intangible assets of the business.

The capitalization rate selected resulted from a buildup of capitalization rate factors. The first factor reflects the basic real rate of interest (risk-free rate) and the expected rate of inflation. This is assumed to be best represented by the yield on longer U.S. government bonds as of the valuation date, which was 8.3%. The risk premium for the industry is expressed as the difference between the rate of return on equity for a group of similar entities and the government bond yield. In this instance that premium is 11.5%. The final rate factor is the growth differential between the subject entity and its industry. In this instance the long-term growth rate in revenue of medical practices is estimated to be about 12%. The five-year revenue growth rate for the subject is 4.3%, or a differential of 7.5%. The foregoing results in an overall capitalization rate of 27.3%.

Long-term Treasury yield	8.3%
Industry risk premium	11.5%
Growth differential premium	7.5%
Capitalization rate	27.3%

When this rate is applied to the weighted before-tax earnings, the result is a business value of *$980,505*. This value is then added to the value of nonoperating assets (such as real estate) for a total entity value indication of *$1,508,255* on December 31, 1990.

Year	Before-Tax Earnings	x	Weighting Factor	=	Extension
1988	$171,908		1		$ 171,908
1989	272,169		2		544,338
1990	296,607		3		889,821
Summary of extensions					$1,606,067
Divided by total weighting					6
Weighted average before-tax earnings					$267,678
Divided by capitalization rate					27.3%
Indicated business value					$980,505
Plus nonoperating assets					$527,750
Total entity combined value					$1,508,255

The excess earnings approach (or IRS formula approach) values the tangible and intangible assets of an entity independently. The two values are then added to obtain the total fair market value of the entity. Tangible assets are comprised of the fair market value of total assets minus total liabilities as of the date of valuation. Intangible assets are estimated by capitalizing any earnings of the entity that exceed the normal rate of return on tangible assets realized by a set of similar entities. Excess earnings represent adjusted net income reduced by an average industry return on net assets.

The excess earnings base is capitalized into perpetuity using a rate of return that reflects the risk that the subject's earnings will remain above the average for that type of investment. Excess earnings are less stable than normal earnings and are anticipatory. They are in "excess" of earnings that are normally expected from a given set of tangible assets in a going concern at a given location. The risks are that excess earnings will attract more competition and, in the absence of pricing freedom, that inflation will diminish the excess earnings over some unknown time period.

To compensate for this higher risk a premium is added to the capitalization rate previously applied to weighted before-tax earnings in the straight capitalization of earnings method. The premium is based on the difference between the industry's median rate of return on assets and the third quartile rate of return on assets. The median rate for the industry group's earnings is 5.6%, say 6%, and the third quartile earnings rate is 26.5%, say 27%, for a risk premium of 21%. When this rate is combined with the earlier capitalization rate, the capitalization rate for excess earnings becomes 48.3%, say 48%. Following this methodology the combined business value of the subject entity is *$718,737* and the combined entity value is *$1,246,487*.

Weighted average before-tax earnings		$ 267,678
Adjusted tangible business assets	$184,085	
	x 6.0%	
Normal earnings		11,045
Excess earnings		256,633
Divided by 48% cap rate for excess earnings		
= total intangible value		534,652
Plus adjusted book value		184,085
Total operating business value		718,737
Plus nonoperating assets		527,750
Total entity combined value		$1,246,487

A second variation for determining entity value based on the excess earnings approach is sometimes used to value a professional medical practice. With this method the weighted before-tax earnings plus the physician's actual salary are calculated. Expected (fair value) physician compensation, as indicated by a set of norm practices, is then deducted to obtain a net adjusted *EBT*. This in turn is reduced by normal earnings on tangible business assets employed, and the excess earnings are then capitalized by an appropriate rate to obtain an indicated intangible value. This method provides an indicated business value of *$673,287* and a total combined value of *$1,201,037*.

Weighted *EBT* plus doctor's actual salary	$ 492,363
Less fair value salary	257,546
Excess earnings	234,817
Divided by 48% cap rate for excess earnings	
= total intangible value	489,202
Plus adjusted book value	184,085
Total indicated business value	673,287
Plus nonoperating assets	$527,750
Total entity combined value	$1,201,037

The discounted future income approach, based on an earnings residual method, estimates the subject's value based on its future income. (The "DFE-asset residual" method is not used as the basis for valuation in this instance because the asset base is not the primary determinant of future earnings in the majority of service businesses or professional practices.) The income levels are projected for the next five years and result from a consideration of both macro-industry factors and the subject's historical and likely future financial performance. The revenue and expense projections reflect a least squares trend projection based on the preceding five years' financial data and a constant percentage of 33.1% (industry norm) of gross revenue for physician salaries in practices having similar levels of gross revenue.

Each year's before-tax earnings are discounted to the valuation date. The fifth year's before-tax earnings are assumed to continue indefinitely at a constant level and are, therefore, capitalized into perpetuity by the required discount rate for a value at the end of the fifth year. The fifth-year perpetuity capitalized value is then discounted back to the valuation date and summed with the individual years' present values. This DFE methodology accounts for all future earnings of the subject in terms of present value as of the date of valuation.

One of the most challenging aspects of DFE methodology is the determination of the appropriate rate of discount. In the discussion above on the capitalized earnings method, a capitalization rate of 27.3% was developed. To recognize that future earnings are less certain, a 5% premium is added to obtain a discount rate of 32.3% for application in this method. Using projected revenues and applying the rate, the business value of the firm was estimated at *$452,371.* The addition of the nonoperating assets of $527,750 obtains a combined entity value of *$980,121.*

Period	Before Tax Operating Earnings	Present Value Before-Tax Operating Earnings
1	$126,803	$95,845
2	$136,076	$77,743
3	$145,350	$62,768
4	$154,623	$50,470
5	$163,897	$40,436
Income residual		$125,109
Business value PV		$452,371
Plus nonoperating assets		$527,750
Total entity value		$980,121

Sales-Based Approaches

In the subject case it was not possible to determine appropriate public financial market multiples for assets, earnings, and book values to derive a market indication of value. There is no ongoing and/or liquid market for medical practice ownership interests as would be the case with an exchange-listed entity's shares, nor are any traded on the over-the-counter market for unlisted securities of comparable entities. While shares of hospital and health provider organizations are traded in the public markets, the lack of comparability between those entities and solo medical practices does not make use of market multiples of value based on such securities a viable method in this case.

Using a direct market comparison approach, however, six private sales transactions of medical practices were located in the Institute of Business Appraisers' database. A weighting was given to each of them on the basis of the type of practice and their respective levels of revenue. The result of this study was a weighted average multiple of transaction price to gross revenue of .2662. When this comparative company multiple is applied to the gross revenue of the subject practice, the business value of *$211,911* is obtained. Because market transaction statistics are based on operating income, however, the subject's nonoperating assets ($527,750) were added to derive an indication of the combined entity value, or *$739,661.*

Value Conclusions

In the evaluation of the subject case a variety of methods were employed. The following is a listing of the specific methods that were considered appropriate for this assignment and their respective indications of both total entity value and the business value element.

	Total Value	Business Value
Book value	$ 374,592	*
Adjusted net assets	794,969	*
Cost-to-create approach	942,599	$414,849
Capitalization of earnings	1,508,255	980,505
Capitalization of excess earnings - A	1,246,487	718,737
Capitalization of excess earnings - B	1,201,037	673,287
Discounted future income (income residual)	980,121	452,371
Direct market comparison approach	739,661	211,911

*Not set forth as a separate item

Based on a review of these valuation indications within the context of the characteristics of the subject, the discounted future earnings (income residual) method is the single method that provides the best representation of the business value. To derive the total entity value, nonoperating assets were added to the business value obtained.

Another consideration before reaching a final conclusion of value for a business concern is recognition that investors have a high degree of preference for investment liquidity. This has been borne out by research findings of the Securities and Exchange Commission and others. With small closely held businesses and private practices there is no ongoing mechanism or institutional arrangement to enable an investor to liquidate his investment in such entities in a very short period of time. A discount for this lack of marketability is, therefore, common to business valuations involving these types of entities. The most representative marketability discount reported by the research has been approximately 30%. In the instant case, however, a potential purchaser of this medical practice would not likely contemplate a near term sale of the practice once it was acquired. At the same time, however, it must be recognized that full value is not likely to be received by the seller in this case. The sale of a medical practice entails additional costs such as brokers, attorneys, appraisers, etc. To recognize this, a discount (called a "transactional discount") of 15% is assigned to the business value element that is established by the above estimates. This so-called transactional discount may not be appropriate if other than the current ownership interest is to be valued for some other purpose.

For the subject case a final combined entity fair market value of $912,333, called *$915,000,* was concluded as of December 31, 1990.

Discounted future income estimate (income-residual method):

Business value	$452,371
Less transactional discount	(67,885)
Net business value	$384,516
Plus nonoperating assets	527,750
Final indicated value, 12/31/90	$912,266
	or $915,000

A P P E N D I X

A

Trends in Hospital Operation
(Data from Health Care Investment Analysts, Inc.)

MAJOR TRENDS IN THE PERFORMANCE OF U.S. HOSPITALS
BY HCIA([1])

The major trends and issues shaping the health care industry over the past few years will continue to have a significant impact on the financial and operating performance of U.S. hospitals. The table at the end of the section illustrates how the nation's hospitals have performed over the past five years, according to *The Sourcebook's* 52 key measures of hospital performance.

Overall, the financial and operating health of the U.S. hospital industry continued to show slight signs of improvement in 1994, despite dramatic marketplace changes. Hospital profitability increased for the fourth consecutive year, with median total profit margins reaching 4.52 percent in 1994, up from 4.25 percent in 1993. Much of the increase in profitability can be attributed to improvements in productivity and efficiency gained through consolidation, downsizing efforts, utilization control and continued reductions in average length of stay, greater use of less costly outpatient services, more efficient use of hospital assets, refinancing of debt, staffing level reductions, and declines in salary and benefit expenses, as well as overhead as a proportion of total operating expenses. As a result of these efficiency gains, hospitals' average revenue per adjusted discharge continued to increase at a faster rate than their average expense per adjusted discharge (between 1993 and 1994 the median operating revenue per adjusted discharge for all U.S. hospitals increased 2.4 percent, while the median operating expense per adjusted discharge increased only 1.8 percent), and hospitals' overall financial and cash position continued to improve.

Uncertainty over the ability of hospitals to remain profitable in the future, however, continues to grow. Despite continued improvements in the overall financial health of the hospital industry in 1994, the nation's hospitals still experienced a number of unfavorable trends. Deductions from gross patient revenue as a percentage of gross patient revenue increased for the fourth consecutive year rising from 30.3 percent in 1990 to 35.7 percent in 1994. Furthermore, Medicare and Medicaid continued to represent a growing proportion of all patients treated at the average hospital, an unfavorable trend in light of the less generous reimbursement patterns under Medicare's Prospective Payment System and most state Medicaid programs. Growth in Medicare and Medicaid payment shortfalls to hospitals in the future, coupled with greater managed care pressures, increased charity care burdens, and a growing number of uninsured patients, could work to reduce hospital profit margins over the next few years.

In the meantime, seven trends in the financial and operating performance of U.S. hospitals have remained particularly noteworthy over the past year. Descriptions of these trends follow.

---

[1] The comparative Performance of U.S. Hospitals: The Sourcebook 1996 HCIA Baltimore Maryland pp. 34-38.

Inpatient Utilization of the Nation's Hospitals Continues to Decline

The median number of total acute care discharges from all U.S. hospitals remained relatively stable in 1994, rising only 1.0 percent to 4,122 discharges from 4,080 discharges in 1993. This slight increase in the median number of discharges follows three years of consecutive declines from a median of 4,224 discharges in 1990. The recent increase in discharges is favorable, and likely the result of overall population growth. At the same time, despite the recent increase in patient discharges, the typical U.S. hospital continued to downsize, reducing its average number of acute care beds in service from 119 in 1993 to 116 in 1994. Downsizing efforts at the typical U.S. hospital also come as a favorable response to continued declines in inpatient utilization rates, as measured, most noticeably, by declines in the median occupancy rate for all U.S. hospitals. In 1994, the median inpatient occupancy rate for all U.S. hospitals fell 0.7 percentage points to 46.6 percent from 47.4 percent in 1993.

Overall, declines in inpatient utilization rates are most likely the result of continued growth in the volume of outpatient services being delivered at most hospitals. In 1994 alone, the median value for outpatient revenue as a percentage of total gross patient revenue increased more than 2.0 percentage points to 35.0 percent, from 33.0 percent in 1993. Declines in the use of hospital inpatient services are expected to continue over the next few years, as changing practice patterns, growth in managed care, a greater emphasis on utilization review, and advances in technology reduce inpatient hospital occupancy rates and average lengths of stay. Between 1993 and 1994, the median average length of stay for all U.S. hospitals fell slightly, from 4.79 to 4.57 days, and the median case mix-adjusted average length of stay also fell, from 3.81 to 3.61 days.

Medicare and Medicaid Patients Continue to Represent a Growing Proportion of All Patients Treated at the Average Hospital

In 1994, the combined proportion of Medicare and Medicaid patients discharged from the typical U.S. hospital reached 55.7 percent in 1990. The percentage of total patient days accounted for by Medicare and Medicaid at the typical U.S. hospital also continued to climb, from 60.9 percent in part to changes in state and federal policies and greater

qualification efforts by hospitals, which have expanded the number of people eligible to participate in the Medicaid program, and in part to an expanded aging population, which has caused growth in the number of Medicare beneficiaries. Continued growth in the proportion of Medicare and Medicaid patients at the typical U.S. hospital is an unfavorable trend for the U.S. hospital industry, especially in light of the fact that future reform will likely bring further cuts in Medicare and Medicaid spending for hospital services.

Recent Increase in Capital Intensity of U.S. Hospitals Not Largely Funded by Additional Debt

The median accounting age of the U.S. hospital industry's fixed assets continued to increase slightly in 1994, to 8.8 years from 8.5 years in 1993. The median amount of net plant, property, and equipment per bed at the typical U.S. hospital also continued to increase, from $92,392 in 1993 to $99,833 in 1994. In contrast to earlier years, however, this recent growth in the capital intensity of U.S. hospitals, which is the combined result of new construction and renovation and the emergence of more sophisticated medical technologies, does not appear to have been largely funded by additional debt, but rather by the favorable refinancing of old debt. For example, although the median ratio of debt per bed continued to increase in 1994, rising 4.8 percent to $97,773 per bed from $93,290 per bed in 1993, the rate of increase was much slower than that experienced in earlier years. (Between 1990 and 1993, the median ratio of debt per bed for all

U.S. hospitals increased at an average rate of 7.3 percent a year.) Furthermore, the median ratio of long-term debt to capitalization at the typical U.S. hospital continued to fall, from 0.39 in 1993 to 0.38 in 1994; the median ratio of long-term debt to net fixed assets continued to fall, from 0.70 to 0.68; and the median ratio of long-term debt to total assets also continued to fall, from 0.33 to 0.32.

At the same time, the median cash flow to total debt ratio for all U.S. hospitals remained relatively stable at 0.25. This is in part due to the fact that along with funding recent increases in capital through the refinancing of old debt, hospitals are also spending a significant portion of their cash profits on infrastructure development. Hospitals are investing money they once spent on "bricks and mortar" projects in areas that bring better returns in terms of profits, savings, and clinical outcomes (i.e., information systems, integration strategies, joint ventures, physician practices, managed care, new programs and services, and outcome management programs, etc.) As a result of reduced spending on "bricks and mortar" capital projects, capital costs as a percentage of total operating expenses at the typical U.S. hospital continued to decline favorably in 1994, falling to 7.41 percent from 7.45 percent in 1993. AT the same time, the median amount of capital costs per adjusted discharge for all U.S. hospitals increased only 0.6 percent in 1994, rising to $346 from $344 in 1993. This compared with an average annual increase for all U.S. hospitals of 5.3 percent a year between 1990 and 1993.

Average Liquidity Level of Typical U.S. Hospital Continues to Rise

Measures of liquidity based on cash and cash equivalents continued to improve for the nation's hospitals in 1994. To illustrate, the median number of days cash on hand for all U.S. hospitals increased 10.7 percent in 1994, to 49.5 days from 44.7 days in 1993. (It is interesting to note, however, that despite the improvement, levels of cash maintained by the typical U.S. hospital are still relatively low, reflective of the fact that hospitals are spending a significant portion of their cash profits on infrastructure development. IF this were not the case, we would expect to see the typical U.S. hospital maintain a level of cash similar to that of an investment grade hospital. In 1994, hospitals with Standard & Poor's bond ratings of BBB or better maintained median figures for days cash on hand of at least 87.1 days.) Along with days cash on hand, the median current ratio for all U.S. hospitals also continued to rise favorably, from 2.64 in 1993 to 2.73 in 1994, as did the median acid test ratio, which increased from 0.78 in 1993 to 0.89 in 1994. At the same time, the median number of days in net accounts receivable for all U.S. hospitals remained relatively stable at 69.0 days in 1994, after falling for three consecutive years from a high of 77.4 days in 1990. This long-term reduction in the median number of days in net accounts receivable, a trend that is expected to continue as hospitals become more efficient through the use of electronic building and automated collection follow-up systems, contributed significantly to improved hospital liquidity. Such favorable trends in liquidity, which appear to be driven by the hospital industry's improved profitability are likely to continue as hospitals continue to build up cash reserves out of fear that future reform will result in increased pressure on prices and cost control measures.

Hospital Profitability Continues to Show Signs of Improvement

All measures of hospital profitability continued to show slight signs of improvement in 1994. The median total profit margin for all U.S. hospitals reached 4.52 percent in 1994, up from 4.25 percent in 1993. The median operating profit margin for all U.S. hospitals, showing greater improvement, increased from 30.6 percent in 1993 to 3.45 percent in 1994. Overall improvements in hospital profitability were primarily the result of hospitals' ability to hold down expenses. Pressured by cost shifting, competition, constrained reimbursement, and reform initiatives, hospitals continued to work to trim inefficiencies from their operations. As a result, the median operating expense per adjusted discharge for all U.S. hospitals, which had been increasing at an average rate of 6.2 percent a year between 1990 and 1993, increased only 1.8 percent in 1994, as compared with an increase in the median operating revenue per adjusted discharge of more than 2.4 percent. As a result of improved profitability, median return on assets and cash flow per bed figures also showed significant signs of improvement for the industry in 1994. The median value for return on assets for all U.S. hospitals increased from 4.4 percent in 1993 to 4.5 percent in 1994, and the median value for cash flow per bed rose from $24,013 to $26,307. Furthermore, the median debt service coverage ratio for all U.S. hospitals increased 5.8 percent to 3.67 times in 1994, mainly as a result of increased growth in industry earnings.

It is interesting to note that while the overall financial condition of hospitals continued to improve across the board in 1994, hospitals in the Western, Central, and Southern regions remained significantly more profitable than their counterpart hospitals in the Northeast. To illustrate, hospitals in New England and the Middle Atlantic region displayed median total profit margins of 2.78 and 2.22 percent, respectively, in 1994. In comparison, median total profit margins for hospitals in the South Atlantic, East North Central, East South Central, West North Central, West South Central, Mountain, and Pacific regions were each above 4.14 percent. Profitability was highest in the Mountain region, where hospitals displayed a median total profit margin of 7.02 percent. The favorable performance of hospitals in the West may be due to a higher penetration of managed care than exists in other regions of the country. Conversely, poorer performance among hospitals in the Northeast could be the result of a higher level of regulation imposing an artificially low cap on profitability.

Deductions from Gross Patient Revenue as a Percentage of Gross Patient Revenue Continue to Increase

Continuing a trend that has lasted more than eight years, deductions from gross patient revenue as a percentage of gross patient revenue increased to 35.7 percent in 1994, from 34.6 percent in 1993. Steady increases in deductions are mainly the result of reduced government subsidies and increasing payer differentials, growth in the size of Medicaid shortfalls to hospitals, and the greater prevalence of HMOs, PPOs, and other managed care organizations, which negotiate discounts from charges. Such continued growth in hospital uncompensated care costs is an unfavorable trend for the industry overall, and could work to reduce hospital profit margins over the next few years.

Hospital Staffing Levels and Proportion of Expenses for Salary and Benefits Begin to Decline

The median number of full-time equivalent personnel (FTEs) per 100 adjusted discharges fell for the second consecutive year in 1994, declining 2.8 percent to 6.29 employees from 6.47 employees in 1993 and 6.48 employees in 1992. In comparison, between 1990 and 1992 the median number of FTEs per 100 adjusted discharges increased at an average annual rate of almost 0.8 percent a year. After adjusting for differences in case mix complexity, the median number of FTEs per 100 adjusted discharges also declined, for the fourth year in a row, from 5.17 employees in 1993 to 5.03 employees in 1994. This continued reduction in hospital staffing levels is a trend that will likely continue over the next few years, as hospitals continue to re-engineer their operations (and increasingly use multi=skilled workers to perform certain non-nursing tasks)in the attempt to further reduce their salary and benefit expenses and overall operating costs, to prepare for future reform. It is interesting to note that between 1993 and 1994, the median salary and benefit expense per full-time equivalent employer for all U.S. hospitals increased a mere 4.3 percent, compared with an average annual increase of more than 6.3 percent between 1990 and 1993.

Looking ahead, it is likely that hospitals will continue to respond to changes currently taking place within the health care and adjust to reform initiatives being undertaken at state and local levels. In particular, hospitals will continue with their attempts to control utilization, reduce average lengths of stay and staffing levels, cut overhead costs, improve productivity and efficiency, and refinance debt. Hospitals will also continue to be more conservative with cash that would otherwise have been spent on new renovations, building projects, and major medical equipment purchases, and will instead continue to re-invest much of this money into consolidation efforts with other hospitals; the development of physician practice settings; managed care infrastructures; ambulatory, outpatient, and other alternative care delivery sites; and eventually the development of integrated delivery networks. Hospitals will also work to improve community services, improve information systems, develop better outcomes measurement programs, and redesign their organizations in order to meet the health care marketplace demands of the future.

HOSPITAL PERFORMANCE OVERVIEW
HPO

Summary

Community Hospital is an efficiently operated and profitable facility. Recent utilization declines will continue to test management's ability to reduce staffing levels while serving a complex mix of patients. On a case-mix adjusted basis, the hospital's staffing levels and costs are below those of similarly situated facilities, and most importantly, well below those of its direct competitor.

Necessary to the hospital's viability is a deceleration of its declines in utilization. With some slowing, Community Hospital should be able to continue to enjoy its market-leading position as a provider of sophisticated medical care.

Market Position

Community Hospital is a 321-bed not-for-profit teaching hospital located in Anytown, New York. Community Hospital, a member of Health System, is one of two major facilities in the eight-hospital Anytown market. Community Hospital and its competitor, County Medical Center, together control more than 75 percent of the market's admissions. With a 41-percent share of the area's admissions, Community Hospital leads its market.

Utilization & Efficiency

As a result of 6.6-percent annualized admissions declines, Community Hospital was forced to close 21 percent of its beds in 1991. The subsequent drop in the hospital's census has caused its per-unit staffing levels to increase abruptly. Community Hospital treats a complex mix of cases. The hospital's Medicare case mix index was 1.7845 in 1991, which ranked in the 96th percentile of all hospitals in the U.S. Despite such a complicated case load, the hospital has an exceptionally short Medicare length of stay. Specifically, its 8.0-day average Medicare stay was 6.0 percent shorter than the typical New York hospital that had 300 to 500 beds, while its Medicare case mix index was 24 percent *higher* than the median of the comparison group. Stated differently, Community Hospital treats a much sicker mix of patients with fewer resources than most New York hospitals in its bed-size range.

The hospital's efficiency is demonstrated by its per-unit cost structure. Case-mix adjusted expenses per unit at Community were equivalent to the median value of the comparison group, and they were more than 25 percent below those at County Medical Center, its chief competitor.

Liquidity & Capital Structure

The physical plant at Community Hospital is relatively young and well-equipped. The hospital's average accounting age was 7.0 years, compared with 7.7 years for the New York comparison group, and Community Hospital had $213,000 in net plant, property and equipment per bed, above the 90th percentile for all U.S. hospitals and more than 80 percent above the median value for the comparison group. Such a sound physical plant should not generate significant demands for new capital in the near future.

The hospital's ratio of long-term debt to capitalization was 57 percent in 1991, compared with 47 percent for other New York hospitals with 300 to 500 beds, indicating the facility's reliance on debt capital for its construction and renovation.

Community Hospital has done an excellent job of collecting accounts receivable. The hospital's days of revenue in accounts receivable have been reduced from 75 days in 1989 to 21 days in 1991. However, with an

Health Care Investment Analysts, Inc. • Baltimore, Maryland • (301) 576-9600

average payment period of 93 days, the hospital is somewhat slow to pay its current liabilities. Furthermore, liquidity may be a serious problem for the hospital, in that its cash on hand fell from 71 days to nine days in 1991, compared with a median value of 83 days for the comparison group in 1991.

Cash Flow & Profitability

Profitability at Community Hospital has risen steadily over the past three years, and in 1991 its total profit margin reached 4.3 percent, compared with 5.5 percent for other New York hospitals in its bed range. Furthermore, cash flow (the sum of net income, depreciation, and interest) at Community Hospital has been consistent during the past several years.

SINGLE HOSPITAL PROFILE

Community Hospital
One Main Street
Anytown, New York 11112

Facility Type:	Acute Care	S&P Rating:	None
Teaching:	Yes	System:	Health System
Ownership:	Not-for-Profit	Distressed:	No

	1991	1990	1989
Beds in Service, Acute Care	321	408	386
Admissions, Total Acute Care	15,233	16,208	17,468
Occupancy Rate, Acute Care (%)	77.56	65.05	74.03
Avg Length of Stay, Medicare	8.00	9.04	11.08
FTEs per 100 Admissions	9.87	8.45	9.61
Expense per Adjusted Admission	6,909	5,847	6,112
Medicare Case Mix Index	1.7845	1.7619	1.7342
Special Care Days (%)	11.37	10.51	9.53
Medicare Days, Acute (%)	51.11	49.34	52.74
Medicaid Days, Acute (%)	9.97	8.14	9.07
Average Age of Plant	7.07	7.57	7.02
Capital Cost Ratio	15.23	9.40	7.51
Net Plt, Prop & Equip per Bed	213,290	159,771	149,978
Debt per Bed	267,788	205,145	208,290
LT Debt to Capitalization	0.57	0.55	0.58
Days in Accts Receivable, Net	21.21	58.60	74.68
Average Payment Period	93.45	69.09	55.47
Days Cash on Hand	8.94	70.85	43.43
Net Avail for Dbt Svc (EBITDA)	14,972,140	17,126,929	12,694,115
Debt Service Coverage Ratio	11.46	2.12	0.86
Cash Flow to Total Debt Ratio	0.14	0.18	0.13
Operating Profit Margin (%)	2.60	1.71	(0.97)
Total Profit Margin (%)	4.31	3.63	0.47
Markup, Tot Ancillary Services	1.78	1.71	1.67

HOSPITAL GROUP MEDIAN PROFILE

New York Hospitals, 300 to 500 Beds

	1991	1990	1989
Beds in Service, Acute Care	369	415	404
Admissions, Total Acute Care	16,064	16,368	17,582
Occupancy Rate, Acute Care (%)	73.70	70.27	68.43
Avg Length of Stay, Medicare	8.51	8.76	8.87
FTEs per 100 Admissions	8.04	8.22	8.35
Expense per Adjusted Admission	5,460	5,080	4,608
Medicare Case Mix Index	1.4388	1.4217	1.3457
Special Care Days (%)	11.08	9.75	9.17
Medicare Days, Acute (%)	48.50	47.66	47.11
Medicaid Days, Acute (%)	9.06	8.24	8.55
Average Age of Plant	7.72	7.57	7.31
Capital Cost Ratio	6.88	6.96	7.26
Net Plt, Prop & Equip per Bed	117,110	107,363	103,872
Debt per Bed	151,332	122,471	145,266
LT Debt to Capitalization	0.47	0.41	0.51
Days in Accts Receivable, Net	61.81	58.60	62.98
Average Payment Period	65.71	62.92	63.22
Days Cash on Hand	82.63	70.85	84.09
Net Avail for Dbt Svc (EBITDA)	15,496,513	15,847,454	12,658,695
Debt Service Coverage Ratio	3.14	2.12	2.30
Cash Flow to Total Debt Ratio	0.25	0.31	0.26
Operating Profit Margin (%)	3.81	5.39	3.17
Total Profit Margin (%)	5.50	6.75	4.62
Markup, Tot Ancillary Services	1.77	1.75	1.69

n=41

Health Care Investment Analysts, Inc. • Baltimore, Maryland • (301) 576-9600

PATIENT ORIGIN & DESTINATION REPORTS

PO&D

PO&D Reports

The Patient Origin & Destination Reports provide a comprehensive picture of patient trends for your hospital and other hospitals in your market area. The Reports give you a detailed profile of where your patients, and your competitors' patients, are located by zip code area.

Information on patient discharges, patient days, average length of stay, average charges per case and total revenues for each hospital or zip code area is in the Reports for your use. This valuable information will help you in the following management areas:

Strategic Planning

The Reports' market-level information identifies patient migration and hospital-use trends for each hospital in your market area.

Marketing

Vital information in the Reports help you identify sources of patients and target your marketing and promotional efforts to neighborhoods where they are the most effective. Also, use the Reports to enhance annual reports, budgets and presentations.

Physician Relations

The Reports pinpoint neighborhoods for you to expand your relationships with practicing physicians and boost referrals. Also, use the Reports to locate out-of-state referral centers to establish transfer relationships or affiliations.

Finance

With the Reports you can compare key financial indicators for each provider in your market area, in addition to the hospital-level data comparisons of financial and operating performance also available from HCIA.

Program and Facilities Planning

The Reports can help you position your hospital's satellite clinics, home care service, mobile services and outreach programs more effectively.

The Reports are prepared from a database of 44 million Medicare discharge records and from the cost reports of each facility. *This is the only comprehensive, nationwide database of patient discharge and cost information.*

Information on your competition is immediately available in HCIA's Patient Origin & Destination Reports. Contact HCIA at 410-576-9600 for more information or to order your Reports.

See reverse side for sample reports

HCIA • Baltimore, Maryland • (410) 576-9600

PO&D SAMPLE REPORTS

■ ■ ■

The Reports provide detailed information on markets, hospitals and patients. Simply select any market, any hospital or any zip code, county or state combination for a comprehensive picture of patient trends.

Admissions

Summary of Admissions by zip code
Different zip codes within market   *Market: Amarillo & Vicinity*

Hospital Name	No. of Beds	79101	79102	79103	79104	79105	79106	79107	79108	79109	79110
High Plains Baptist Hospital	302										
Total Admissions		51	152	63	36	19	481	256	70	560	186
% of Total		1.3	3.9	1.6	0.9	0.5	12.4	6.6	1.8	14.4	4.8
Northwest Texas Hospital	350										
Total Admissions		58	133	82	68	27	424	364	48	355	119
% of Total		2.2	5.2	3.2	2.6	1.0	16.4	14.1	1.9	13.8	4.6
St. Anthony's Hospital	310										
Total Admissions		63	130	78	41	38	324	252	71	373	104
% of Total		1.6	3.3	2.0	1.0	1.0	8.2	6.4	1.8	9.5	2.6
Market Total:											
Total Admissions		172	415	223	145	84	1,229	872	189	1,286	409
% of Total		1.7	4.0	2.1	1.4	0.8	11.8	8.4	1.8	12.4	3.9

Hospital Performance

Summary of Admissions by zip code
Different zip codes within market   *Market: Amarillo & Vicinity*

Zip Code	Hospital Name	Total Admission	Total Inpatient Days	Avg. Length of Stay	Total Inpatient Charges	Avg. Daily Charges	Avg. Total Charges
79101	High Plains Baptist Hospital	51	495	9.7	$ 305,412	617.0	$5,988
	Northwest Texas Hospital	58	515	8.9	402,308	781.2	6,936
	St. Anthony's Hospital	63	418	6.6	366,972	877.9	5,825
79102	High Plains Baptist Hospital	152	1,543	10.2	1,085,745	703.7	7,143
	Northwest Texas Hospital	133	1,058	8.0	743,708	702.9	5,592
	St. Anthony's Hospital	130	884	6.8	872,481	987.0	6,711

Provider Analysis

Zip Code 79101 Provider Analysis   *Market: Amarillo & Vicinity*

Provider	Total Admission	Total Charges	Average Length of Stay	Average Charges
St. Anthony's Hospital	63	$366,972	6.6	$5,825
Northwest Texas Hospital	58	402,308	8.9	6,936
High Plains Baptist Hospital	51	305,412	9.7	5,988
Family Hospital Center	6	36,500	5.7	6,083
Coronado Hospital	2	4,872	5.0	2,436
St. Rose Dominican Hospital	2	12,445	4.5	6,222

≡HCIA • Baltimore, Maryland • (410) 576-9600

NURSING HOME
DATA BASE

NURSING HOME PROFILE
Golden Age Nursing Home
342 Maple Street
Hollywood, Florida 12345

Certification: Medicare and Medicaid
Ownership: Proprietary
System: Nursing Corp. of America

	1990	1989	1988
Beds	67	67	67
Occupancy Rate (%)	90.92	93.16	92.83
Medicaid Resident Days (%)	44.73	40.09	33.75
FTEs per Average Daily Census	0.80	0.82	0.80
Salaries & Benefits per FTE	15,285	14,576	14,192
Net Revenue per Resident Day	74.46	67.77	65.39
Cost per Resident Day, Total	72.16	62.79	62.15
Direct Patient Care Cost per Resident Day	26.11	22.41	19.63
Indirect Patient Care Cost per Resident Day	12.36	11.58	11.07
Cost per Resident Day, Administrative	20.00	18.82	17.22
Cost per Resident Day, Depreciation & Interest	8.44	7.63	7.74
Total Profit Margin (%)	4.38	8.82	6.50
Days in Accounts Receivable	79.27	64.56	58.11
Days in Accounts Payable	18.59	16.95	11.55
Current Ratio	2.58	2.43	2.93
Average Age of Plant (years)	4.55	4.12	3.79
Long-Term Debt to Total Assets	0.35	0.42	0.48
Debt Service Coverage Ratio	2.45	3.15	2.51

Select any 15 elements from the data element listing (see reverse side).
Additionally, nursing home group medians or averages are available by:
State
Ownership Type
Census Division
Bed Size Category

HCIA • Baltimore, Maryland • (410) 576-9600

CAPACITY & UTILIZATION

- ❑ Avg Beds, ICF
- ❑ Avg Beds, SNF Non-Participating
- ❑ Avg Beds, SNF Participating
- ❑ Average Daily Census
- ❑ Average Length of Stay, Medicaid
- ❑ Average Length of Stay, Medicare
- ❑ Average Length of Stay, Total
- ❑ Beds, Participating
- ❑ Beds, Total Facility
- ❑ Dischgs, Medicaid Total Facility
- ❑ Dischgs, Medicare Total Facility
- ❑ Dischgs, Other Total Facility
- ❑ Dischgs, Total Facility
- ❑ FTEs per Avg Daily Census
- ❑ Full-Time Equivalent Personnel(FTEs)
- ❑ Occupancy Rate
- ❑ Percent Medicaid Discharges
- ❑ Percent Medicaid Resident Days
- ❑ Percent Medicare Discharges
- ❑ Percent Medicare Resident Days
- ❑ Percent Other Discharges
- ❑ Resident Days, ICF
- ❑ Resident Days, Medicaid ICF
- ❑ Resident Days, Medicaid SNF Participating
- ❑ Resident Days, Medicaid Total
- ❑ Resident Days, Medicare SNF Participating
- ❑ Resident Days, Medicare Total
- ❑ Resident Days, SNF Non-Participating
- ❑ Resident Days, SNF Participating
- ❑ Resident Days, Other, SNF Non-Participating
- ❑ Resident Days, Other, SNF Participating
- ❑ Resident Days, Other, Total Facility
- ❑ Resident Days, Total Facility

REVENUES, EXPENSES & PROFITABILITY

- ❑ Admin & General Exp, Res Day
- ❑ Costs, Admin & General
- ❑ Costs, Cafeteria
- ❑ Costs, Central Svcs & Supply
- ❑ Costs, Dietary
- ❑ Costs, Employee Benefits
- ❑ Costs, Housekeeping
- ❑ Costs, Lndry & Linen
- ❑ Costs, Maintenance & Repairs
- ❑ Costs, Medical Records
- ❑ Costs, Nursing Administration
- ❑ Costs, Other General Services
- ❑ Costs, Pharmacy
- ❑ Costs, Plant Operations
- ❑ Costs, Social Services
- ❑ Costs per Day, Admin & Gen
- ❑ Costs per Day, Cafeteria
- ❑ Costs per Day, Cntrl Svcs & Supp
- ❑ Costs per Day, Dietary
- ❑ Costs per Day, Employee Bens
- ❑ Costs per Day, Housekeeping
- ❑ Costs per Day, Lndry & Linen
- ❑ Costs per Day, Maint & Repairs
- ❑ Costs per Day, Med Records
- ❑ Costs per Day, Nursing Admin
- ❑ Costs per Day, Other Gen Svcs
- ❑ Costs per Day, Pharmacy
- ❑ Costs per Day, Plant Operations
- ❑ Costs per Day, Social Services
- ❑ Costs per Day, Total
- ❑ Depreciation & Interest Expense, Res Day
- ❑ Direct Care Expense, Res Day
- ❑ Indirect Care Expense, Res Day
- ❑ Gross Patient Revenue
- ❑ Net Income
- ❑ Net Income per Resident Day
- ❑ Net Patient Revenue
- ❑ Net Patient Rev per Res Day
- ❑ Operating Expenses, Total
- ❑ Operating Profit Margin
- ❑ Return on Assets
- ❑ Return on Equity
- ❑ Salaries & Benefits per FTE
- ❑ Salaries, Admin & General
- ❑ Salaries, Cafeteria
- ❑ Salaries, Cntrl Svcs & Supply
- ❑ Salaries, Dietary
- ❑ Salaries, Employee Benefits
- ❑ Salaries, Housekeeping
- ❑ Salaries, Lndry & Linen
- ❑ Salaries, Maint & Repairs
- ❑ Salaries, Medical Records
- ❑ Salaries, Nursing Admin
- ❑ Salaries, Other Gen Services
- ❑ Salaries, Pharmacy
- ❑ Salaries, Plant Operations
- ❑ Salaries, Social Services
- ❑ Salaries, Total
- ❑ Salaries per Day, Admin & Gen
- ❑ Salaries per Day, Cafeteria
- ❑ Salaries per Day, Cntrl Svcs & Supp
- ❑ Salaries per Day, Dietary
- ❑ Salaries per Day, Employee Benefits
- ❑ Salaries per Day, Housekeeping
- ❑ Salaries per Day, Lndry & Linen
- ❑ Salaries per Day, Maint & Repairs
- ❑ Salaries per Day, Medical Records
- ❑ Salaries per Day, Nursing Admin
- ❑ Salaries per Day, Other Gen Svcs
- ❑ Salaries per Day, Pharmacy
- ❑ Salaries per Day, Plant Operations
- ❑ Salaries per Day, Social Services
- ❑ Salaries per Day, Total
- ❑ Total Profit Margin
- ❑ Uncollectible Ratio

LIQUIDITY & CAPITAL STRUCTURE

- ❑ Accounting Age, All Assets
- ❑ Accounts Payable
- ❑ Accounts Receivable
- ❑ Accumulated Depreciation
- ❑ Allowances from Receivables
- ❑ Balance of Depreciation Fund
- ❑ Capital Cost Ratio
- ❑ Capital Costs, Bldgs & Fixtures
- ❑ Capital Costs, Movable Equipment
- ❑ Cash
- ❑ Cash & Cash Equivalents
- ❑ Current Assets
- ❑ Current Liabilities
- ❑ Current Ratio
- ❑ Days Cash on Hand
- ❑ Days in Accounts Payable
- ❑ Days in Accounts Receivable
- ❑ Debt Service Coverage Ratio
- ❑ Fund Balance or Equity
- ❑ Interest Expense
- ❑ Long-Term Debt to Equity
- ❑ Long-Term Debt to Total Assets
- ❑ Net Plant, Property & Equipment per Bed
- ❑ Notes & Loans Payable, Short-Term
- ❑ Notes Receivable
- ❑ Temporary Investments
- ❑ Total Assets
- ❑ Total Liabilities
- ❑ Total Long-Term Liabilities
- ❑ Total Plant, Property & Equipment

HCIA • Baltimore, Maryland • (410) 576-9600

HOSPITAL ■ ■ ■ ■ ■ ■ ■
DATA BASE

HOSPITAL PROFILE
Community Hospital
Main Street
Anytown, Maryland 21112

Facility Type:	Acute Care		System Affiliation:	Health System, Inc.
Teaching:	Yes		S&P Rating History:	None
Ownership:	Not-for-Profit		HCIA Distressed List:	No

	1991	1990	1989
Beds in Service, Acute Care	296	296	274
Occupancy Rate, Acute Care (%)	73.88	72.21	74.59
Average Length of Stay, Acute Care	5.62	5.89	6.52
Average Length of Stay, Medicare	8.83	8.60	8.79
Medicare Admissions (%)	33.69	35.31	38.07
FTEs per Adjusted Average Daily Census	4.24	4.44	4.26
Current Ratio	1.94	1.52	1.60
Days in Accounts Receivable, Net	55.79	51.20	55.85
Days Cash on Hand	23.06	8.67	28.09
Average Payment Period	61.94	67.84	64.89
Long-Term Debt to Equity	0.76	0.95	1.33
Net Plant, Property & Equipment per Bed	95,324	91,099	106,421
Debt Service Coverage Ratio	3.73	2.70	2.01
Operating Profit Margin (%)	5.42	3.30	5.55
Total Profit Margin (%)	6.22	4.00	6.45

Select any 15 elements from the data element listing (see reverse side).
Additionally, hospital group medians or averages are available by:
State
Ownership Type
Census Division
Bed Size Category
Bond Rating
Custom Groups

Health Care Investment Analysts, Inc. • Baltimore, Maryland • (410) 576-9600

UTILIZATION & PAYOR MIX

- ❑ Adj Admissions, Total Facility
- ❑ Adjusted Admissions, Acute
- ❑ Adjusted Days, Acute
- ❑ Adjusted Days, Total Facility
- ❑ Admissions, ICF
- ❑ Admissions, Other LTC
- ❑ Admissions, SNF
- ❑ Admissions, Subprovider I
- ❑ Admissions, Subprovider II
- ❑ Admissions, Total Acute Care
- ❑ Admissions, Total Facility
- ❑ Average Daily Census, ICF
- ❑ Average Daily Census, OLTC
- ❑ Average Daily Census, SNF
- ❑ Average Daily Census, Sub I
- ❑ Average Daily Census, Sub II
- ❑ Average Daily Census, Tot Fac
- ❑ Average Length of Stay, ICF
- ❑ Average Length of Stay, OLTC
- ❑ Average Length of Stay, SNF
- ❑ Average Length of Stay, Sub I
- ❑ Average Length of Stay, Sub II
- ❑ Avg Daily Census, Acute Care
- ❑ Avg Length of Stay, Acute Care
- ❑ Avg Length of Stay, Medicaid
- ❑ Avg Length of Stay, Medicare
- ❑ Avg Length of Stay, Tot Fac
- ❑ Beds in Service, Acute Care
- ❑ Beds in Service, CCU
- ❑ Beds in Service, Gen Service
- ❑ Beds in Service, ICF
- ❑ Beds in Service, ICU
- ❑ Beds in Service, Nursery
- ❑ Beds in Service, Other Acute
- ❑ Beds in Service, Other LTC
- ❑ Beds in Service, SNF
- ❑ Beds in Service, Subprovider I
- ❑ Beds in Service, Subprovider II
- ❑ Beds in Service, Tot Facility

- ❑ Case-mix Adj ALOS, Acute
- ❑ CCU Days (%)
- ❑ Days, Medicaid CCU
- ❑ Days, Medicaid Gen Service
- ❑ Days, Medicaid ICU
- ❑ Days, Medicaid Other Acute
- ❑ Days, Medicare CCU
- ❑ Days, Medicare Gen Service
- ❑ Days, Medicare ICU
- ❑ Days, Medicare Other Acute
- ❑ FTE Interns & Residents
- ❑ FTE Personnel, Hospital
- ❑ Government Admiss, Acute
- ❑ Government Admiss, Acute (%)
- ❑ Government Days, Acute
- ❑ ICU Days (%)
- ❑ Inpat Days, Medicaid Nursery
- ❑ Inpat Days, Medicare Nursery
- ❑ Inpatient Days, Acute Care
- ❑ Inpatient Days, CCU
- ❑ Inpatient Days, Gen Service
- ❑ Inpatient Days, ICF
- ❑ Inpatient Days, ICU
- ❑ Inpatient Days, Nursery
- ❑ Inpatient Days, Other Acute
- ❑ Inpatient Days, Other LTC
- ❑ Inpatient Days, SNF
- ❑ Inpatient Days, Sub I
- ❑ Inpatient Days, Sub II
- ❑ Inpatient Days, Total Facility
- ❑ LTC Admissions (%)
- ❑ LTC Avg Length of Stay
- ❑ LTC Days (%)
- ❑ LTC Revenues (%)
- ❑ Medicaid Admiss, Sub II (%)
- ❑ Medicaid Admiss, Total Acute
- ❑ Medicaid Admiss, Total Acute (%)
- ❑ Medicaid Admissions, ICF (%)
- ❑ Medicaid Admissions, OLTC (%)

- ❑ Medicaid Admissions, SNF (%)
- ❑ Medicaid Admissions, Sub I (%)
- ❑ Medicaid Days, ICF (%)
- ❑ Medicaid Days, OLTC (%)
- ❑ Medicaid Days, Sub I (%)
- ❑ Medicaid Days, Sub II (%)
- ❑ Medicaid Days, Total Acute
- ❑ Medicaid Days, Total Acute (%)
- ❑ Medicare Admiss, Sub II (%)
- ❑ Medicare Admiss, Total Acute
- ❑ Medicare Admiss, Total Acute (%)
- ❑ Medicare Admissions, ICF (%)
- ❑ Medicare Admissions, OLTC (%)
- ❑ Medicare Admissions, SNF (%)
- ❑ Medicare Admissions, Sub I (%)
- ❑ Medicare Days, ICF (%)
- ❑ Medicare Days, OLTC (%)
- ❑ Medicare Days, SNF (%)
- ❑ Medicare Days, SNF (%)
- ❑ Medicare Days, Sub I (%)
- ❑ Medicare Days, Sub II (%)
- ❑ Medicare Days, Total Acute
- ❑ Medicare Days, Total Acute (%)
- ❑ Non-acute Admissions (%)
- ❑ Non-acute Avg Length of Stay
- ❑ Non-acute Beds
- ❑ Non-acute Days (%)
- ❑ Non-Gov Admiss, Acute (%)
- ❑ Non-Government Admiss, Acute
- ❑ Non-Medicare Avg Lgth of Stay
- ❑ Nursery Days (%)
- ❑ Occupancy Rate, Acute Care (%)
- ❑ Occupancy Rate, ICF (%)
- ❑ Occupancy Rate, OLTC (%)
- ❑ Occupancy Rate, SNF (%)
- ❑ Occupancy Rate, Sub I (%)
- ❑ Occupancy Rate, Sub II (%)
- ❑ Occupancy Rate, Total Facility
- ❑ Special Care Days (%)

PRODUCTIVITY, EFFICIENCY & PRICING

- ❑ Adjustment Factor
- ❑ Adjustment Factor, Tot Fac
- ❑ Admissions per Bed, Acute Care
- ❑ Admissions per Bed, Tot Fac
- ❑ Anesthesiology, Charge
- ❑ Anesthesiology, Cost
- ❑ Blood Storage, Charge
- ❑ Blood Storage, Cost
- ❑ EEG, Charge
- ❑ EEG, Charge
- ❑ EEG, Cost
- ❑ EKG, Cost
- ❑ FTEs per 100 Admiss, Cmix Adj
- ❑ FTEs per 100 Admissions
- ❑ FTEs per Adj Avg Daily Census
- ❑ FTEs Per Avg Daily Cen, ICF
- ❑ FTEs Per Avg Daily Cen, OLTC
- ❑ FTEs Per Avg Daily Cen, SNF
- ❑ FTEs Per Avg Daily Cen, Sub I
- ❑ FTEs Per Avg Daily Cen, Sub II
- ❑ I-V Therapy, Charge
- ❑ I-V Therapy, Cost
- ❑ Labor & Delivery Room, Charge
- ❑ Labor & Delivery Room, Cost
- ❑ Laboratory, Charge
- ❑ Laboratory, Cost

- ❑ Markup, Anesthesiology
- ❑ Markup, Diagnostic Radiology
- ❑ Markup, I-V Therapy
- ❑ Markup, Labor & Delivery
- ❑ Markup, Laboratory
- ❑ Markup, Med Supplies Sold
- ❑ Markup, Operating Room
- ❑ Markup, Outpatient
- ❑ Markup, Oxygen Therapy
- ❑ Markup, Pharmacy
- ❑ Markup, Physical Therapy
- ❑ Markup, Tot Ancillary Services
- ❑ Medical Supplies Sold, Charge
- ❑ Medical Supplies Sold, Cost
- ❑ Medicare Case Mix Index
- ❑ Occupational Therapy, Charge
- ❑ Occupational Therapy, Cost
- ❑ Operating Room, Chg
- ❑ Operating Room, Cost
- ❑ Outpatient Clinic, Charge
- ❑ Outpatient Clinic, Cost
- ❑ Outpatient Emergency, Charge
- ❑ Outpatient Emergency, Cost
- ❑ Overhead Expense (w/ Capital)
- ❑ Overhead/Op Exp (w/Capital)
- ❑ Oxy Inhalation Therapy, Charge

- ❑ Oxy Inhalation Therapy, Cost
- ❑ Pat Care Square Feet per Bed
- ❑ Pct Patient Care Square Feet
- ❑ Pharmacy, Charge
- ❑ Pharmacy, Cost
- ❑ Physical Therapy, Charge
- ❑ Physical Therapy, Cost
- ❑ Radioisotope, Charge
- ❑ Radioisotope, Cost
- ❑ Radiology Diagnostic, Charge
- ❑ Radiology Diagnostic, Cost
- ❑ Radiology Therapy, Charge
- ❑ Radiology Therapy, Cost
- ❑ Recovery Room, Charge
- ❑ Recovery Room, Cost
- ❑ Renal Dialysis, Charge
- ❑ Renal Dialysis, Cost
- ❑ Salary & Benefits Per FTE
- ❑ Speech Pathology, Charge
- ❑ Speech Pathology, Cost
- ❑ Total Ancillary Svcs, Charge
- ❑ Total Ancillary Svcs, Cost
- ❑ Whole Blood, Charge
- ❑ Whole Blood, Cost

LIQUIDITY & CAPITAL STRUCTURE

- ❑ Accounts Payable
- ❑ Accounts Receivable, Gross
- ❑ Accounts Receivable, Net
- ❑ Accts Rec Collection Ratio
- ❑ Accumulated Depreciation
- ❑ Acid Test Ratio
- ❑ Allowances From Receivables

- ❑ Annual Debt Service
- ❑ Average Age of Plant
- ❑ Average Payment Period
- ❑ Buildings & Fixtures
- ❑ Buildings & Fixtures Accum Dep
- ❑ Capital Cost Ratio
- ❑ Capital Costs, Bldg & Fixtures

- ❑ Capital Costs, Maj Mov Equip
- ❑ Capital Costs, Total
- ❑ Capital Costs per Adj Admiss
- ❑ Capital Csts per Admiss, Bldgs
- ❑ Capital Csts per Admiss, Equip
- ❑ Cash
- ❑ Cash & Cash Equivalents

LIQUIDITY & CAPITAL STRUCTURE (cont.)

- ❏ Current Assets
- ❏ Current Liabilities
- ❏ Current Portion of LT Debt
- ❏ Current Ratio
- ❏ Cushion Ratio
- ❏ Days Cash on Hand
- ❏ Days in Accts Receiv, Gross
- ❏ Days in Accts Receivable, Net
- ❏ Dbt Svc as a Pct of Net Rev
- ❏ Debt per Bed
- ❏ Debt Service Coverage Ratio
- ❏ Depreciation Fund Balance
- ❏ Equity Financing Ratio
- ❏ Fixed Asset Turnover Ratio
- ❏ Index of Predictive Credit
- ❏ Interest Exp to Lt Debt Ratio

- ❏ Liabilities, Total
- ❏ Long-Term Debt to Equity
- ❏ Long-Term Debt to Net PP&E
- ❏ Long-Term Debt to Total Assets
- ❏ Long-term Liabilities
- ❏ LT Debt to Capitalization
- ❏ Net Capital Acquisitions
- ❏ Net Plant, Property & Equip
- ❏ Net Plt, Prop & Equip per Bed
- ❏ Notes Payable, Current
- ❏ Notes Receivable
- ❏ Other Receivables, Gross
- ❏ Patient Accts Receivable, Gross
- ❏ Payroll Taxes Payable
- ❏ Plant Square Feet, Gen Svc
- ❏ Plant Square Feet, Nonreimb

- ❏ Plant Square Feet, Total
- ❏ Quick Ratio
- ❏ Return on Assets (%)
- ❏ Return on Equity (%)
- ❏ Salaries, Wages & Fees Payable
- ❏ Temporary Investments
- ❏ Times Interest Earned Ratio
- ❏ Total Asset Turnover Ratio
- ❏ Total Assets
- ❏ Total Assets, Begin Balance
- ❏ Total Capital Acquisitions
- ❏ Total Capital Disposals
- ❏ Total Fund Balance or Equity
- ❏ Total Plant, Prop & Equip

REVENUES, EXPENSES & PROFITABILITY

- ❏ Admin & Gen Exp, Direct Cost
- ❏ Administrative Expense (%)
- ❏ Ancillary Revenue
- ❏ Ancillary Revenue (%)
- ❏ Anesthesiology Revenue (%)
- ❏ Approved Intern & Resident Exp
- ❏ Blood Storage Revenue (%)
- ❏ Cafeteria, Direct Cost
- ❏ Cafeteria Expense (%)
- ❏ Cash Flow Margin (%)
- ❏ Cash Flow per Bed
- ❏ Cash Flow to Total Debt Ratio
- ❏ Central Svc & Sup, Direct Cost
- ❏ Central Svc & Supp Expense (%)
- ❏ Cmix Adj Exp per Adj Day
- ❏ Cmix Adj Gross Rev per Adj Day
- ❏ Cmix Adj Net Rev per Adj Day
- ❏ Cmix Wage Adj Exp per Adj Adm
- ❏ Cmix Wage Gr Rev per Adj Adm
- ❏ Cmix Wage Net Rev per Adj Adm
- ❏ Depreciation & Amortization
- ❏ Dietary, Direct Cost
- ❏ Dietary Expense (%)
- ❏ DRG Amount, Excluding Outlier
- ❏ DRG Amount, Outlier Payments
- ❏ Employee Benefits Expense
- ❏ Exp per Adj Admiss, Cmix Adj
- ❏ Expense per Adj Patient Day
- ❏ Expense per Adjusted Admission
- ❏ Expense per Admission, ICF
- ❏ Expense per Admission, OLTC
- ❏ Expense per Admission, SNF
- ❏ Expense per Admission, Sub I
- ❏ Expense per Admission, Sub II
- ❏ Expense per Pat Day, ICF
- ❏ Expense per Pat Day, OLTC
- ❏ Expense per Pat Day, SNF
- ❏ Expense Per Pat Day, Sub I
- ❏ Expense per Pat Day, Sub II
- ❏ Gen Svc Costs, Adult/Ped
- ❏ Gen Svc Costs, ASC
- ❏ Gen Svc Costs, CCU
- ❏ Gen Svc Costs, Clinic
- ❏ Gen Svc Costs, Emergency
- ❏ Gen Svc Costs, Hospice
- ❏ Gen Svc Costs, ICF
- ❏ Gen Svc Costs, ICU
- ❏ Gen Svc Costs, LTC
- ❏ Gen Svc Costs, Nursery
- ❏ Gen Svc Costs, Other Routine
- ❏ Gen Svc Costs, SNF
- ❏ Gen Svc Costs, Sub I
- ❏ Gen Svc Costs, Sub II
- ❏ Gr Rev per Adj Adm, Cmix Adj
- ❏ Gross Inpatient Revenue
- ❏ Gross Outpatient Revenue
- ❏ Gross Pat Rev per Adj Admiss
- ❏ Gross Pat Rev per Adj Pat Day
- ❏ Gross Patient Revenue, Total
- ❏ Gross Rev per Admiss, ICF

- ❏ Gross Rev per Admiss, OLTC
- ❏ Gross Rev per Admiss, SNF
- ❏ Gross Rev per Admiss, Sub I
- ❏ Gross Rev per Admiss, Sub II
- ❏ Gross Revenue, Acute Care Svcs
- ❏ Gross Revenue, Acute Care (%)
- ❏ Gross Revenue per Day, ICF
- ❏ Gross Revenue per Day, OLTC
- ❏ Gross Revenue per Day, SNF
- ❏ Gross Revenue per Day, Sub I
- ❏ Gross Revenue per Day, Sub II
- ❏ Housekeeping, Direct Cost
- ❏ Housekeeping Expense (%)
- ❏ ICF Revenue (%)
- ❏ Indirect GME Adjustment
- ❏ Indirect GME as Pct Net Rev
- ❏ Inp Rev / Gr Rev, Tot Facility
- ❏ Inpatient Revenue (%)
- ❏ Inpatient Routine Revenue
- ❏ Interest Exp as Pct Oper Exp
- ❏ Interest Expense
- ❏ Intern & Resident Exp per Bed
- ❏ Intern & Resident Expense
- ❏ I-V Therapy Revenue (%)
- ❏ Labor & Del Room Revenue (%)
- ❏ Laboratory Revenue (%)
- ❏ Laundry & Linen, Direct Cost
- ❏ Laundry & Linen Expense (%)
- ❏ Main of Personnel Exp (%)
- ❏ Maint of Personnl, Direct Cost
- ❏ Maintain & Repair, Direct Cost
- ❏ Maintenance % Repair Exp (%)
- ❏ Malprac Prem as Pct Op Exp
- ❏ Malprac Premiums & Paid Losses
- ❏ Malpractice Loss, Total
- ❏ Medical Records, Direct Cost
- ❏ Medical Records Expense (%)
- ❏ Medical Supplies Revenue (%)
- ❏ Medicare Coinsurance
- ❏ Medicare Deducibles
- ❏ Medicare Deducibles & Coinsur
- ❏ Medicare PPS Rev per Admission
- ❏ Medicare PPS Revenue
- ❏ Net Avail for Dbt Svc (EBITDA)
- ❏ Net Income
- ❏ Net Income before Depreciation
- ❏ Net Income Margin
- ❏ Net Income per Adj Admiss
- ❏ Net Income per Adj Day
- ❏ Net Pat Rev per Adj Admission
- ❏ Net Pat Rev per Adj Pat Day
- ❏ Net Patient Revenue
- ❏ Net Rev Per Adj Adm, Cmix Adj
- ❏ Nonphysician Anesths, Cost
- ❏ Non-acute, Total Cost
- ❏ Non-acute Costs (%)
- ❏ Non-acute Rev (%)
- ❏ Non-op Revenue, Invest Inc
- ❏ Non-op Revenue, Philanthropy
- ❏ Non-operating Revenue, Total

- ❏ Non-operating Revenue Ratio
- ❏ Nursing Admin, Direct Cost
- ❏ Nursing Admin Expense (%)
- ❏ Nursing School, Cost
- ❏ Oper Exp, Less Deprec & Int
- ❏ Oper Margin (w/o Other Op Rev)
- ❏ Operating Exp, Cmix Wage Adj
- ❏ Operating Exp, Less Deprec
- ❏ Operating Expense, Total
- ❏ Operating Income
- ❏ Operating Profit Margin (%)
- ❏ Operating Ratio
- ❏ Operating Revenue
- ❏ Operating Room Revenue (%)
- ❏ Other Expense, Total
- ❏ Other General Service Cost
- ❏ Other Income Ratio
- ❏ Other LTC Revenue (%)
- ❏ Other Operating Revenue
- ❏ Other Revenue, Total
- ❏ Outpatient Cost Ctrs, Clinic
- ❏ Outpatient Cost Ctrs, Emerg
- ❏ Outpatient Revenue (%)
- ❏ Oxygen Therapy Revenue (%)
- ❏ Paramedical Education Expense
- ❏ Pass Through Costs
- ❏ Pass Through Costs, Ancillary
- ❏ Pass Through Costs, Routine
- ❏ Patient Operating Income
- ❏ Pct Dir Intern & Resident Exp
- ❏ Pharmacy, Direct Cost
- ❏ Pharmacy Expense (%)
- ❏ Pharmacy Revenue (%)
- ❏ Plant Operations, Direct Cost
- ❏ Plant Operations Expense (%)
- ❏ Radiology Revenue (%)
- ❏ Recovery Room Revenue (%)
- ❏ Routine Revenue (%)
- ❏ Sal & Ben Exp, Pct of Oper Exp
- ❏ Salary Expense, Total
- ❏ Salary & Benefits
- ❏ SNF Revenue (%)
- ❏ Social Service, Direct Cost
- ❏ Social Service Expense (%)
- ❏ Sub I Rev as Pct Gross Rev
- ❏ Sub II Rev as Pct Gross Rev
- ❏ Teaching Physicians, Cost
- ❏ Tot Gen Inp Rout Svc Charge
- ❏ Tot Malpractice Loss (Current)
- ❏ Total Ancillary Revenue (%)
- ❏ Total Profit Margin (%)
- ❏ Total Revenue, ASC
- ❏ Total Revenue, CORF
- ❏ Total Revenue, Home Health Agy
- ❏ Total Revenue, ICF
- ❏ Total Revenue, Other LTC
- ❏ Total Revenue, SNF
- ❏ Total Revenue, Subprovider I
- ❏ Total Revenue, Subprovider II
- ❏ Uncollectible Ratio (%)

HCIA ON-LINE SERVICES

Name: Community Hospital	**SINGLE PROFILE**		
	1991	1990	1989
Beds in Service, Acute Care	296	296	274
Occupancy Rate, Acute Care (%)	73.88	72.21	74.59
Avg Length of Stay, Acute Care	5.62	5.89	6.52
Avg Length of Stay, Medicare	8.83	8.60	8.79
Medicare Admissions (%)	33.69	35.31	38.07
FTEs per Adj Avg Daily Census	4.24	4.44	4.26
Current Ratio	1.94	1.52	1.60
Days in Accts Receivable, Net	55.79	51.20	55.85
Days Cash on Hand	23.06	8.67	28.09
Average Payment Period	61.94	67.84	64.89
Long-Term Debt to Equity	0.76	0.95	1.33
Net Plt, Prop & Equip per Bed	95,324	91,099	106,421
Debt Service Coverage Ratio	3.73	2.70	2.01
Operating Profit Margin (%)	5.42	3.30	5.55
Total Profit Margin (%)	6.22	4.00	6.45

Market Area: Anywhere, USA	**MARKET SHARE DATA**		
	Market Share		
Hospital Name	1991	1990	1989
Community Hospital	43.38	41.63	41.78
Mercy Medical Center	41.15	41.95	41.69
Southside General Hospital	7.84	7.44	7.52
St. Luke's Health Center	7.63	8.98	9.02

Market Area: Anywhere, USA	**COMPETITOR DATA**		
Hospital Name	Beds	Occ Rate	Total Profit Margin	1991 Market Share
Community Hospital	296	73.88	6.22	43.38
Mercy Medical Center	320	71.82	6.85	41.15
Southside General Hospital	101	38.29	5.79	7.84
St. Luke's Health Center	68	49.95	2.90	7.63

SINGLE HOSPITAL PROFILE

Display the three most recent years of utilization and financial data for any one of over 6,000 hospitals.

- Use a Standard Profile or a user-defined Custom Profile.
- Choose from over 500 data elements.
  Choose from any U.S. hospital.
- Data on-line within six months of hospital's fiscal year end.
- Print to local printer or disk file.

MARKET AREA PROFILE

Display the three most recent years of market share data and most recent year of competitor data for any hospital in the U.S.

- Market share based on hospital's percentage of market area admissions.
- Market area defined by geographic proximity.
- Competitor data provide overview of other hospitals in the market area.

S & P Rating: A Beds: 250 to 399 n=99	**GROUP PROFILE**		
	1991	1990	1989
Beds in Service, Acute Care	327	309	322
Occupancy Rate, Acute Care (%)	64.89	64.60	65.79
Avg Length of Stay, Acute Care	5.93	5.87	6.09
Avg Length of Stay, Medicare	8.43	8.58	8.73
Medicare Admissions (%)	32.00	31.44	33.87
FTEs per Adj Avg Daily Census	4.35	4.21	4.33
Current Ratio	3.03	3.04	3.20
Days in Accts Receivable, Net	78.46	74.08	77.39
Days Cash on Hand	70.49	79.58	70.43
Average Payment Period	55.26	56.85	57.90
Long-Term Debt to Equity	0.70	0.73	0.87
Net Plt, Prop & Equip per Bed	105,136	105,969	109,722
Debt Service Coverage Ratio	3.00	3.03	2.85
Operating Profit Margin (%)	2.54	2.95	3.87
Total Profit Margin (%)	4.74	4.89	5.63

Name: Community Hospital	**COMPARATIVE PROFILE**			
Comparison Group: S & P Rating: A Beds: 250 to 399 n=99				
	Hospital		Group	
	1991	1990	1991	1990
Beds in Service, Acute Care	296	296	327	309
Occupancy Rate, Acute Care (%)	73.88	72.21	64.89	64.60
Avg Length of Stay, Acute Care	5.62	5.89	5.93	5.87
Avg Length of Stay, Medicare	8.83	8.60	8.43	8.58
Medicare Admissions (%)	33.69	35.31	32.00	31.44
FTEs per Adj Avg Daily Census	4.24	4.44	4.35	4.21
Current Ratio	1.94	1.52	3.03	3.04
Days in Accounts Receivable, Net	55.79	51.20	78.46	74.08
Days Cash on Hand	23.06	8.67	70.49	79.58
Average Payment Period	61.94	67.84	55.26	56.85
Long-Term Debt to Equity	0.76	0.95	0.70	0.73
Net Plt, Prop & Equip per Bed	95,324	91,099	105,136	105,969
Debt Service Coverage Ratio	3.73	2.70	3.00	3.03
Operating Profit Margin (%)	5.42	3.30	2.54	2.95
Total Profit Margin (%)	6.22	4.00	4.74	4.89

GROUP HOSPITAL PROFILE & COMPARATIVE HOSPITAL PROFILE

The Group Hospital Profile displays the median values for any one of over 1,000 different groups of hospitals.
The Comparative Hospital Profile selects a hospital and a comparative group to be viewed side-by-side on the screen.

- Use a Standard Profile or a user-defined Custom Profile.
- Select any hospital or group, by choosing a state, Standard & Poor's bond rating, industry-standard national group, user-defined Custom Group, Metropolitan Statistical Area (MSA), or multihospital system.
- Narrow the group by choosing an optional bed-size range.
- View the group medians for several years.

NO ADDITIONAL CHARGE FOR ON-LINE SERVICE. YOU ONLY PAY FOR DATA ACCESSED.

ALABAMA

Alabama had a moratorium on new bed construction which ended in June 1989. Current policy gives priority to the conversion of hospital beds to long-term care beds where it is more economical and where the existing structure can meet licensure and certification requirements. Nursing homes exist in all but one county. In 1992, the statewide average occupancy rate was 97 percent, and 65 percent of the residents were Medicaid beneficiaries.

The state had a Provider Privilege Tax which taxed Medicaid beds with a hold harmless provision until May 1992. At that time Alabama changed to a tax of $1,000 per bed, thus eliminating the hold harmless provision which did not meet new federal tax requirements. This new tax is expected to produce about one-half of the state's Medicaid matching funds for long-term care.

Certificate of Need

Alabama requires a CON for the following: to acquire or construct a nursing home; to acquire medical equipment costing more than $500,000; to provide a new service with an annual cost of $500,000 or more; to incur any other capital expense of $1.5 million or more; and to change the total bed capacity or to move beds from one site to another. New freestanding facilities must have at least 50 beds.

Bed Need Methodology

The state calculates the number of long-term care beds needed from the projected population age 65 and older, an occupancy factor of 97 percent, and current utilization figures, which are subject to a ceiling of 40 beds per 1,000 population age 65 and older. Alabama employs a three-year planning horizon and applies ceilings to each county separately. The recently amended state plan indicates a shortage of 205 beds, but only two counties have a shortfall of more than 50 beds.

Medicaid

Medicaid reimbursement rates are prospective without a final settlement. However, during the first six months of the rate year (July 1 to December 31) facilities are paid an interim rate, which is the lower of the previous year's approved rate and the previous year's ceiling, after each has been trended forward for inflation. After desk audits of a facility's cost reports and the recalculation of allowable costs and ceilings, adjustments are made so that the rates paid during the final six months of the year are such that the average per diem paid for the whole year is at the appropriate level. Alabama employs four components in calculating rates: management and administrative costs, direct patient care, indirect patient care, and property costs. The component ceiling for the first category equals the median plus ten percent for two groups of facilities: those with 75 beds or less and those with more than 75 beds. Ceilings for the year ending June 30, 1992 were $7.65 and $6.70 for these two groups, respectively. The ceiling for the direct patient care component, set equal to the median cost per resident day plus 20 percent, was $43.67 during this time period. The ceiling for the indirect patient care component equals the median component cost plus ten percent, which was $16.57 for the most recent period. The median

1992 Statewide Statistics	Total
No. of Nursing Facilities	229
No. of Beds	22,765
No. of Beds per 1,000, Age 65+	43.53
No. of Beds per 1,000, Age 75+	102.65

value of the indirect care component was $16.97 for the same period. There is an incentive available for this component equal to 50 percent of the difference between allowable component costs and the ceiling. The allowable costs of the three non-property components are trended forward and added to the property component to establish the overall rate. The Alabama Medicaid Inflation Index, based on the DRI Market Basket Index of Operating Costs—Skilled Nursing Facility, is then applied to the overall rate. For the year ended June 30, 1992, the operating components ceiling was $67.89 for facilities with fewer than 76 beds, and $66.94 for all other facilities.

A Fair Rental method of paying for property costs was adopted in September 1991. It is based on the current asset value per bed, calculated as $25,000 per bed less 1 percent for each year of age, not to exceed a 50 percent reduction. The $25,000 value is re-based each year using information from the Marshall-Swift Evaluation Service. The depreciated value is multiplied by a gross rental factor to determine the rental value of the facility. The rate of return on the current value of the property is calculated by subtracting the amount due on notes incurred to purchase all land, buildings and equipment from the current asset value of the facility, and then multiplying the difference by the current yield of 30-year U.S. Treasury Bonds as of June 30 of each year. The product of the current asset value multiplied by a risk premium of 1.5 percent is then added to the rate of return figure. Interest expense related to debt incurred to purchase land, buildings, and equipment is also an allowable property expense, as are property taxes and property insurance costs. The property component is the total of the rental value, rate of return, interest, property taxes, and property insurance.

The previous practice of stepping up the asset value of a facility following a sale will no longer be employed. The allowable basis to a purchaser will be the current asset value of the previous owner. Renovations with a value greater than one percent of the current asset value will be considered for adjusting the current asset value.

The allowable per diem rate equals the total allowable costs of the four components divided by the number of resident days in the prior year. There is a mechanism for paying for the costs of nurse aide training and competency testing in addition to the per diem. For the fiscal year ended June 30, 1992, the average Medicaid reimbursement rate was $68.04. The lowest rate was $53.73, and the highest was $85.54. The state believes that about 90 percent of the facilities are paid rates that are at least equal to their allowable Medicaid costs.

ALL	Median Values		
	1990	1989	1988
Beds	102	104	103
Occupancy Rate (%)	97.91	97.00	96.96
Medicaid Resident Days (%)	72.28	69.57	67.14
FTEs per Average Daily Census	0.80	0.81	0.81
Salaries and Benefits per FTE ($)	12,288	11,216	10,136
Per Resident Day ($)			
Net Patient Revenue	46.84	45.63	41.10
Expenses			
Total Operating	50.17	46.79	42.82
Direct Care	19.95	16.16	15.39
Indirect Care	10.63	10.09	9.60
Administrative and General	13.63	13.07	12.46
Depreciation and Interest	9.09	8.44	7.03
Total Profit Margin (%)	2.13	3.35	1.24
Days in Accounts Receivable	36.96	39.98	32.64
Days in Accounts Payable	8.83	7.40	8.85
Current Ratio	1.63	1.72	1.74
Average Age of Plant (years)	6.20	5.09	4.16
Long-Term Debt to Total Assets	0.59	0.57	0.60
Debt Service Coverage Ratio	1.07	1.17	1.09

FOR-PROFIT	1990	1989	1988
Beds	103	104	105
Occupancy Rate (%)	97.86	96.99	97.07
Medicaid Resident Days (%)	71.98	68.45	66.23
FTEs per Average Daily Census	0.81	0.81	0.81
Salaries and Benefits per FTE ($)	12,258	10,726	9,979
Per Resident Day ($)			
Net Patient Revenue	46.93	45.97	40.94
Expenses			
Total Operating	50.03	46.49	42.72
Direct Care	19.79	15.81	15.27
Indirect Care	10.56	10.05	9.54
Administrative and General	13.42	12.99	12.35
Depreciation and Interest	9.98	8.82	7.84
Total Profit Margin (%)	2.25	3.67	1.44
Days in Accounts Receivable	36.72	35.98	32.62
Days in Accounts Payable	8.77	7.23	8.45
Current Ratio	1.61	1.70	1.72
Average Age of Plant (years)	5.82	5.06	4.13
Long-Term Debt to Total Assets	0.61	0.58	0.63
Debt Service Coverage Ratio	1.07	1.19	1.12

ALL OTHER	1990	1989	1988
Beds	60	60	60
Occupancy Rate (%)	98.93	97.48	95.13
Medicaid Resident Days (%)	73.88	70.92	72.49
FTEs per Average Daily Census	0.75	0.77	0.77
Salaries and Benefits per FTE ($)	14,618	12,651	11,211
Per Resident Day ($)			
Net Patient Revenue	46.02	42.97	42.37
Expenses			
Total Operating	55.41	47.98	44.84
Direct Care	24.95	20.09	17.17
Indirect Care	12.38	12.03	9.63
Administrative and General	16.54	17.00	16.94
Depreciation and Interest	6.55	6.45	5.62
Total Profit Margin (%)	1.45	(0.52)	(1.37)
Days in Accounts Receivable	41.41	43.48	32.92
Days in Accounts Payable	10.17	9.37	11.74
Current Ratio	1.91	2.08	2.04
Average Age of Plant (years)	10.95	9.45	7.91
Long-Term Debt to Total Assets	0.47	0.53	0.57
Debt Service Coverage Ratio	1.08	1.02	0.85

Median values are not additive.

Percentile Values for the 52 Performance Measures, All Hospitals

Percentile	1994 75th	1994 50th	1994 25th	1993 75th	1993 50th	1993 25th	1992 75th	1992 50th	1992 25th	1991 50th	1990 50th
CAPACITY & UTILIZATION											
Beds in Service, Acute Care	232	116	55	236	119	56	238	119	57	120	122
Total Discharges, Acute Care	9,389	4,122	1,655	9,409	4,080	1,648	9,448	4,149	1,666	4,190	4,224
Occupancy Rate (%)	61.49	46.57	30.21	62.80	47.29	30.70	65.27	49.08	32.26	50.31	51.36
Average Length of Stay	5.45	4.57	3.81	5.81	4.79	3.97	5.97	4.95	4.12	5.08	5.19
ALOS, Case Mix Adjusted	4.26	3.61	3.09	4.49	3.81	3.23	4.67	3.96	3.38	4.13	4.27
ALOS, Medicare	7.41	6.26	5.11	7.84	6.62	5.35	8.21	6.93	5.62	7.14	7.29
ALOS, Non-Medicare	4.17	3.39	2.80	4.42	3.56	2.95	4.60	3.68	3.04	3.81	3.91
PATIENT & PAYER MIX											
% Medicare Discharges	51.11	41.91	33.51	49.95	40.72	32.28	48.85	39.52	31.30	38.40	37.65
% Medicaid Discharges	21.67	13.80	8.06	21.62	13.87	7.95	21.09	13.84	7.60	12.29	10.78
% Medicare Acute Care Days	64.74	57.53	47.96	63.46	56.16	47.15	62.95	55.29	45.99	53.67	52.59
% Medicaid Acute Care Days	16.02	10.20	6.00	16.02	10.15	6.08	15.94	10.06	5.88	9.32	8.34
% Special Care Days	12.12	8.58	5.56	11.93	8.42	5.46	11.45	8.18	5.40	7.94	7.69
Medicare Case Mix Index	1.3911	1.2422	1.1130	1.3829	1.2357	1.1117	1.3588	1.2258	1.1056	1.2139	1.2012
% Outpatient Revenue	42.96	35.01	27.33	40.54	33.00	25.57	38.25	31.07	24.35	29.02	26.58
CAPITAL STRUCTURE											
Average Age of Plant	11.04	8.80	7.06	10.70	8.52	6.78	10.38	8.36	6.60	8.21	8.07
Net PP&E per Bed	154,537	99,833	52,538	144,414	92,392	49,500	136,131	87,643	47,230	84,228	79,584
Debt per Bed	176,408	97,773	38,264	169,798	93,290	37,031	158,533	87,995	35,840	82,271	75,475
% Capital Costs	9.67	7.41	5.52	9.88	7.45	5.56	9.97	7.45	5.58	7.59	7.80
Capital Costs per Adj. Discharge ($)	512	346	218	518	344	216	495	326	205	308	294
LT Debt to Total Assets	0.46	0.32	0.16	0.49	0.33	0.16	0.49	0.33	0.16	0.34	0.34
LT Debt to Net Fixed Assets	1.02	0.68	0.35	1.04	0.70	0.34	1.04	0.70	0.35	0.70	0.69
LT Debt to Capitalization	0.56	0.38	0.19	0.59	0.39	0.19	0.60	0.40	0.20	0.40	0.41
Cash Flow to Total Debt	0.43	0.25	0.15	0.43	0.25	0.15	0.43	0.25	0.16	0.24	0.23
Debt Service Coverage Ratio	6.78	3.67	2.01	6.46	3.47	1.86	6.21	3.40	1.82	2.90	2.63
LIQUIDITY											
Current Ratio	4.18	2.73	1.77	3.99	2.64	1.71	4.02	2.65	1.72	2.66	2.66
Acid Test Ratio	2.08	0.89	0.22	1.94	0.78	0.17	1.90	0.75	0.16	0.69	0.65
Days in Net Accounts Receivable	83.29	68.97	57.17	83.07	68.76	57.28	85.13	71.65	58.95	75.56	77.44
Average Payment Period	73.09	54.73	41.34	72.79	54.61	40.64	72.58	53.97	40.53	55.71	55.28
Days Cash on Hand	112.38	49.45	13.41	103.30	44.66	10.91	100.78	42.67	10.81	39.32	38.38
REVENUES & EXPENSES											
Gross Revenue per Adj. Disch. ($)	10,420	7,204	5,145	10,072	6,924	4,952	9,169	6,401	4,526	5,778	5,164
Gross Revenue per Adj. Disch., Case Mix- and Wage-Adj. ($)	7,822	6,233	5,055	7,574	5,984	4,813	6,991	5,604	4,500	5,069	4,614
Operating Revenue per Adj. Disch. ($)	6,201	4,720	3,643	6,089	4,609	3,575	5,754	4,358	3,370	4,038	3,713
Expense per Adj. Disch. ($)	5,951	4,542	3,518	5,872	4,460	3,465	5,575	4,246	3,259	3,944	3,635
Expense per Adj. Disch., Case Mix- and Wage-Adj. ($)	4,545	3,924	3,365	4,500	3,862	3,339	4,331	3,696	3,198	3,464	3,226
% Deductions from Gross Revenue	44.12	35.72	27.68	43.14	34.55	26.87	41.25	32.92	25.31	31.58	30.32
Operating Profit Margin (%)	7.13	3.45	0.18	6.53	3.06	(0.21)	6.55	2.88	(0.40)	2.42	2.17
Total Profit Margin (%)	8.37	4.52	1.22	7.88	4.25	0.95	8.09	4.20	0.77	4.00	3.77
Return on Assets (%)	8.12	4.50	1.37	8.00	4.40	1.06	8.25	4.39	0.82	3.96	3.70
Cash Flow per Bed ($)	44,053	26,307	12,417	40,185	24,013	11,175	37,871	23,021	10,829	20,558	17,841
PRODUCTIVITY & EFFICIENCY											
FTE Personnel per Adj. Avg. Daily Census	5.98	5.09	4.35	5.80	4.97	4.25	5.60	4.80	4.12	4.66	4.52
FTE Personnel per 100 Adj. Disch.	7.63	6.29	5.26	7.86	6.47	5.41	7.82	6.48	5.41	6.43	6.38
FTE Personnel per 100 Adj. Disch., Case Mix-Adj.	5.90	5.03	4.29	6.10	5.17	4.43	6.11	5.22	4.48	5.26	5.30
Salary & Benefits Expense per FTE Personnel ($)	42,182	36,643	31,722	40,762	35,133	30,424	38,732	33,327	28,912	31,409	29,280
% Salary and Benefits Expense	55.99	51.15	45.98	56.13	51.07	45.89	56.42	51.43	46.00	51.86	52.36
% Overhead Expense	37.56	33.85	30.61	38.22	34.21	30.79	38.49	34.63	31.11	35.07	35.65
Discharge per Bed	44.25	35.96	25.76	43.30	34.95	24.92	43.24	34.81	25.09	34.57	33.58
Total Assets Turnover Ratio	1.27	0.98	0.78	1.30	1.01	0.80	1.29	1.01	0.80	0.98	0.96
PRICING STRATEGIES											
Markup, All Ancillary Services	2.73	2.29	1.96	2.68	2.25	1.91	2.57	2.18	1.84	2.07	1.94
Markup Ratio, Medical Supplies	3.86	2.68	1.94	3.76	2.64	1.91	3.64	2.55	1.86	2.48	2.38
Markup Ratio, Drugs Sold	3.83	2.94	2.24	3.85	2.94	2.22	3.76	2.85	2.17	2.81	2.74
Markup Ratio, Laboratory	3.05	2.42	1.91	3.04	2.36	1.86	2.92	2.29	1.82	2.21	2.13
Markup Ratio, Diagnostic Radiology	2.53	2.07	1.68	2.43	2.00	1.62	2.35	1.94	1.58	1.91	1.84

The Sourcebook

A P P E N D I X

B

Claritas Senior Life Report Reference Guide

DESCRIPTION

The "Graying of America" is one of the most noted and discussed demographic trends. Americans are growing older and as the country matures, new opportunities are constantly emerging for marketing products and services. Developed by Claritas, the Senior Life Report provides essential demographics on the population 55 years and older. 1990 U.S. Census data and Claritas' current year estimates and five year projections* are combined to present a format that offers detailed information on population, race, income, housing value, detail on household type, owner costs, renter information, and more. Data for the Senior Life report can be retrieved at the following geographic levels:

Census	**U.S. Postal**	**Other**
U.S.	3-Digit ZIP	Congressional District
State	ZIP Code	
Metropolitan Statistical Area (MSA)		
County	**Media**	
Place	Area of Dominant Influence (ADI)	
Minor Civil Division (MCD)	Designated Market Area (DMA)	
Census Tract	Cabletrack	
Block Group	Exchange	
	Yellow Page Directory (YPD)	

HOW TO USE THIS GUIDE

Explanations of data and definitions of key terminology used on the Senior Life Report are provided in this guide. Pages 1 through 4 provide overview information and the remaining pages are related to specific sections of the report. Three columns of data are provided for tables 1 through 5 on the Senior Life Report: 1990, 19cy, and 19xx,

---

*Detailed information on the methodology used by Claritas Inc. to determine current year estimates and five-year projections is available in *UPDATE: precision demographics, How Claritas updates local demographic data.* To obtain a copy, contact Claritas Technical Support at 800-234-5629.

1 of 15

---

where cy is current year for current year estimates, and xx is current year plus five for five year projections. Tables 6 through 11 reflect only 1990 data. Since all data on the Senior Life report, with the exception of median values, are shown in both counts and percentages, description of how the data are structured pertains to both.

Throughout this document, we provide examples using actual numbers. Unless specified otherwise, the data used in the examples are taken from the 1990 column of the table being described.

Population by Age and Sex	1990		1993 Estimate		1998 Proj.	
Population Age 55 +......	2728	100.0%	2811	100.0%	3217	100.0%
55 to 59...............	1156	42.4%	1174	41.8%	1436	44.6%
60 to 64...............	689	25.3%	671	23.9%	689	21.4%
65 to 69...............	398	14.6%	395	14.1%	396	12.3%
70 to 74...............	233	8.5%	263	9.4%	279	8.7%
75 to 79...............	124	4.5%	138	4.9%	171	5.3%
80 to 84...............	84	3.1%	101	3.6%	131	4.1%
85 + ...	44	1.6%	69	2.5%	115	3.6%

EXAMPLE: "...*adding the seven age breaks equals the total population age 55+. For example, 2728 = 1156 + 689 + 398 + 233 + 124 + 84 + 44.*"

Although the numbers used in this example refer to the 1990 column of the table above, the same formula applies to the 1993 estimate and 1998 projected columns.

COMMON TERMS

The following list of definitions are "common" terms, meaning they apply to several sections of the Senior Life report. Instead of listing the same definition in each segment for which it applies, this list has been compiled in reference to all sections. Definitions provided in this document are derived from the *Technical Documentation, Census of Population and Housing 1990: Summary Tape Files 1 and 3.*

Household - All persons who occupy a housing unit.

Household Income - Total money received in the stated calendar year by all household members 15 years old and over, tabulated for all households. Household income differs from family household income by including income from all persons age 15 years and older in all households, including persons living alone and other non-family households. The income is presented in terms of current dollars for the particular year in question.

Householder - The person who was reported in column 1 on the census questionnaire was to be the person or one of the persons in whose name the home was owned or rented. If there was no such person, any adult household member at least 15 years old and over could be designated as the householder.

Median - The median divides a distribution (income, for example) into two equal parts, one half of the values being above the median and the other being below the median.

OWNER/RENTER-OCCUPIED VERSUS SPECIFIED OWNER/RENTER-OCCUPIED

A housing unit is *owner-occupied* if the owner or co-owner lives in the unit, even if it is mortgaged or not fully paid for.

All *occupied* housing units which are not *owner-occupied*, whether they are rented for cash rent or occupied without cash rent, are classified as *renter-occupied*.

An *occupied* housing unit is also a *specified occupied* housing unit if it is a single family house on fewer than 10 acres without a business or medical office on the property and not a mobile home.

Mobile homes or houses with a business or medical office, houses on 10 or more acres and housing units in multi-unit buildings, such as condominiums, can still be *occupied* but not *specified occupied*.

SAMPLE DATA VERSUS 100% DATA

One of two questionnaires are distributed to every household in the country. A short-form questionnaire is distributed to the majority of households. This questionnaire asks 14 questions, 7 questions of each person in the household and 7 questions concerning the household as a whole.

The long-form questionnaire is called a sample as it is distributed to only 17 percent of all households. The long-form includes all the questions included on the short-form, in addition to another 19 questions on housing and 26 on each person of the household. The data are then weighted to 100 percent to represent the total population.

Summary Tape File 1 (STF1) - from the Census Bureau contains the information obtained from the *short-form* of the census and the first 14 questions of the long-form which are identical to the questions on the short-form.

Summary Tape File 3 (STF3) - is a sample count and contains the information obtained from the long-form of the census which was distributed to only 17 percent of the population. The data were then weighted to 100 percent using the Census Bureau's methodology.

UPDATE - A database developed by Claritas Inc. which provides 1980, 1990, current-year and five-year projected demographic data based on the 1980 and 1990 Census' STF1 and STF3. All 1990 data in this database have been adjusted to be consistent with the 100% counts from STF1. Detailed information on the methodology used by Claritas to determine current year estimates and five-year projections is available in *UPDATE: precision demographics, How Claritas updates local demographic data.*

DATA SOURCE

1990 - For tables 1 through 5, the 1990 data come from UPDATE and have been adjusted to be consistent with the 100% counts from STF1. Tables 6 through 11 reflect only 1990 data, taken from STF3.

Current-year estimates and five-year projections - For tables 1 through 5, data are taken from UPDATE. No current-year estimates or five-year projections are available for tables 6 through 11.

Population by Age and Sex

Population by Age and Sex	1990		1993 Estimate		1998 Proj.	
Population Age 55 +......	2728	100.0%	2811	100.0%	3217	100.0%
55 to 59...............	1156	42.4%	1174	41.8%	1436	44.6%
60 to 64...............	689	25.3%	671	23.9%	689	21.4%
65 to 69...............	398	14.6%	395	14.1%	396	12.3%
70 to 74...............	233	8.5%	263	9.4%	279	8.7%
75 to 79...............	124	4.5%	138	4.9%	171	5.3%
80 to 84...............	84	3.1%	101	3.6%	131	4.1%
85 + ...	44	1.6%	69	2.5%	115	3.6%
Males Age 55 +..........	1308	47.9%	1355	48.2%	1556	48.4%
55 to 59...............	612	22.4%	625	22.2%	759	23.6%
60 to 64...............	347	12.7%	339	12.1%	349	10.8%
65 to 69...............	184	6.7%	185	6.6%	186	5.8%
70 to 74...............	98	3.6%	114	4.1%	124	3.9%
75 to 79...............	31	1.1%	38	1.4%	50	1.6%
80 to 84...............	21	0.8%	28	1.0%	41	1.3%
85 + ...	15	0.5%	26	0.9%	47	1.5%
Female Age 55 +..........	1420	52.1%	1456	51.8%	1661	51.6%
55 to 59...............	544	19.9%	549	19.5%	677	21.0%
60 to 64...............	342	12.5%	332	11.8%	340	10.6%
65 to 69...............	214	7.8%	210	7.5%	210	6.5%
70 to 74...............	135	4.9%	149	5.3%	155	4.8%
75 to 79...............	93	3.4%	100	3.6%	121	3.8%
80 to 84...............	63	2.3%	73	2.6%	90	2.8%
85 + ...	29	1.1%	43	1.5%	68	2.1%

Table 1

This section provides population data in two ways: the total population over age 55 divided into age breaks, and the population over age 55 divided into age by sex breaks (Table 1). Key points are:

- The combined sum of the seven age breaks listed under each category equal the total for that category. For example, 2728 = 1156 + 689 + 398 + 233 + 124 + 84 + 44.

- Adding the male total to the female total equals the total population of the study area. For example, 2728 = 1420 + 1308.

Population by Age and Race

Page 1

```
Population by Age & Race       1990          1993 Estimate      1998 Proj.
-------------------------  ---------------   ---------------   ---------------
Total Population.........   47170  100.0%     49082  100.0%     53277  100.0%
    White Population......   36772   78.0%     37660   76.7%     39780   74.7%
    Age 65 and Over.......     707    1.5%       764    1.6%       853    1.6%
    Black Population......    8355   17.7%      9106   18.6%     10699   20.1%
    Age 65 and Over.......     122    0.3%       136    0.3%       165    0.3%
    Asian Population......    1869    4.0%      2127    4.3%      2590    4.9%
    Age 65 and Over.......      51    0.1%        62    0.1%        69    0.1%
    Am. Indian Population.     174    0.4%       189    0.4%       208    0.4%
    Age 65 and Over.......       3    0.0%         4    0.0%         5    0.0%
Hispanic Population.....     2498    5.3%      2906    5.9%      3705    7.0%
    Age 65 and Over.......      43    0.1%        49    0.1%        81    0.2%
```
Table 2

Data on the population by race and of Hispanic origin are provided in this section. A count of the population age 65+ is given by race and of Hispanic origin (Table 2). Key points are:

- The total population figure listed represents the entire population of the study area, regardless of age.

- Adding the totals of the four race categories (White, Black, Asian, American Indian) equals the total population. For example, 47170 = 36772 + 8355 + 1869 + 174.

- Sub-categories "Age 65 and Over" reflect the count of the senior population for its respective race, and are already counted into its race total. For example, 707 is included in 36772.

- The Census Bureau considers Hispanic as an ethnicity, not a race. Therefore, a total count of the Hispanic population is listed. This figure reflects all persons, regardless of race, who claimed Hispanic origin. Adding the Hispanic population total to the total population will result in a double-count of Hispanics.

5 of 15

Household Income by Age of Householder	--- Households with Householder Age 55 and Over ----					
	1990		1993 Estimate		1998 Proj.	
Householder Age 55 to 64.	1074	100.0%	1103	100.0%	1279	100.0%
Under $5,000........	7	0.7%	7	0.6%	6	0.5%
$5,000-$9,999........	19	1.8%	21	1.9%	17	1.3%
$10,000-$14,999........	14	1.3%	12	1.1%	16	1.3%
$15,000-$24,999........	50	4.7%	30	2.7%	25	2.0%
$25,000-$34,999........	105	9.8%	79	7.2%	63	4.9%
$35,000-$49,999........	249	23.2%	212	19.2%	193	15.1%
$50,000-$74,999........	331	30.8%	362	32.8%	396	31.0%
$75,000-$99,999........	200	18.6%	201	18.2%	284	22.2%
$100,000-$149,999.......	83	7.7%	156	14.1%	219	17.1%
$150,000-$249,999.......	13	1.2%	17	1.5%	51	4.0%
$250,000-$499,999.......	2	0.2%	5	0.5%	8	0.6%
$500,000 or More.......	1	0.1%	1	0.1%	1	0.1%
Median Income............	57024		63156		70170	

Table 3

Provides a count of households by the householder's age (55+), dividing each age category total into 12 income brackets (Table 3). Key points are:

- Tables are provided for the following age breaks: 55-64, 65-69, 70-74, 75-79, 80-84, and 85+.

- A median income figure is listed at the bottom of each column. The median income for households is based on the distribution of the total number of households, including those with no income.

Household Income

Household Income	1990 Census		1993 Estimate		1998 Proj.	
Total....................	14268	100.0%	15013	100.0%	16637	100.0%
Under $5,000..........	108	0.8%	83	0.6%	67	0.4%
$5,000 to $9,999....	158	1.1%	145	1.0%	135	0.8%
$10,000 to $14,999....	171	1.2%	176	1.2%	161	1.0%
$15,000 to $24,999....	921	6.5%	622	4.1%	447	2.7%
$25,000 to $34,999....	1830	12.8%	1324	8.8%	1055	6.3%
$35,000 to $49,999....	3649	25.6%	3237	21.6%	2659	16.0%
$50,000 to $74,999....	5097	35.7%	5464	36.4%	5466	32.9%
$75,000 to $99,999....	1682	11.8%	2582	17.2%	3851	23.1%
$100,000 to $124,999....	482	3.4%	951	6.3%	1745	10.5%
$125,000 to $149,999....	110	0.8%	310	2.1%	648	3.9%
$150,000 to $249,999....	47	0.3%	96	0.6%	351	2.1%
$250,000 to $499,999....	12	0.1%	20	0.1%	45	0.3%
$500,000 or More........	1	0.0%	3	0.0%	7	0.0%
Median Household Income..	51026		58539		67542	

Table 4

This section follows the same format as described for "Household Income by Age of Householder" (Table 3). The difference is that this section reflects the total count of households in the study area, regardless of the householder's age (Table 4).

Housing Value	1990 Census		1993 Estimate		1998 Proj.	
Total Units..............	10342		10874		12033	
Less than $15,000....	6	0.1%	6	0.1%	6	0.0%
$15,000 to $19,999....	7	0.1%	7	0.1%	2	0.0%
$20,000 to $24,999....	6	0.1%	5	0.0%	7	0.1%
$25,000 to $29,999....	0	0.0%	1	0.0%	5	0.0%
$30,000 to $34,999....	0	0.0%	0	0.0%	1	0.0%
$35,000 to $39,999....	7	0.1%	0	0.0%	0	0.0%
$40,000 to $44,999....	2	0.0%	7	0.1%	0	0.0%
$45,000 to $49,999....	4	0.0%	2	0.0%	3	0.0%
$50,000 to $59,999....	9	0.1%	6	0.1%	7	0.1%
$60,000 to $74,999....	45	0.4%	34	0.3%	16	0.1%
$75,000 to $99,999....	1414	13.7%	969	8.9%	522	4.3%
$100,000 to $124,999....	4078	39.4%	2815	25.9%	1546	12.8%
$125,000 to $149,999....	3320	32.1%	3464	31.9%	2752	22.9%
$150,000 to $174,999....	913	8.8%	2332	21.4%	3157	26.2%
$175,000 to $199,999....	264	2.6%	725	6.7%	2198	18.3%
$200,000 to $249,999....	205	2.0%	333	3.1%	1349	11.2%
$250,000 to $299,999....	38	0.4%	121	1.1%	291	2.4%
$300,000 to $399,999....	13	0.1%	32	0.3%	135	1.1%
$400,000 to $499,999....	4	0.0%	7	0.1%	22	0.2%
$500,000 and over.......	7	0.1%	8	0.1%	14	0.1%
Median Housing Value....	122505		136439		159103	

Table 5

A count of specified owner-occupied housing units is provided in this section. The housing units are distributed accordingly among twenty housing "value" categories (Table 5).

Specified owner-occupied housing unit - A housing unit is *owner-occupied* if the owner or co-owner lives in the unit, even if it is mortgaged or not fully paid for.

A *specified owner-occupied* housing unit is a single family house on fewer than 10 acres without a business or medical office on the property and not a mobile home.

Value - The respondent's estimate of the dollar worth of the property, including the house and the lot on which it stands.

NOTE: The total count of specified owner-occupied housing units *does not* match the total count listed under the heading "Monthly Owner Costs as a Percent of 1989 HH Income" described later in this guide (see Table 7 on page 9). The data source of "Housing Value" is Claritas' UPDATE and the data source of "Monthly Owner Costs..." is STF3.

Household Type and Relationship	Population 65+		Household Type and Relationship	Population 65+	
Total.............	780	100.0%			
In Family Households	635	81.4%	In Nonfamily Hhlds...	145	18.6%
Householder........	222	28.5%	Male Householder....	31	4.0%
Spouse.............	130	16.7%	Living Alone.......	31	4.0%
Other Relative.....	246	31.5%	Not Living Alone...	0	0.0%
Nonrelative........	37	4.7%	Female Householder..	112	14.4%
			Living Alone.......	101	12.9%
In Group Quarters...	0	0.0%	Not Living Alone...	11	1.4%
Institutionalized..	0	0.0%	Nonrelative.........	2	0.2%
Other.............	0	0.0%			

Table 6

This section provides 1990 data on the population age 65+ by household type and relationship (Table 6). Key points are:

- This table is divided into the three parts - "Family Households", "Group Quarters", and "Nonfamily Households". Adding the total of these parts equals the "Total" population figure. For example, 780 = 635 + 0 + 145.

- "Family Households" is divided into four categories - "Householder", "Spouse", "Other relative", and "Nonrelative". Adding the four categories equals the total for "Family Households". For example, 635 = 222 + 130 + 246 + 37.

- "Groups Quarters" is divided into two categories - "Institutionalized" and "Other". Adding the two categories equals the total for "Group Quarters".

- "Nonfamily Households" is divided into three categories - "Male Householder", "Female householder", and "Nonrelative". Adding the three categories equals the total for "Nonfamily Households". For example, 145 = 31 + 112 + 2.

- "Female Householder" and "Male Householder" are each divided into two sub-categories - "Living Alone" and "Not Living Alone". Adding the two sub-categories equals the total. For example, 112 = 101 + 11.

- The two "Nonrelative" categories are defined separately.

Family Households
Family household - A household with persons related by birth, marriage, or adoption. The householder and all persons in the household related to him or her are family members. A family household may also include non-relatives living with the family.

Spouse - A person married to and living with a householder. This category includes persons in formal marriages, as well as persons in common-law marriages.

Other relative - Includes any household member not listed in a reported category (parent, brother/sister, grandchild) who is related to the householder by birth, marriage, or adoption (brother/sister-in-law, grandparent, nephew, aunt, mother-in-law, daughter-in-law, cousin, etc...).

Nonrelative (family households) - Includes any household member, including foster children not related to the householder by birth, marriage, or adoption.

Group Quarters
Group Quarters - All persons not living in households are classified by the Census Bureau as living in group quarters..

Institutionalized - Includes persons under formally authorized, supervised care or custody in institutions at the time of enumeration. Such persons are considered "inmates or patients" of an institution regardless of the availability of nursing or medical care, the length of stay, or the number of persons in the institution.

Other (group quarters) - Includes all persons who live in group quarters other than institutions. Living quarters with less than ten unrelated persons living in the unit are classified as housing units.

Nonfamily Households
Nonfamily household - A household consisting of a person living alone or of a householder living with persons not related.

Nonrelative (nonfamily households) - Includes persons 65+ living in nonfamily households who are not householders. This number does not equal the added total of Male and Female Householders Not Living Alone, since the number of persons in the Not Living Alone categories may be living with nonrelatives under age 65, and those nonrelatives would not be counted in the "Nonrelatives" category.

Monthly Owner Costs as a Percent of 1989 Household Income

Monthly Owner Costs as a Percent of 1989 HH Inc.	Spec. Owner-Occ Units by Age of Householder			
	Total Units		65 Yrs +	
Total.....................	10573	100.0%	335	100.0%
Less than 20%............	3442	32.6%	201	60.0%
20 - 24%.................	1879	17.8%	33	9.9%
25 - 29%.................	1880	17.8%	46	13.7%
30 - 34%.................	1356	12.8%	0	0.0%
35% or More.............	1997	18.9%	55	16.4%
Not computed............	19	0.2%	0	0.0%

Table 7

This section provides a count of specified owner-occupied housing units by monthly owner costs as a percent of 1989 household income. Key points are:

- Adding the percentage categories equals the total units of the study area. For example, 10573 = 3442 + 1879 + 1880 + 1356 + 1997 + 19.

- The figures in the "65 Yrs +" column have been included in the "Total Units" column. Adding the two columns together will result in a double count of all specified owner-occupied housing units in which the householder is age 65+.

Selected monthly owner costs - The sum of payments for mortgages, deeds of trust, contracts to purchase, or similar debts on the property (including payments for the first mortgage, second or junior mortgages, and home equity loans); real estate taxes; fire, hazard, flood insurance on the property; utilities (electricity, gas, and water); and fuels (oil, coal, kerosene, wood, etc.).

Selected monthly owner costs as a percentage of 1989 household income - The computed ratio of selected monthly owner costs to monthly household income in 1989. The ratio was computed separately for each unit and rounded to the nearest whole percentage.

NOTE: The total count of specified owner-occupied housing units *does not* match the total count listed under the heading "Housing Value" described previously (see Table 5 on page 7). The data source of "Monthly Owner Costs..." is STF3 and the data source of "Housing Value" is Claritas' UPDATE.

Gross Rent as Percent of 1989 Household Income Page 5

Gross Rent as Percent of 1989 HH Income	----- Spec. Renter-Occ Units ----- by Age of Householder		
	Total Units		65 Yrs +
Total......................	3329	100.0%	28	100.0%
Less than 20%............	701	21.1%	0	0.0%
20 - 24%.................	658	19.8%	10	35.7%
25 - 29%.................	640	19.2%	0	0.0%
30 - 34%.................	337	10.1%	0	0.0%
35% or More.............	956	28.7%	18	64.3%
Not computed............	37	1.1%	0	0.0%

Table 8

This section provides a count of specified renter-occupied housing units by monthly owner costs as a percent of 1989 household income (Table 8). Key points are:

- Adding the percentage categories equals the total units of the study area. For example, 3329 = 701 + 658 + 640 + 337 + 956 + 37.

10 of 15

- The figures in the "65 Yrs +" column are included in the "Total Units" column. Adding the two columns together will result in a double count of all specified owner-occupied housing units with the householder's age 65+.

Gross Rent as a Percentage of Household Income - a computed ratio of monthly gross rent to monthly household income (total household income in 1989 divided by 12). The ratio was computed separately for each unit and was rounded to the nearest whole percentage. Units for which no cash rent is paid and units occupied by households that reported no income or a net loss in 1989 comprise the category "Not Computed".

Specified Renter-Occupied Housing Unit - All *occupied* housing units which are not *owner-occupied*, whether they are rented for cash rent or occupied without cash rent, are classified as *renter-occupied*.

A *specified renter-occupied* housing unit is a single family house on fewer than 10 acres without a business or medical office on the property and not a mobile home.

Occupied Housing Units   **page 5**

Attribute	----- Occupied Housing Units -----		
	Total		Hhldr 65 +	
Owner Occupied Units.....	10939	76.7%	356	92.7%
Renter Occupied Units.....	3329	23.3%	28	7.3%
Complete Plumbing Facil..	14254	99.9%	384	100.0%
Lacking Plumbing Facil...	14	0.1%	0	0.0%
With Telephone...........	14094	98.8%	376	97.9%
No Telephone.............	174	1.2%	8	2.1%
One or More Vehicles.....	14009	98.2%	329	85.7%
No Vehicles Available....	259	1.8%	55	14.3%

Table 9

Table 9 provides 1990 data for occupied housing units including both owner and renter-occupied. Key points are:

- Adding owner and renter occupied housing units totals together equals the total count of occupied housing units.

- The categories for plumbing, telephone, and vehicles reflects counts for all occupied housing units in the study area, regardless of status (renter or owner occupied).

- The total count of owner-occupied housing units does include the count of specified owner-occupied housing units, as does the count of renter-occupied housing units include specified renter-occupied.

11 of 15

- The figures in the "65 Yrs +" column are included in the "Total Units" column. Adding the two columns together will result in a double count of all owner-occupied housing units in which the householder is age 65+.

Owner-occupied housing unit - A housing unit is *owner-occupied* if the owner or co-owner lives in the unit, even if it is mortgaged or not fully paid for.

Renter-occupied housing unit - All *occupied* housing units which are not *owner-occupied*, whether they are rented for cash rent or occupied without cash rent, are classified as *renter-occupied*.

Poverty Status by Household Type

Poverty Status by Household Type	------ 1990 Households by Age of Householder ------					
	Total		Age 65-74		Age 75 +	
Total...................	14360	100.0%	262	100.0%	103	100.0%
Married Couple Family..	10748	74.8%	159	60.7%	31	30.1%
Other Family...........	1630	11.4%	19	7.3%	13	12.6%
Male Householder.....	447	3.1%	7	2.7%	7	6.8%
Female Householder...	1183	8.2%	12	4.6%	6	5.8%
Nonfamily..............	1982	13.8%	84	32.1%	59	57.3%
HHer Living Alone.....	1368	9.5%	73	27.9%	59	57.3%
HHer Not Living Alone.	614	4.3%	11	4.2%	0	0.0%
Above Poverty..........	14072	98.0%	255	97.3%	95	92.2%
Married Couple Family..	10686	74.4%	159	60.7%	23	22.3%
Other Family...........	1457	10.1%	12	4.6%	13	12.6%
Male Householder.....	424	3.0%	7	2.7%	7	6.8%
Female Householder...	1033	7.2%	5	1.9%	6	5.8%
Nonfamily..............	1929	13.4%	84	32.1%	59	57.3%
HHer Living Alone.....	1337	9.3%	73	27.9%	59	57.3%
HHer Not Living Alone.	592	4.1%	11	4.2%	0	0.0%
Below Poverty..........	288	2.0%	7	2.7%	8	7.8%
Married Couple Family..	62	0.4%	0	0.0%	8	7.8%
Other Family...........	173	1.2%	7	2.7%	0	0.0%
Male Householder.....	23	0.2%	0	0.0%	0	0.0%
Female Householder...	150	1.0%	7	2.7%	0	0.0%
Nonfamily..............	53	0.4%	0	0.0%	0	0.0%
HHer Living Alone.....	31	0.2%	0	0.0%	0	0.0%
HHer Not Living Alone.	22	0.2%	0	0.0%	0	0.0%

Table 10

This section provides a count of households by age of householder showing poverty status by household type (Table 10). Key points are:

- Table 10 has three parts: "Total", "Above Poverty", and "Below Poverty". Adding the totals for "Above Poverty" and "Below Poverty" equals the "Total" count. For example, 14360 = 14072 + 288.

- Each part is divided into three categories: "Married Couple Family", "Other Family", and "Nonfamily". Adding the totals of these three categories equals the total for their respective part. For example, 14360 = 10748 + 1630 + 1982.

- Each "Other Family" category is divided into 2 sub-categories - "Male Householder" and "Female Householder". Adding the two sub-categories equals the total for "Other Family". For example, 1630 = 447 + 1183.

- Each "Nonfamily" category is divided into two sub-categories - "HHer Living Alone" and "HHer Not Living Alone". Adding the two sub-categories equals the total for "Nonfamily". For example, 1982 = 1368 + 614.

- The figures in the "Age 65 -74" and "Age 75+" columns have been included in the "Total" column. Adding these two columns to the "Total" will result in a double count of households in which the householder is age 65+.

Poverty Status - Households are classified below the poverty level when the total 1989 income of the family or of the nonfamily householder is below the appropriate poverty threshold. The income of persons living in the household who are unrelated to the householder is not considered when determining the poverty status of a household, nor does their presence affect the household size in determining the appropriate poverty threshold.

NOTE: The total count of households at the top of this table *does not* match the total count of households listed under Household Income (see Table 4 on page 6). The source of the data on "Poverty Status" is STF3 and the data source of "Household Income" is Claritas' UPDATE.

Mobility and Disability   **Page 7**

Mobility and Disability	Civilian Noninstitutionalized Persons Age 16+					
	Total		Age 65+		Age 75 +	
Persons.................	30814	100.0%	780	100.0%	223	100.0%
With Mblty or Care Lmts.	2200	7.1%	259	33.2%	117	52.5%
Mobility Limits Only...	1723	5.6%	205	26.3%	72	32.3%
Self Care Limits Only..	303	1.0%	7	0.9%	0	0.0%
Both Limits............	174	0.6%	47	6.0%	45	20.2%
No Mblty or Care Limits.	28614	92.9%	521	66.8%	106	47.5%
With a Work Disability..	1912	6.2%	267	34.2%		
In Labor Force.........	1107	3.6%	50	6.4%		
Employed..............	1001	3.2%	45	5.8%		
Unemployed............	106	0.3%	5	0.6%		
Not in Labor Force.....	805	2.6%	217	27.8%		
Prevented from Working	628	2.0%	206	26.4%		
Not Prevented from Wrk	177	0.6%	11	1.4%		
No Work Disability......	28902	93.8%	513	65.8%		
In Labor Force.........	24519	79.6%	122	15.6%		
Employed..............	23764	77.1%	108	13.8%		
Unemployed............	755	2.5%	14	1.8%		
Not in Labor Force.....	4383	14.2%	391	50.1%		

Table 11

This table has two parts: Mobility and Work Disability. Each part is broken into two categories, which in turn are broken into sub-categories. It is important to remember that the only things these parts share in common are the universe in which they study

13 of 15

(civilian noninstitutionalized persons age 16+), and the source of the data (STF3). Data for each part do not cross reference one another. The key points of this table are listed by part.

Mobility - "With Mobility or Care Limits" and "No Mobility or Care Limits"

- Adding the total of the two categories equals the count of "Total Persons". For example, 2200 + 28614 = 30814.

- Adding the sub-categories "Mobility Limits Only", "Self Care Limits Only", and "Both Limits" equals the total for "With Mobility or Care Limits".

- The three columns at the top of the table follow a hierarchical succession. "Age 75+" is reflected in the "Age 65+" column, which is reflected in the "Total" column.

Work Disability - "With a Work Disability" and "No Work Disability"

- Adding the total of the two categories equals the count of "Total Persons". For example, 1912 + 28902 = 30814.

- "With a Work Disability" is divided into the "In Labor Force" and "Not In Labor Force" sub-categories, which are each divided up into two more categories. Adding "Employed" and "Unemployed" equals "In Labor Force", and adding "Prevented from Working" and "Not Prevented From Work" equals "Not In Labor Force". For example, 628 + 177 = 805, 1001 + 106 = 1107, and 805 + 1107 = 1912 (the total for "With A Work Disability"). The category "No Work Disability" follows the same structure.

- There are no Work Disability data available for the age break 75+. The count of persons who fall into this age break is reflected in the "Age 65+" column, and the "Total" column.

- The counts listed in the " Age 65 Yrs +" column are included in the "Total" column. Adding the two columns together will result in a double count of all civilian noninstitutionalized persons age 65+.

Civilian Noninstitutionalized Person age 16+ - All persons age 16+ who are not on active duty with the U.S. Armed Forces and are not living in institutionalized group quarters.

Mobility Limitation Status - A health condition (mental and/or physical) that has lasted for 6 or more months and which makes it difficult to go outside the home alone. This excludes any temporary health conditions, such as a broken bone that is expected to heal normally.

Self-Care Limitation Status - A health condition (mental and/or physical) that has lasted for 6 or more months and which makes it difficult for a person to take care of their own personal needs, such as dressing, bathing, or getting around inside the home. This excludes any temporary health conditions, such as a broken bone that is expected to heal normally.

Work Disability Status - A health condition (mental and/or physical) that has lasted for 6 or more months which limits the kind or amount of work a person can do at a job or business. This excludes any temporary health conditions, such as a broken bone that is expected to heal normally.

APPENDIX

C

Summary of State Requirements/Regulations for Assisted Living Facilities

Alabama: Facilities provide room, board, meals, laundry, and at least 24 hours per week of personal care and other services. Classified according to number of residents served. 205/240-3508.

Alaska: Under new statute, homes may provide nursing and assistance with activities of daily living in residential settings that do not need to be private apartments. 24-hour skilled care may not exceed 45 consecutive days. 907/563-5654.

Arizona: Assisted living type of facilities licensed as "unclassified health care institutions," with minimal physical plant requirements. Pilot program known as "supportive residential living centers" underway in Maricopa County. 602/255-1177.

Arkansas: Licensed by Department of Human Services as "residential care facilities" to provide room and board to individuals with impaired functioning who do not require hospital or nursing home care. 501/682-8468.

California: Licensed by Department of Social Services as "residential care facilities for the elderly," must provide basic services including meals, transportation arrangements, recreational activities, personal care, and assistance with ADL and medications. 916/327-2459.

Colorado: Typically licensed by Department of Health as "personal care boarding homes" under set of core regulations applicable to all residential care facilities. 303/866-5907.

Connecticut: Department of Public Health and Addiction Services licenses only delivery of services, not residential setting where services are provided. 203/566-5758.

Delaware: No regulations specifically for assisted living facilities. Regulations for "rest (residential) homes" apply to facilities that provide personal care services to persons who can normally manage their activities of daily living. 202/995-6674.

Florida: Most AL facilities licensed as "adult congregate living facilities," which may assist with ADL and supervise self-administered medications. Not appropriate for residents requiring 24-hour nursing supervision or bedridden for over seven days. 904/487-2515.

Georgia: Falls under regulations for "personal care homes," which provide or arrange for the provision of housing, food service, and one or more personal services. Private apartments are not required. 404/657-6527.

Hawaii: No regulations specifically for AL. Rules for "adult residential care homes" apply to facilities providing 24-hour living accommodations to residents requiring minimal assistance with ADL. 808/586-4100.

Idaho: State officials considering a regulatory category for AL. License currently required for "residential care facilities" that provide nonmedical personal care or services to elderly or disabled residents who need assistance or supervision to sustain ADL. 208/334-3577.

Illinois: No residential model for AL. Regulations for "sheltered care" apply; may not admit or retain residents with serious mental or emotional problems. 217/782-2913.

Indiana: No residential model for AL. "Residential care facility" regulations apply. AL facilities must also fulfill food service, pharmaceutical service, activities program, and medical record requirements applicable to nursing homes. 317/633-8442.

Iowa: Legislation pending (1996). Current regulations apply to "residential care facilities" that provide personal assistance to persons who are "unable to sufficiently or properly care for themselves but who do not require the services of a licensed nurse except on an emergency basis." 515/281-4115.

Kansas: Legislation pending (1996). Most AL providers licensed as "intermediate personal care homes," a dwindling minority of others as "residential care facilities." 913/296-1246.

Kentucky: AL legislation proposed but not enacted (1994). Regulations for "personal care homes" apply to facilities providing continuous supervision, health-related services, personal care, and recreational activities for residents who can manage most ADL. 502/564-2800.

Louisiana: Task force established to draft AL regulations, intends to use current "adult residential care home" regulations as starting point. 504/922-0015.

Maine: "Boarding home" regulations adapted to assisted living; most significant modification allows for provision of nursing services. Another option is certification as "congregate housing services program." 207/624-5250.

Maryland: Office on Aging oversees two types of AL facilities: "multifamily senior housing" and "group sheltered housing for the elderly" (or group senior assisted housing). 410/225-1118.

Massachusetts: Legislation defines an AL residence as any entity providing room and board that either directly provides or arranges for provision of assistance with ADL. 617/727-7750.

Michigan: No residential model for AL. "Home for the aged" regulations apply to facilities providing room and board, protection, supervision, assistance, and supervised personal care to residents who are 60 and older. 517/373-8562.

Minnesota: Industry opposing attempts to adopt regulations for "residential care homes." Some AL facilities licensed as "board and lodging homes" with special services. 612/643-2100.

Mississippi: No residential model for AL. Regulations for "personal care homes" apply to facilities providing assistance to residents who do not need nursing care. 601/981-3775.

Missouri: No regulations specifically for AL. Rules apply to facilities that provide residents with shelter, board, and protective oversight. Incapacitated residents may remain in facility with physician's written approval for up to 45 days. 314/751-3082.

Montana: Proposal to establish separate licensure category defeated in 1993. Most AL facilities licensed under "personal care facilities," which provide residential services, personal assistance services, recreational activities, and supervision of self-medication. 406/444-2868.

Nebraska: Department of Health licenses "residential care facilities," which may provide assistance with ADL to four or more unrelated individuals. 402/471-2946.

Nevada: Division of Health licenses "residential facilities for groups" to provide assistance with ADL and to oversee taking of medication. Two categories: those with fewer than seven residents and those with seven or more residents. 702/687-4475.

New Hampshire: "Residential care home facilities" provide supervision and physical assistance with ADL. Must also provide protective services, access to community services, and supervision of self-administered medications. 603/271-4592.

New Jersey: Licensing for "assisted living facilities" covers apartment-style housing, congregate dining, and coordinated array of supportive personal and health services, available 24 hours per day. 609/588-7728.

New Mexico: Residential care provided pursuant to license for "adult residential shelter care homes," which provide assistance with ADL, periodic professional nursing care, and supervision of self-administered medication. 505/827-4225.

New York: Complex scheme for "assisted living program" that uses existing licensure categories. Provider must hold license as an adult home or enriched housing program and as a home care services agency, certified home health agency, or a long-term home health program. 518/432-2986.

North Carolina: Department of Human Resources reviewing a recommendation for AL; legislation was to have been introduced in 1995-96 session. Currently, "homes for the aged" licensed to provide personal care and supervision. 919/733-3983.

North Dakota: "Basic care facilities" are licensed to provide an atmosphere conducive to achieving the highest level of self-sufficiency and quality of life possible. Staff may provide assistance with ADL. 701/224-2352.

Ohio: Licensed AL facilities may provide or arrange for the provision of noncontinuous skilled nursing care, personal care services, homemaker services, and therapy services. 614/752-2761.

Oklahoma: Department of Health likely to propose licensure category for "geriatric assisted living facilities." Currently, "residential care homes" are licensed to provide supportive assistance for residents who are ambulatory and capable of managing their affairs. 405/271-6868.

Oregon: "Assisted living" is a program approach within a physical structure that provides or coordinates a range of services available on a 24-hour basis to support resident independence. Aging in place is encouraged. 503/945-6411.

Pennsylvania: "Personal care homes" are licensed to care for residents who require assistance but do not need hospitalization or skilled or intermediate nursing care. Immobile residents may be admitted if the home complies with certain requirements. 717/783-8975.

Rhode Island: AL services are provided by "residential care and assisted living facilities" that are licensed to provide personal assistance, lodging, and meals to adults who do not require medical or nursing care but may require assistance with medication. 401/277-2566.

South Carolina: "Community residential care facilities" are licensed to provide assistance with ADL and to monitor residents' activities. Not open to any person who needs hospitalization or nursing home care, or who needs the daily attention of a licensed nurse. 803/737-7202.

Tennessee: Licensed "homes for the aged" provide personal services, including assistance with ADL. Residents must be able to evacuate the home, with staff assistance, in under 13 minutes. 615/367-6316.

Texas: Licensed "personal care facilities," in order to receive Medicaid funds for AL services, must provide personal care services, home management, social and recreational activities and more. 512/450-4971.

Utah: Legislation passed for licensure category for "assisted living facilities" during 1993-94 session. Regulations for three categories of facilities: "large" (17 or more residents), "small" (6 to 16 residents), and "limited capacity" (no more than 5 residents). 801/538-6152.

Vermont: "Residential care homes" are licensed to provide care to persons unable to live wholly independently but not in need of the level of care provided in a nursing home. 802/241-2400.

Virginia: Regulations for "assisted living facilities" require them to satisfy all of the regulations for "residential living facilities" plus additional requirements. 804/692-1787.

Washington: Department of Social and Health Services may contract with licensed "boarding homes" to provide AL services to residents. Contracted services must include personal care, nursing services, medication administration, and supportive services. 206/493-2556.

West Virginia: "Personal care homes" are licensed to provide custodial services to aged or infirm persons; medical care is only occasional or incidental. 304/558-0050.

Wisconsin: Legislation will be proposed to create a new licensure level; would have to deny admission to persons who are bed-bound 24 hours a day or are dangerous to themselves or others. 608/266-5456.

Wyoming: Statutes amended in 1993 to create a new Department of Health licensure category for "assisted living facilities." Proposed regulations allow provision of boarding, personal, and limited nursing care. 307/777-7121.

APPENDIX

D

Glossary of Terms

acid test ratio. A measure of liquidity, in which the sum of a hospital's cash, temporary investments, and the balance of its depreciation fund is divided by total current liabilities; a more stringent measure of liquidity than the current ratio because it includes in the numerator only those items that are immediately and unquestionably liquid. (See *current ratio.*)

activities of daily living (ADL). The most frequent and basic activities of human life such as bathing, dressing, going to the toilet, eating, and ambulation.

acute care. Comprehensive inpatient care (diagnostic and therapeutic services) designed for those who have had an acute illness, injury, or exacerbation of a disease process.

acute care hospital. An institution that is primarily engaged in providing diagnostic and therapeutic services for medical diagnosis, treatment, and care, by or under the supervision of physicians, to injured, disabled, or sick persons or rehabilitation services for injured, disabled, or sick persons.

actuary. An insurance professional who mathematically analyzes and prices the risks associated with providing insurance coverage.

adjusted average daily census. An expression of all of a hospital's patient services—inpatient and outpatient—as equivalent to the average number of acute care inpatients in the hospital. Calculated by multiplying the hospital's average daily census by its adjustment factor. (See also *adjustment factor, average daily census, acute care.*)

adjusted discharges. An expression of all of a hospital's patient services—inpatient and outpatient—as acute care discharge equivalents. Calculated by multiplying the number of the hospital's acute care discharges by its adjustment factor. (See also *adjustment factor, average daily census, acute care.*)

adjustment factor. Calculated as the ratio of gross patient revenue to gross inpatient acute care revenue. The adjustment factor is used to transform all of a hospital's revenue-generating activities, including inpatient acute care services, inpatient nonacute care services, and outpatient services, into units expressed in terms of inpatient acute care services. The transformation is applied by multiplying the adjustment factor times a measure of inpatient acute care output, e.g., discharges or inpatient days of care.

administrative services only. A contract with an insurer to perform only administrative services for a self-insured organization. (See also *self insurance.*)

admissions (inpatient). Persons admitted or readmitted to inpatient services as well as persons returned from long-term leave or transferred from non-inpatient (e.g., outpatient or partial care) components of organizations.

affiliated provider. A practitioner or organization subcontracted by a health maintenance organization (HMO) to provide services to the HMO's members.

all-payer system. A rate-setting program whereby all third-party payers pay the same rates, set by the government, for the same medical services.

alternative delivery systems. Alternatives to traditional health care financing and processes for providing medically necessary services in a more cost-effective manner; e.g., an HMO or PPO.

Alzheimer's care facilities. Assisted living facilities (ALFs) or skilled nursing facilities (SNFs) or a portion thereof that provide specialized care for patients suffering from Alzheimer's disease or related forms of dementia.

ambulatory care. Health care services or medical procedures performed on an outpatient basis whereby the patient is able to return home without an overnight stay in a medical facility.

ambulatory surgical center (ASC). A freestanding facility certified by Medicare that performs limited types of procedures on an outpatient basis. (See also *ASC-approved procedure, surgery center,* and *surgery recovery center.*)

ancillary services. Supplemental services provided to patients other than room and board and nursing; e.g., X-ray, laboratory work, MRI, cardiac testing, physical therapy, occupational therapy, and speech therapy.

ASC-approved procedure. A procedure performed on an outpatient basis approved for payment by Medicare. A procedure is approved if it can be performed safely in the outpatient setting, if it was performed in the inpatient setting at least 20% of the time when it was approved, and if it is performed in physicians' offices no more than 50% of the time.

assisted living facility (ALF). Licensed care facilities for the frail elderly who need assistance with one or more activities of daily living (ADLs). Also called residential care facilities (RCFs), personal care units, retirement hotels, rest homes, and board and care facilities.

at risk. The profit-or-loss burden placed on a hospital due to a set reimbursement rate.

average age of plant. A measure of the average accounting age of a hospital's capital assets such as buildings, fixtures, and major movable equipment. Calculated by dividing total accumulated depreciation on all of a hospital's property, plant, and equipment by total current depreciation.

average daily census, acute care. A measure of the average number of inpatients occupying acute care beds in a hospital on any given day. Calculated by dividing the total number of acute care inpatient days in a hospital by 365.

average length of stay (ALOS), acute care. The total number of acute care inpatient days in a hospital divided by the total number of acute care discharges from the hospital. A hospital's acute care ALOS is a key indicator of utilization and clinical management and is predictive of the average resources used by the hospital per patient discharge.

average length of stay, acute care, Medicare. The total number of Medicare acute care inpatient days in a hospital divided by the total number of Medicare acute care discharges from the hospital. Specifically relevant to the hospital's Medicare caseload, Medicare ALOS is predictive of the average acute care resources used per Medicare discharge.

average payment period. A hospital's total current liabilities times 365, divided by its total operating expenses less depreciation. A measure of the average amount of time that elapses before current liabilities are met.

balance billing. Physician charges in excess of Medicare-allowed amounts, for which Medicare patients are responsible, subject to a limit.

basic DRG payment rate. The payment rate a hospital will receive for a Medicare patient in a particular diagnosis-related group (DRG). The payment rate is calculated by adjusting the standardized amount to reflect wage rates (and non-wage cost of living differences) in the hospital's geographic area and the costliness of the DRG. (See also *diagnosis-related group* and *standardized amount.*)

beds in service, total acute care. The total number of beds set up and staffed for use in a hospital's inpatient acute care units at the end of its fiscal year. A measure of the capacity or size of a hospital.

beneficiary. A person enrolled in the Medicare program. (See also *enrollee, member.*)

beneficiary liability. The amount beneficiaries must pay providers for Medicare-covered services including copayments, deductibles, and balance billing amounts. Beneficiaries also are responsible for paying the Medicare program for their share of the Part B premium. (See also *balance billing, copayment,* and *Part B.*)

benefits. The money or services provided under the terms of an insurance policy.

board certified. A physician who has passed the examinations of a professional association that regulates the physician's specialty.

bundling. The use of a single payment for a group of related services. (See also *capitation, fee for service, per diem,* and *rate setting.*)

capital costs. Defined by Medicare as depreciation, interest, leases and rentals, and taxes and insurance on tangible assets such as physical plant and equipment.

capital costs as a percentage of operating expense. The sum of capital-related operating costs (e.g., depreciation, interest, and capital leases) expressed as a percentage of total operating expense. A measure of the relative amount of a hospital's fixed costs that can indicate the amount of risk it may face from changes in Medicare's reimbursement of capital costs. Favorable values are below the median.

capital costs per adjusted discharge. A measure of the amount of capital-related expense per unit of hospital utilization. Calculated by dividing capital-related operating costs (e.g., depreciation, interest, and capital leases) by the number of adjusted discharges from a hospital.

capitation. A method of paying health care providers or insurers in which a fixed amount is paid per enrollee to cover a defined set of services over a specified period, regardless of actual services provided. (See also *bundling, fee for service, per diem,* and *rate setting.*)

carrier. An organization, typically an insurance company, that has a contract with the Health Care Financing Administration to administer claims processing and make Medicare payments to health care providers for most Medicare Part B benefits. (See also *fiscal intermediary* and *Part B.*)

case management. The monitoring and coordinating of treatment for specific diagnosis, particularly high-cost or extensive services.

case mix. The mix of patients treated within a particular institutional setting such as a hospital. Patient classification systems (e.g., DRG system) can be used to measure hospital case mix. (See also *diagnosis-related groups* and *case-mix index.*)

case-mix index. The average diagnosis-related group weight for all cases paid under a prospective payment system. A measure of the relative costliness of treatment in each hospital or group of hospitals. (See also *diagnosis-related groups.*)

cash flow per bed, total facility. An indicator of the amount of cash available at a hospital that can be used for debt-service payments and other purposes. Calculated by dividing the total cash flow (the sum of net income, depreciation, and interest) by the number of beds in the facility.

cash flow to total debt. The sum of net income, current depreciation expense, and interest expense divided by total liabilities. A measure of the proportion of a hospital's total debt obligations that could be met with available cash flow if demanded by creditors within one year. One measure of a hospital's debt repayment ability or creditworthiness.

charges. The posted prices of services provided by a facility. Medicare requires hospitals to apply the same schedule of charges to all patients, regardless of the expected sources or amount of payment.

claim. A statement of health services and their costs provided by a hospital, physician's office, or other provider facility.

coalitions. Associations of health care sponsors that pool resources to gather information on and negotiate with insurers and other health care providers.

coinsurance. The percentage of the costs of medical care that a patient pays.

community rating. Premiums based on the average cost of providing medical services to all people in a geographic area without adjusting for an individual's medical history or likelihood of using such services.

concurrent review. A review of a procedure to ensure that medically necessary and appropriate care is delivered during a patient's hospital stay.

continuing care retirement center (CCRC). A community established to provide a continuum of care to people of retirement age. This type of community offers housing, health care, and various residential supportive services depending on a resident's level of independence.

continued stay review. A review that monitors the continued appropriateness of a patient's hospital stay.

coordination of benefits. A cost-control measure to prevent an insured person from receiving duplicate benefits.

copayment. A cost-sharing arrangement in which an HMO enrollee pays a specified fee for a specific service.

cost-based reimbursements. A method of paying providers an amount based on the cost to the provider of delivering services.

cost contract. An arrangement between a managed health care plan and the Health Care Financing Administration under Section 1876 or 1833 of the Social Security Act, in which the health plan provides health services and is reimbursed its costs. The beneficiary can use providers outside the plan's provider network. (See also *health care prepayment plan* and *risk contract*.)

cost shifting. Increasing revenues from or charges to some payers to offset uncompensated care losses and lower net payments from other payers.

current ratio. The ratio of a hospital's total current assets, including the balance of the depreciation fund, to its total current liabilities. An indicator of a hospital's liquidity and ability to meet short-term (i.e., due within one year) obligations. (See also *acid test ratio*.)

day/evening care. Mental health treatment programs that focus on sustainment, maximization, or socialization through recreational and/or occupational activities, etc. (See also *partial care*.)

day/evening treatment. Mental health treatment programs that place heavy emphasis on intensive short-term therapy and rehabilitation. (See also *partial care*.)

days' cash on hand. The sum of cash, temporary investments, and the balance of the depreciation fund at a hospital multiplied by 365 and divided by the hospital's total operating expenses less depreciation. A measure of the number of days a hospital could operate if no further revenues were received.

days in net accounts receivable. A hospital's net patient accounts receivable divided by its net patient revenue times 365. The number of days of net patient revenue that a hospital has due from its patient billings after all deductions.

debt per bed, total facility. One measure of the amount of debt of a hospital in relation to its size. Calculated as the ratio of total liabilities (both long-term and short-term) to the total number of beds in service in a facility.

debt service coverage ratio. The sum of a hospital's net income, current depreciation, and interest expense, divided by the same year's debt service payments. Debt service coverage measures the ratio of a hospital's funds available for the payment of debt service to the same year's principal and interest payments. As such, it is an important measure of a hospital's creditworthiness or ability to repay debt.

deductible. The amount of money an insured person must pay before the payer begins reimbursement.

deductions from gross patient revenue as a percentage of gross patient revenue. Calculated as total deductions from gross patient revenue divided by gross patient revenue, expressed as a percentage. Total deductions from gross patient revenue consist of contractual allowances and discounts, bad debts, and charity care.

Department of Health and Human Services. The cabinet agency of the United States government that administers most federal health programs.

diagnosis-related groups (DRGs). A system for determining case mix used for payment under Medicare's Prospective Payment System (PPS) and by some other payers. The DRG system classifies patients into groups based on the principal diagnosis, the presence and type of surgical procedure, presence or absence of significant comorbidities or complications, and other relevant criteria. DRGs are intended to categorize patients into groups that are clinically meaningful and homogeneous with respect to resource use. There are currently 490 mutually exclusive DRGs in Medicare's PPS, each of which is assigned a relative weight that compares its costliness to the average for all DRGs. (See also *case mix.*)

discharges per bed, acute care. A ratio of total acute care discharges from a hospital divided by the number of acute care beds in service. A measure of the number of patients who use a hospital's acute care beds during a year; varies directly with occupancy rate and inversely with average length of stay. Because it indicates the relationship between inputs (beds) and outputs (discharges), acute care discharges per bed is another measure of productivity.

discharge planning. A review process in which health care professionals identify and evaluate the anticipated needs of a patient following discharge from the hospital.

disproportionate share adjustment. A payment adjustment under Medicare or Medicaid for hospitals that serve a relatively large volume of low-income patients.

DRGs. See *diagnosis-related groups.*

education and training. Treatment programs that focus on change through an integration of education, habilitation, and training, including special education classes, therapeutic nursery schools, and vocational training.

enrollee. A person who is covered by health insurance. (See also *beneficiary.*)

enrollment. The number of members in a health maintenance organization (HMO), preferred provider organization (PPO), or other health care organization.

excluded hospitals and distinct-part units. Hospitals and hospital units that are specifically excluded from Medicare's Prospective Payment System such as children's, cancer, long-term, rehabilitation, and psychiatric hospitals. Rehabilitation and psychiatric units of acute care hospitals are exempt if they meet certain criteria specified by the Secretary of Health and Human Services. Hospitals located in U.S. territories, federal hospitals, and Christian Science sanatoria are also excluded from PPS. Excluded facilities remain under cost-based reimbursement, subject to rate of increase limits, established in accordance with the Tax Equity and Fiscal Responsibility Act of 1982. (See also *Tax Equity and Fiscal Responsibility Act of 1982.*)

exclusions. Specific conditions listed for exclusion in a contract.

exclusive provider organization (EPO). Similar to a preferred provider organization (PPO) in structure and purpose; however, enrollees are limited to receive all of their covered services from providers that participate in the EPO.

fee for service. A method of reimbursing health care providers in which payment is made for each unit of service rendered. (See also *bundling, capitation, per diem,* and *rate setting.*)

fee reimbursement. The payment received by a provider from an HMO or similar entity for services rendered to patients after the care has been provided.

fee schedule. A list of charges or established benefits for specific medical or dental procedures.

fiscal intermediary. An entity, usually an insurance company, having a contract with the Health Care Financing Administration to determine and make Part A Medicare payments and certain Part B benefits to hospitals and other providers of services and to perform related functions.

fiscal year. A 12-month period for which an organization plans the use of its funds, e.g., the federal government's fiscal year is October 1 to September 30. Fiscal years are referred to by the calendar year in which they end; for example, the federal fiscal year 1995 began October 1, 1994, and ended September 30, 1995. Individual providers can designate their own fiscal years, which is reflected in differences in the time periods covered by Medicare cost reports. (See also *PPS year.*)

flat percent rates. The percent discount applied to full service provided to all patients.

full-time equivalent (FTE) personnel per adjusted average daily census. The total number of FTE personnel in a hospital divided by its adjusted average daily census. A measure of the staffing level of a hospital or of the labor inputs being used to provide a day of hospital care. (See also *adjusted average daily census.*)

full-time equivalent (FTE) personnel per 100 adjusted discharges. The total number of FTE personnel divided by the number of adjusted discharges, multiplied by 100. A staffing ratio that uses discharges as the measure of output. It is less affected by differences in length of stay than a staffing ratio based on the hospital's average daily census.

gatekeeper. The primary care physician or manager (case manager) who authorizes all medical services.

global budget. Term used to place a nationwide limit on overall spending for health care services.

grace period. A period of time after a premium is due during which coverage must be provided and the premium paid without penalty.

gross domestic product. The value of all goods and services produced within the United States' boundaries during a given period.

gross patient revenue per adjusted discharge. Total charges for hospital services divided by the number of adjusted discharges from a hospital. One measure of the inpatient price per unit (per case) in a hospital, although not equivalent to the unit revenue actually received. As such, it measures a hospital's pricing policies, although it is less revealing in markets in which few third-party payers are charge-based. (See also *adjusted discharge.*)

group HMO. A health maintenance organization that contracts with one or more independent group practices to provide services in one or more locations, in which the physicians of the group are paid on a capitated basis.

Group I, II, and III classifications. Hospital equipment classifications. Group I equipment is permanent equipment, installed in or attached to the building, part of the general contract. Group II equipment is equipment often installed and becoming part of the real property, but typically not part of the general contract, such as autoclaves, permanent surgical lights, and other equipment. Group III equipment is movable personal property such as furniture, fixtures, instruments, etc.

Health Care Financing Administration (HCFA). The agency within the Department of Health and Human Services that administers federal health financing and related regulatory programs, principally the Medicare and Medicaid programs.

health care prepayment plans. Plans that receive payment for their reasonable costs of providing Medicare Part B services to Medicare enrollees. (See also *cost contract* and *risk contract.*)

health insurance purchasing cooperatives. Purchasing agents for large groups of employers in a region that shop for the highest quality health plan at the lowest price, per President Clinton's restructured health care system.

health maintenance organization (HMO). A managed care plan that integrates financing and delivery of a comprehensive set of health care services to an enrolled population. HMOs may contract with, directly employ, or own participating health care providers. Enrollees are usually required to choose from among these providers and in return have limited copayments. Providers may be paid through capitation, salary, per diem, or prenegotiated fee-for-service rates. (See also *capitation, fee for service, managed care, managed care plan, per diem,* and *preferred provider organization.*)

home health care. Medical care provided in the home by certified professionals for patients who no longer need the extensive treatment provided by a hospital or skilled nursing facility.

hospice care. An organized program that provides palliative and supportive care for terminally ill patients at home or in a hospice rather than a hospital.

incurred but not reported. A loss, claim, or expense that occurred within a fixed period and for which an insurance company or medical provider becomes liable whether or not yet reported, adjusted, and paid.

indemnity. Protection against loss. Also in reference to private insurance.

independent physician association. Contracts with individual physicians who see patients for a set rate, as well as their own patients, in their own private offices.

individual practice association. One of four models that is a mixture of physicians or health care professionals from solo and group practices.

instrumental activities of daily living (IADL). Activities such as doing housework, preparing meals, shopping, and performing other tasks considered to be essential to the ability to live alone.

insured services. Special procedures or tests performed on a patient which are considered part of the services to be covered.

inpatient care. Provision of 24-hour care in a hospital setting.

intensity of services. The number and complexity of patient care services used per hospital admission or outpatient visit, nursing home day, home health visit, or dialysis treatment. Examples of services contributing to an admission or outpatient visit include nursing care, surgeries, and radiological procedures.

intermediate care facility (ICF). See *nursing facility* and *skilled nursing facility.*

large urban area. A metropolitan statistical area with a population of one million or more, or a New England County Metropolitan Area with a population of 970,000 or more. (See also metropolitan statistical area and other urban area.)

licensed bed capacity. Official maximum number of inpatient hospital beds authorized by state licensure.

long-term care. Ongoing health and social services provided for individuals who need assistance on a continuing basis because of physical or mental disability. Services can be provided in an institution, the home, or the community, and include informal services provided by family or friends as well as formal services provided by professionals or agencies.

long-term debt to capitalization. The ratio of a hospital's long-term liabilities to the sum of its long-term liabilities and fund balance or equity capital. A measure of the proportion of a hospital's total capitalization provided by debt.

long-term debt to net fixed assets. The ratio of a hospital's long-term liabilities to its property, plant, and equipment (net of accumulated depreciation). A measure of the proportion of a hospital's net fixed assets financed through the use of long-term debt. As such, a measure of financial leverage.

long-term debt to total assets. The ratio of a hospital's long-term liabilities to its total assets. Frequently used as a measure of the degree of financial leverage employed by a hospital.

major teaching hospital. A hospital with an approved graduate medical education program and a ratio of interns and residents to beds of 0.25 or greater.

managed care. Any payment or delivery arrangement used by a health plan or provider to control or coordinate use of health services to contain health expenditures, improve quality, or both. Utilization review is a common example of a managed care technique. (See also *managed care plan* and *utilization review.*)

managed care plan. A health plan that uses managed care arrangements and has a defined system of selected providers that contract with the plan. Enrollees have a financial incentive to use participating providers that agree to furnish a broad range of services to them. Providers may be paid on a prenegotiated fee-for-service, capitated, per diem, or salaried basis. (See also *health maintenance organization, point-of-services plan,* and *preferred provider organization.*)

market basket index. An index of the annual change in the prices of goods and health services providers; also referred to as an input price index. There are separate market baskets for prospective payment system (PPS) hospital operating inputs, PPS hospital capital inputs, PPS-excluded facility operating inputs, skilled nursing facilities, home health agencies, and renal dialysis facility operating and capital inputs.

Medicaid. State programs of public assistance to persons whose resources are insufficient to pay for medical care.

Medicare. A federally funded nationwide hospital and medical care insurance program for citizens over age 65 and for disabled people of all ages. (See also *Part A* and *Part B.*)

Medicare cost report. An annual report required of all institutions participating in the Medicare program. A record of each institution's total costs and charges associated with providing services to all patients, the portion of those costs and charges allocated to Medicare patients, and the Medicare payments received. (See also *PPS year.*)

Medicare provider analysis and review (MedPAR) file. A data file of the Health Care Financing Administration that contains charge data and clinical characteristics such as diagnoses and procedures for every hospital inpatient bill submitted to Medicare for payment.

Medicare supplement. An insurance program that specifically covers those costs not covered by Medicare.

Medigap policy. A privately purchased insurance policy that supplements Medicare coverage and meets specified requirements set by federal statute and the National Association of Insurance Commissioners.

member. A person eligible to receive benefits from an insurance policy. (See also *beneficiary* and *enrollee.*)

metropolitan statistical area (MSA). A geographic area that includes at least one city with 50,000 or more inhabitants, or a Census Bureau-defined urbanized area of at least 50,000 inhabitants and a total MSA population of at least 100,000 (75,000 in New England).

morbidity. An actuarial concept that shows the average incidence of illness occurring in a large group of people.

multispecialty group. A group of doctors who represent various medical specialties and who work together in a practice.

national practitioner data bank. A computerized data bank maintained by the federal government that contains information on physicians and other practitioners against whom malpractice claims have been paid or certain disciplinary actions have been taken.

negotiated fee schedule. A payment system in which providers work for a fixed portion of their usual fee.

negotiated rates. Rates that vary by patient type and/or payer.

net property, plant, and equipment per bed, total facility. A measure of the degree of investment by a hospital in the capital assets of property, plant, and major movable equipment in relation to its size. Calculated as total property, plant, and equipment less accumulated depreciation, divided by the total number of beds in service in the facility.

network HMO. A type of health maintenance organization that contracts with two or more independent group practices to provide health services.

nursing facility. An institution that provides skilled nursing care and rehabilitation services to injured, functionally disabled, or sick persons. Formerly, distinctions were made between intermediate care facilities (ICFs) and skilled nursing facilities (SNFs). The Omnibus Budget Reconciliation Act of 1987 eliminated this distinction effective October 1, 1990, by requiring ICFs to meet SNF certification requirements. (See also *skilled nursing facility.*)

occupancy rate, acute care. The ratio of a hospital's average daily census of inpatients in acute care beds to the average number of acute care beds in service, expressed as a percentage. A measure of the utilization of the capacity of the hospital.

open enrollment. The annual period during which people can choose from health plans being offered.

operating profit margin. A measure of a hospital's profitability with respect to its patient care services and operations. The difference between a hospital's total operating revenue and total operating expense, expressed as a percentage of its total operating revenue. Total operating revenue is the sum of net patient revenue plus other operating revenue.

operating expense per adjusted discharge. A measure of a hospital's average cost of delivering inpatient care per unit (per case). Calculated by dividing total operating expenses by the number of adjusted discharges.

operating revenue per adjusted discharge. An indicator of a hospital's ability to generate revenues from its patient care operations. Calculated by dividing total operating revenue by the number of adjusted discharges from the hospital. Total operating revenue is defined as the sum of net patient revenue (payments actually received or expected to be received) plus other operating revenue.

other urban area. A metropolitan statistical area with a population of less than one million, or a New England County Metropolitan Area with fewer than 970,000 people. (See also *large urban area* and *metropolitan statistical area.*)

out-of-area. Refers to the treatment given an HMO member outside the geographical limits of the HMO.

outliers. Under the Prospective Payment System, cases with extremely long lengths of stay (day outliers) or extraordinarily high costs (cost outliers) compared with others in the same diagnosis-related group. Hospitals receive additional payment for these cases.

outpatient care. Health services to ambulatory patients on an individual, group, or family basis, generally provided in less than three hours at a single visit, in a hospital, clinic, or similar organization. Included are emergency care on a walk-in basis as well as care provided by mobile teams who visit patients outside the hospital. All "hotline" services are excluded.

outpatient gross revenue as a percentage of gross patient revenue. Approximates the proportion of a hospital's revenue that is attributable to services provided to outpatients.

outpatient surgery. Minor ambulatory surgery.

overhead expense as a percentage of operating expense. A measure of the relative amount of total overhead (or administrative and general) expense in a hospital; as such, a measure of the relative amount of fixed expenses at a hospital. Calculated by dividing a hospital's total overhead expense by its total operating expense, expressed as a percentage.

Part A. Medicare Hospital Insurance (HI) (Part A of Title XVIII of the Social Security Act), which covers beneficiaries for inpatient hospital, home health, hospice, and limited skilled nursing facility services. Beneficiaries are responsible for deductibles and copayments. Part A services are financed by the Medicare HI Trust Fund, which consists of Medicare tax payments. (See also *fiscal intermediary* and *Part B.*)

Part B. Medicare Supplementary Medical Insurance (SMI) (Part B of Title XVIII of the Social Security Act), which covers Medicare beneficiaries for physician services, medical supplies, and other outpatient treatment. Beneficiaries are responsible for monthly premiums, copayments, deductibles, and balance billing. Part B services are financed by a combination of enrollee premiums and general tax revenues. (See also *carrier* and *Part A.*)

partial care. A planned program of mental health treatment services generally provided to groups of patients in sessions lasting three or more hours. Includes day/evening treatment and day/evening care. (See also *day/evening treatment* and *day/evening care.*)

peer review. A cost- and quality-control system in which physicians review or evaluate the work of other physicians using predetermined standards.

peer review organization. An organization that contracts with the Health Care Financing Administration to investigate the quality of health care furnished to Medicare beneficiaries and to educate beneficiaries and providers. Also conducts limited review of medical records and claims to evaluate the appropriateness of care provided.

penetration. The percentage of business an insurer is able to capture in the market areas as a whole.

per diem payments. Fixed daily payments that do not vary with the level of services used by the patient. Generally used by managed care plans to pay institutional providers (e.g., hospitals and nursing facilities). (See also *capitation.*)

per member per month (pmpm). The fee paid under a capitated contract to the provider for members enrolled in a plan and which is paid on a monthly basis.

point-of-service (POS) plan. A health plan with a network of providers whose services are available to enrollees at a lower cost than the services of nonnetwork providers. POS enrollees must receive authorization from a primary care physician to use network services. POS plans typically do not pay for out-of-network referrals for primary care services. (See also *preferred provider organization.*)

PPO. See *preferred provider organization.*

PPS. See *prospective payment system.*

PPS year. Refers to hospital cost reporting periods that begin during a given federal fiscal year, reflecting the number of years since the initial implementation of the prospective payment system (PPS). For example, PPS 1 refers to a hospital fiscal year that began during federal fiscal year 1984, which was the first year of PPS. (See also *fiscal year.*)

pre-existing medical condition. A physical and/or mental condition that a patient has before applying for insurance coverage.

preferred provider organization (PPO). A health plan with a network of providers whose services are available to enrollees at lower cost than the services of nonnetwork providers. PPO enrollees may self-refer to any network provider at any time. (See also *fee for service, health maintenance organization, managed care, managed care plan,* and *point-of-service plan.*)

preventive health care. Care aimed at the prevention of disease and concentrated on keeping patients well in addition to healing them when they are sick.

primary care physician. A physician who assumes continuing responsibility for the comprehensive care of an individual.

principal diagnosis. A condition determined to be chiefly responsible for the admission of a patient to an inpatient hospital setting.

productivity. The ratio of outputs (goods and services produced) to inputs (resources used in production). Increased productivity implies that the hospital or health care organization is either producing more output with the same resources or the same output with fewer resources.

program. In mental health care, an organized set of therapeutic activities which, under psychiatric guidance, are aimed at reducing an impairment resulting from a psychiatric disorder.

ProPac (Prospective Payment Assessment Commission). A commission of private industry medical participants established by Congress to report on national health care spending trends and related matters of the health care financing environment.

prospective payment. A method of paying health care providers at established rates regardless of the costs they actually incur.

prospective payment system (PPS). Medicare's payment method for acute hospital inpatient care. Prospective per-case payment rates are set for given diagnosis-related groups at levels intended to cover operating costs of treating a typical inpatient in an efficient hospital. Payments for each hospital are adjusted for differences in area wages, teaching activity, care to the poor, and other factors. Hospitals may also receive additional payments to cover extra costs associated with atypical patients (outliers) in each DRG. Capital costs, originally excluded from PPS, are being phased into the system. By 2001, capital payments will be made on a fully prospective, per-case basis. (See also *capital costs, diagnosis-related groups, outliers,* and *prospective payment.*)

quality assurance. A set of activities to assure the quality of services provided. (See also *concurrent review* and *peer review.*)

rate setting. A method of paying health care providers at rates established by the federal or state government for one or more payers for various categories of health services.

registered nurse turnover rate. The number of full-time equivalent (FTE) registered nurse terminations for a reporting period divided by the number of FTE registered nurses on the rolls at the end of the reporting period.

reinsurance. The purchasing of insurance by one insurance company from another insurance company to protect itself against part or all of the losses incurred in honoring the claims of policy holders.

relative value scale. An index that assigns weights to medical services; the weights represent the relative amount to be paid for each service. The relative value scale used in developing the Medicare Physician Fee Schedule consists of three cost components: physician work, practice expense, and malpractice expense. (See also *resource-based relative value scale.*)

residential assisted Alzheimer's living facility (RAALF). A facility that provides assisted living or a residential care environment to persons suffering from Alzheimer's disease.

residential care facility (RCF). A facility that provides persons with shelter and food and a limited amount of other services.

residential treatment care. Overnight care in conjunction with an intensive treatment program in a setting other than a hospital.

resource-based relative value scale. A system for determining the level of payments to physicians based on the amount of work involved in the treatment. (See also *relative value scale.*)

return on assets. A measure of the overall profitability of a hospital. Calculated by dividing a hospital's net income by its total assets. Compares total revenue over total expense (i.e., net income) in relation to the assets controlled by the hospital.

risk adjustment. Increases or reductions in the amount of payment made to a health plan on behalf of a group of enrollees to compensate for health care expenditures that are expected to be higher or lower than average. (See also *risk selection.*)

risk contract. An arrangement between a managed health care plan and the Health Care Financing Administration under Section 1876 of the Social Security Act, in which the enrolled Medicare beneficiary must use the plan's network of providers and payment to the plan is made on a capitated basis using the adjusted average per capita cost. (See also *adjusted average per capita cost, capitation, cost contract,* and *health care prepayment plan.*)

risk selection. Enrollment choices made by health plans or enrollees on the basis of perceived risk relative to the premium to be paid. (See also *risk adjustment.*)

safety net provider. One that provides services to the medically indigent and special needs segments of a state's population.

salary and benefits expense as a percentage of operating expense. A measure of the proportion of a hospital's costs attributable to employee labor costs. Calculated by dividing the sum of salaries and employee benefits expense by total operating expense, expressed as a percentage.

salary and benefits expense per full-time equivalent (FTE) personnel. Measures a hospital's average direct labor expense per employee. Calculated by dividing the sum of salaries and employee benefits expense by the total number of FTE personnel.

self insurance. A health benefits program in which a business pays the cost of employees' medical benefits up to a certain amount.

senior plan. A benefits package to the nonworking person over the age of 65, often under Medicare through a contract with the federal government.

service area. The geographic area served by an insurer or health care provider.

shared risk pool. An incentive program for controlling the cost of selected services when actual incurred costs are favorable compared to a predetermined budget; the savings may be shared with the physician, the hospital, and others.

single payer. A system whereby one entity pays for all health care.

skilled nursing facility (SNF). An institution that has a transfer agreement with one or more hospitals, provides primarily inpatient skilled nursing care and rehabilitative services, and meets other specific certification requirements. (See also *nursing facility*).

sole community hospital. One designated for special treatment under the Prospective Payment System as the only provider of hospital care in its market area. Under PPS, sole community hospitals benefit from payment provisions intended to ensure their financial viability and access to hospital services for Medicare beneficiaries.

specialty HMO. A health maintenance organization organized around a specific medical specialty.

staff-based HMO. A health maintenance organization that delivers services at one or more locations by doctors who are employed by the HMO.

staffed bed capacity. Actual number of inpatient psychiatric beds set up, staffed, and available for service.

standardized amount. Used as the basis for payment under the Prospective Payment System; intended to represent the national average operating cost of inpatient treatment for a typical Medicare patient in a reasonably efficient hospital in a large urban or other area. Standardized amounts are based on costs reported by hospitals to Medicare for reporting periods ending in 1982 and adjusted for geographic location and certain hospital characteristics (e.g., teaching activity). The adjusted amounts are updated to the year of payment by an annual update factor. (See also *update factors.*)

stop-loss. The practice of an insurance company protecting itself or its contracted medical groups against part or all losses above specified dollar amounts.

subacute care. Good oriented treatment rendered immediately after, or instead of, acute hospitalization to treat one or more specific active complex medical conditions or to administer one or more technically complex treatments in an environment that does not depend heavily on high-technology monitoring or complex diagnostic procedures.

supplemental health services. Optional services that an insurer might provide in addition to the basic care, usually at additional cost.

supplemental insurance. Any private health insurance plan held by a Medicare beneficiary, including Medigap policies and post retirement health benefits.

surgery center (SC). A specifically designed single-purpose building or a unit in a medical building providing same-day surgical procedures outside of the traditional hospital setting.

surgery recovery center (SRC). A surgery center with inpatient beds allowing the facility to conduct procedures that usually require a short-term hospital stay of one to three days.

swing-bed hospital. One participating in the Medicare swing-bed program; allows rural hospitals with fewer than 100 beds to provide skilled post-acute care services in acute care beds.

targeted case management. Project involving intensive case management of high-cost or high-risk beneficiaries aimed at positively impacting patient outcomes.

Tax Equity and Fiscal Responsibility Act of 1982 (TEFRA). Legislation that established target rate of increase limits on reimbursements for inpatient operating costs per discharge under Medicare. A facility's target amount is derived from costs in a base year and updated to the current year by the annual allowable rate of increase. Medicare payments for operating costs generally may not exceed the facility's target amount. These provisions still apply to hospitals and units excluded from PPS. (See also *excluded hospitals and units.*)

third-party administrator. An organization or person who provides certain administrative services to group benefits plans, including premium accounting, claims review, and payments.

third-party payment. Payment for health care services by someone other than the individual who received the care or administered it.

Title XVIII of the Social Security Act. Established Medicare.

total charity cost. The total expense not billed to patients for the specific purpose of providing charity to these cases.

total dietary cost. The total of food, supplies, salaries and benefits, contract labor, and management fees.

total discharges, acute care. The total number of patients discharged from a hospital's acute care beds in a year. A measure of the utilization of acute care inpatient services at a hospital.

total margin. A measure that compares total hospital revenue and expenses for inpatient, outpatient, and nonpatient care activities. Calculated by subtracting total expenses from total revenue and dividing by total revenue.

total profit margin. The difference between a hospital's total revenue and total expense (i.e., net income) to its total revenue, expressed as a percentage. Includes philanthropic contributions, endowment revenue, government grants, investment income, and other revenue and expense not related to patient care operations. A measure of the overall profitability of a hospital.

unbundled services. The provision of a wide range of health care services that may be purchased separately.

uncompensated care. Care rendered by hospitals or other providers without payment from the patient or a government-sponsored or private insurance program. Includes both charity care, which is provided without the expectation of payment, and bad debts, for which the provider has made an unsuccessful effort to collect payment from the patient.

utilization review. The review of services delivered by a health care provider to evaluate the appropriateness, necessity, and quality of the prescribed services. Can be performed on a prospective, concurrent, or retrospective basis.

volume performance standard. A mechanism to adjust updates to fee-for-service payment rates based on how actual aggregate expenditure increases compare to predetermined target rates of increase. (See also *fee-for-service.*)

withhold. The portion of the monthly capitation payment to providers withheld until the end of the year to create an incentive for efficient care.

worker's compensation. A state-operated insurance program that protects employees who are injured on the job against loss of income .

wraparound. A supplementary plan designed to pay for benefits not provided under the basic plan.

A P P E N D I X

E

Bibliography

American Association of Retired Persons and Stein Gerontological Institute. *Life-Span Design of Residential Environments for an Aging Population.* Washington, DC: 1993.

American Hospital Association/American Society for Hospital Engineering. *1993 International Conference and Exhibition on Health Planning, Design and Construction: Proceedings Manual.* Chicago, 1993.

American Institute of Architects, Committee on Architecture for Health. *Guidelines for Construction and Equipment of Hospital and Medical Facilities.* Washington, DC: 1993.

———. *Design for Aging: 1992 Review.* Washington, DC: AIA Press, 1993.

American Seniors Housing Association and Coopers & Lybrand LLP. *The State of Seniors Housing 1995.* Washington, DC.

Burda, David. "Changing Ownership." *Modern Healthcare* (May 7, 1988).

Clipp, JoAnn. "Pursuing the Frail Elderly." *Assisted Living Today* (1995).

Dahl, Robert J. "Elements of a Site Evaluation." *Transitions* (November/December 1994).

Desmond, Glenn, and John Marcello. *Handbook of Small Business Valuation Formulas.* Marina del Rey, Calif.: Valuation Press, 1988.

Gulak, Morton B. "Architectural Guidelines for State Psychiatric Hospitals." *Hospitals and Community Psychiatry* (July 1991), 706.

Hansen, James M. *Guide to Buying or Selling a Business,* Mercer Island, WA: Grenadier Press, 1979.

Havlicek, Penny L. *Medical Groups in the United States, 1984.* Chicago: American Medical Association, 1985.

Health Care Investment Analysts, Inc., and Deloitte & Touche. *The Comparative Performance of U.S. Hospitals: The Sourcebook.* Baltimore, MD.

Healthcare Merger and Aquisition Report. New Canaan, CT.: Irving Levin Associates.

Hiatt, Lorraine G. *Nursing Home Renovation Designed for Reform.* Butterworth Architecture, 1991.

Hyatt, Laura. *Subacute Care.* Chicago: Richard D. Irwin, 1995.

Jones, Jeffrey D. "Rule of Thumb Formulas for Small Businesses," *Business Valuation News* (December 1982).

Jesudason, Victor. "Changing Characteristics of Elderly Nursing Home Residents, Wisconsin 1980-90." *Health Data Review,* Wisconsin Department of Health and Social Services, vol. 5, no. 8 (August 1991).

Larkin, Howard. "Managed Mental Health Moves Patients Out." *Hospitals* (April 20, 1989), 64.

Marshall Valuation Service. Marshall & Swift. Los Angeles.

McDowell, Tim, and Harvey Brown. "Integrated Delivery Systems," *Transitions,* vol. 1, no. 1 (July/August 1994), 10-11.

Miller, Richard L, and Earl S. Swensson. *New Directions in Hospital and Healthcare Facility Design.* New York: McGraw-Hill, Inc., 1995.

Pol, Louis G., and Richard K. Thomas. *The Demography of Health and Health Care.* New York: Plenum Press, 1992.

"Psych Chains Had Another Tough Year." *Modern Healthcare* (May 22, 1995).

Regnier, Victor. *Assisted Living for the Elderly.* New York: Van Nostrand Reinhold, 1994.

Reinhardt, Uwe. "A Production Function for Physician Services." *The Review of Economics & Statistics,* February 1972.

Reynold, Roger A., and Daniel J. Duann, eds. *1985 Socioeconomic Characteristics of Medical Practice.* Chicago: American Medical Association, 1985.

Roberts, Joe R., and Eric Roberts. "Nursing Homes: Government Influence." *The Appraisal Journal* (July 1989), 309-316.

The Senior Care Acquisition Report. New Canaan, CT.: Irving Levin Associates, Inc., 1996.

SMG Marketing Group, Inc. *Market Letter* (January 1995).

SMG Marketing Group, Inc. *Market Letter* (June 1994).

"Special Report: Survey of Small Business and Professional Practice Transaction Prices." Contained in *Valuing Small Businesses and Professional Practices,* by Shannon Pratt. Homewood, IL: Dow Jones-Irwin, 1986.

"Subacute Care: Halfway Between Sick and Well." *The Genesis Report* (November 1994).

Thomas, Richard K. *Health Care Consumers in the 1990s,* Ithaca, NY: American Demographics Books, 1993.

Walton, John B. *Business Profitability Data.* Dallas, TX: Weybridge Publishing Co., 1990.

Periodicals

American Demographics, P.O. Box 68, Ithaca, NY 14851

The Construction Specifier, Construction Specifications Institute, 601 Madison St., Alexandria, VA 22314

Healthcare Financial Management, 2 Westbrook Corporate Center, Ste. 700, Westchester, IL 60154

Healthcare Forum Journal, 425 Market St., 16th Floor, San Francisco, CA 94105

Health Care Strategic Management

Health Facilities Management, American Hospital Publishing Inc., 737 N. Michigan Avenue, Ste. 700, Chicago, IL 60611-2615

Health Marketing Quarterly

Hospitals, American Hospital Publishing Inc., 737 N. Michigan Avenue, Ste. 700, Chicago, IL 60611-2615

Hospitals and Health Networks, American Hospital Publishing Inc., 737 N. Michigan Avenue, Ste. 700, Chicago, IL 60611-2615

Hospital Management International

Hospitality Design

Journal of Ambulatory Care Management

Journal of Healthcare Design

Medical Clinics of North America

Modern Healthcare, Crain Communications, 740 N. Rush, Chicago, IL 60611

Association and Government Agency Sources

American Association of Homes & Services for the Aging, 901 E St., N.W., Ste. 500, Washington, DC 20004-2037. (202)783-2242

American Health Association, 13701 State Rd., Ste. 535, Orlando, FL 32821-6367. (407)422-2404

American Health Care Association, 1201 L St., N.W., Washington, DC 20005. (202)842-4444

American Hospital Association, 1 N. Franklin, #27, Chicago, IL 60606. (312)422-3000

American Institute of Architects, Committee on Architecture for Health, 1735 New York Ave., N.W., Washington, DC 20006. (202)626-7300

American Medical Association, 515 N. State St., Chicago, IL 60610-0174. (312)464-4470

American Society of Healthcare Engineering, c/o American Hospital Association, 1 N. Franklin, Chicago, IL 60606. (312)422-3800

American Subacute Care Association, 1440 Kennedy Causeway, Ste. 421, North Bay Village, FL 33141. (305)864-0396

Assisted Living Facilities Association of America, 9411 Lee Hwy., Ste. J, Fairfax, VA 22031. (703)691-8100

Council on Tall Buildings & Urban Habitat, Lehigh University, Fritz Engineering Lab, 13 E. Packer Ave., Bethlehem, PA 18015. (215)758-3515

Institute of Business Appraisers, Inc., P.O. Box 1447, Boynton Beach, FL 33435. (407)732-3202

Joint Commission on the Accreditation of Healthcare Organizations, 1 Renaissance Blvd., Oakbrook Terrace, IL 60181. (630)916-5600

National Association of Private Psychiatric Health Systems, 1319 F St., N.W., Ste. 1000, Washington, DC 20004. (202)393-6700

National Institute of Senior Housing, c/o National Council on the Aging, 409 3rd St., S.W., 2nd Flr., Washington, DC 20024. (202)479-6680

United States Bureau of the Census (*County and City Data Book; Statistical Abstract of the United States*)

United States Department of Commerce

United States Department of Health & Human Services

Private Data Sources and Consultants

Arthur Andersen & Company (214)741-8300

Arthur Gimmy International (415)781-6262

Business Trend Analysts (http://www.users.aol.com/compadvant/bta.html)

Claritas (800)234-5629

Health Care Investment Analysts, Inc. (410)576-9600

The Comparative Performance of U.S. Hospitals: The Sourcebook

Inforum, Inc. (800)829-0600

Institute for Health and Aging

Irving Levin Associates, Inc. (800)248-1668

The Health Care M&A Report

The Hospital Acquisition Report

The Senior Care Investor

The Senior Care Acquisition Report

MACRO International (info@macroint.com)

Marshall & Swift (800)544-2678

Mergers & Aquisitions Database, Philadelphia, PA (1-800-ADP-DATA).

National Center for Health Statistics (301)436-8500

National Research Corporation (402)475-2525

Health Care Market Guide

Professional Research Corporation (402)592-5656

SMG Marketing Group, Inc. (312)642-3026